CW00602536

Hove Tongourc
01273 242010.

Cochlear Implants for Young Children

Second Edition

SPEECH & LANGUAGE THERAPY
A3, BRIGHTON GENERAL HOSPITAL
ELM GROVE, BRIGHTON BN2 3EW
TEL: 01273 - 242074
FAX: 01273 - 242116

Dedication

This page is dedicated to our families for their patience during the preparation of this book and to our entire team who make this work possible.

Special thanks are due to Lynne Ansell for her secretarial help.

Cochlear Implants for Young Children

The Nottingham Approach to Assessment and Rehabilitation

Second edition

Edited by

BARRY MCCORMICK OBE, PhD

and

SUE ARCHBOLD MPhil

both of the Nottingham Paediatric Cochlear Implant Programme

W

WHURR PUBLISHERS

LONDON AND PHILADELPHIA

© 2003 Whurr Publishers

First Edition Published 1994
Second Edition Published 2003
Whurr Publishers Ltd
19b Compton Terrace, London N1 2UN, England and
325 Chestnut Street, Philadelphia PA19106, USA

All rights reserved. No part of this publication may be
reproduced, stored in a retrieval system, or transmitted
in any form or by any means, electronic, mechanical,
photocopying, recording or otherwise, without the prior
permission of Whurr Publishers Limited.

This publication is sold subject to the conditions that it
shall not, by way of trade or otherwise, be lent, resold,
hired out, or otherwise circulated without the
Publisher's prior consent, in any form of binding or
cover other than that in which it is published, and without a similar condition including this condition being
imposed upon any subsequent purchaser.

British Library Cataloguing in Publication Data

A catalogue record for this book is available from the
British Library.

ISBN 1 86156 218 7

Printed and bound in the UK by Athenaeum Press Limited,
Gateshead, Tyne & Wear.

Contents

Contributors

Sue Archbold MPhil, Nottingham Paediatric Cochlear Implant Programme

Yvonne Cope MSc, Nottingham Paediatric Cochlear Implant Programme

Dee Dyar LCSLT, Nottingham Paediatric Cochlear Implant Programme

Sarah Flynn MSc, South of England Cochlear Implant Programme, Southampton

Kevin P Gibbin FRCS, Nottingham Paediatric Cochlear Implant Programme

Steve Mason PhD, Medical Physics Department, Queen's Medical Centre, Nottingham

Barry McCormick OBE, PhD, Nottingham Paediatric Cochlear Implant Programme

Thomas P Nikolopoulos MD, DM, PhD, Nottingham Paediatric Cochlear Implant Programme

Gerard M O'Donoghue FRCS, Nottingham Paediatric Cochlear Implant Programme

Hazel Lloyd-Richmond BEd, Nottingham Paediatric Cochlear Implant Programme

Margaret Tait PhD, Nottingham Paediatric Cochlear Implant Programme

Catherine L Totten MSc, Nottingham Paediatric Cochlear Implant Programme

Foreword

The cochlear implant field has seen great advances in the last 20 years, no more so than in the management of children with a profound hearing loss. These advances were facilitated by a number of studies in children that commenced using a single-electrode system in 1980, and a multiple-electrode system in 1985. Since those studies there have been significant developments internationally in the management of children. These have included improved speech processing strategies and their adaptation to children. Greater experience has shown that children who undergo operations at a young age will achieve better speech and language skills than older children. The important relation between speech perception and production, language, and educational methods, is now appreciated. The implant has also been the stimulus for a greater knowledge of neuropsychology, learning, and other areas of cognition. The wider question of human communication is being addressed, and the implications of implants for auditory-oral, sign language of the deaf, and total communication are now being brought into focus. The benefits offered by the implant are the motivation behind research to develop special psychophysical, speech feature, and speech tests in very young children, and measures to better assess the psychosocial and economic benefits.

Although the results for children are now good they still do not achieve near normal hearing especially in background noise, and there is considerable variability in performance. For this reason more research is needed and a further refinement of clinic procedures.

The Nottingham clinic was the first to be established in the UK to manage children. The team is an interdisciplinary team of surgeons, audiologists, speech pathologists and educators. The members of the team have written extensively on their experience and studies and they encapsulated their early work in the first edition of their book *Cochlear Implants for Young Children*. This book outlined their goals, objectives and achievements and provided a great resource of material for both the specialist and the generalist. It gave a clear and thorough explanation of the management of the clinic, the audiological and medical aspects of selection, and the post-operative testing, fitting and programming of the device. It concluded with a detailed discussion of language and its development, as well as family issues. It combined a depth of experience and wide knowledge of the implant field. Since the first edition there has been continued progress in the design of electrodes, the type of speech processing strategy used, and methods of monitoring the thresholds and comfortable levels. The new edition is very timely considering the expanding nature of the field, and will provide an excellent base for further research and clinical studies. The authors are to be congratulated for their efforts in bringing this edition to fruition.

Graeme Clark AO
The University of Melbourne/The Bionic Ear Institute

Preface

There can be no doubt that the advent of cochlear implantation marks the most significant new trend to have influenced the progress of profoundly deaf children. We are extremely fortunate to have witnessed such advances during our lifetime and it is a particular honour to have a foreword from one of the pioneers of the technique, Professor Graeme Clarke, in this new volume.

The preface to the first edition of this book stated that cochlear implantation had grown at an exceptional pace. No one could have predicted that the pace would step up to such an extent in subsequent years that the previous growth would be viewed as pedestrian in comparison. When the first edition was published, paediatric cochlear implant programmes were, on the whole, in their infancy and, just like the children they serve, they have matured considerably with the passage of time. Armed with long-term follow-up data we are much wiser now than we were then and this second edition contains a wealth of cumulative results on the 350 children so far implanted in the Nottingham programme.

The intention of the first edition was to offer guidance and encouragement to other teams who were considering the implantation of very young children. Enthusiasm has been out there in abundance with desire for implantation and for the setting up of new programmes often outstripping available resources. This has attracted the attention of health economists and forced the need for programmes to justify their very existence and their every step with outcome measures.

The first edition offered a practical guide to techniques that had been adopted in the evolving programme at Nottingham. If that text proved useful to readers then this latest volume should prove to be even more valuable containing, as it does, a mass of data on children in addition to extending coverage of the 'how we do it' approach. Although primarily aimed at professionals already working in the area the book should also be of interest to students and parents of deaf children.

Barry McCormick OBE
Senior Editor
October 2002

Chapter 1
Current trends in paediatric cochlear implantation

THOMAS P NIKOLOPOULOS, SUE ARCHBOLD, BARRY McCORMICK

Cochlear implantation now ranks as one of the most successful forms of management enabling profoundly deaf individuals to gain a sense of hearing and to develop and maintain spoken language skills. The introduction of a new healthcare technology such as cochlear implantation demands a close scrutiny of benefits and eventual outcomes to justify both the investment of resources and the risks associated with any medical and surgical intervention. In the case of children the responsibility for making decisions rests with their parents and it is vital that, prior to considering implantation for their children, they should be informed of a full range of risks, benefits and outcomes so that they can make an informed choice based on evidence.

There are complex issues surrounding the assessment of benefit in young deaf children. Benefit may be defined differently by parents, purchasers of healthcare, representatives of the deaf community and eventually by the children themselves as they become teenagers and adults. Progress for deaf children could, of course, be influenced by a wide range of variables including duration of deafness, age at implantation or hearing-aid fitting, degree of residual hearing, etiology, efficiency of hearing aid or cochlear implant use, mode of communication, educational management, degree of home support and commitment, to name just a few. These variables and their complex interactions pose challenges to investigators in their search for definitive predictions of benefit for individual cases. It is necessary, therefore, to consider observable trends in order to

1

enlighten our knowledge about cochlear implantation and its success or failure. It is instructive to consider these trends under various headings.

Audiological trends

The availability of long-term outcomes from cochlear implantation has produced an interesting dilemma. Early candidates, for whom the long-term outcomes are now available, often outperform their profoundly deaf peers who continue to use hearing aids and many now function on a par with severely deaf hearing-aid users (a full discussion is given in Chapter 4). Performance and progress can be assessed using a wide variety of measures that will be outlined in later chapters of this book but the most obvious changes are seen in spoken language perception and speech production skills, described in more detail in Chapter 10. The limitations of hearing aids for different groups of children now need to be considered in the light of the strong evidence of the benefits of cochlear implantation. The early candidates for cochlear implantation tended to be deafer, with longer durations of deafness, and tended to be older at the time of implantation than children who have received cochlear implants in more recent years. Each of these factors could militate against optimum performance with the devices and yet many of these children have still often outperformed their hearing-aided peers. What sort of long-term performance might we expect from children for whom all factors are working in their favour? Present cochlear implant systems are more sophisticated than the older devices and the application of the latest technology to children who have greater levels of neural survival (associated with significant amounts of residual hearing), and who receive their implants at more optimum times, should produce far better results.

Cochlear implant selection criteria have gradually relaxed over the years as a direct consequence of the documented high level of performance of the users, giving rise to the trend to implant children with greater amounts of residual hearing. The improvement of speech intelligibility and of access to telephone use are now very real possibilities. These were not envisaged as outcomes in the very early days of cochlear implantation when the expectation was to impart some basic and rather rudimentary stimulation of the auditory system. The significant changes in the audiological selection criteria that have taken place will be detailed in Chapter 4.

Trends in implantation age

At the beginning of the new millennium early implantation has become a factor of great importance in paediatric cochlear implantation and serious debate has taken place about the most appropriate age to implant a young deaf child. Auditory discrimination abilities have been demonstrated in human subjects very early in life, as normally hearing neonates have a preference for the voice to which they were mostly exposed *in utero* (DeCasper and Prescott, 1984). Infants with hearing are becoming linguistically sophisticated by one year of age, although this may not be clearly visible to naïve observers. During this period of time, the neurones in the auditory pathways are maturing and billions of major neural connections are being formed. The auditory system appears to adapt in response to psychophysical and electrophysiological stimuli over time (Ruben, 1997). When sensory input to the auditory nervous system is interrupted, especially during early development, the morphology and functional properties of neurones in the central auditory system can break down (Sininger, Doyle and Moore, 1999). It seems that the ability of neuroplasticity in the developing auditory system declines as children grow older and therefore early implantation could result in shorter auditory deprivation and better spoken language acquisition.

When reviewing the literature with regard to age at implantation there have been conflicting conclusions in the past. This may arise from studies which contain small numbers of children, and widely heterogeneous groups, and which have only comparatively short-term results. (Nikolopoulos et al, 1999). Shea, Domico and Lupfer, (1994) for example, found that age at implantation was positively correlated with outcomes in pre-lingually and peri-lingually deafened children. This earlier study may be thought to support later, rather than earlier, implantation. However, only 26 children were studied with ages at implantation ranging from two to 16 years old, and more than half of them had been implanted before less than 1.5 years. Children older at implantation may initially do better than younger children, because of their better language levels and ability to carry out testing, but when one follows the younger implanted children over a longer time-scale, the better outcomes in these younger children become apparent, as the following study shows.

Outcomes in terms of speech perception and production were measured on open and closed-set measures of speech perception and on two hierarchical scales of auditory perception and speech intelligibility (Nikolopoulos et al, 1999). The hierarchical scale of auditory perception was Categories of Auditory Performance (see Chapter 3; Archbold et al, 1998) and the scale for speech intelligibility was the Speech Intelligibility Rating (see Chapter 10; Allen et al, 1998). Results were reported on 126 congenitally or pre-lingually deaf children. Up to two years after implantation, a positive correlation between these outcomes and age at implantation was found. However, at three and four years after implantation, a negative correlation was found (all statistically significant, p< 0.5). This study demonstrated the importance of long-term follow-up in those children implanted early. Although the results support early implantation, older children should not be excluded from assessment on the basis of age alone, and may do well.

The effect of age at implantation on the long-term functional outcome is illustrated in Figures 1.1 and 1.2. Figure 1.1 illustrates the comparative percentages of children achieving either of the two top categories of the rating scale, Categories of Auditory Performance (Archbold, Lutman and Nikolopoulos, 1998). Significantly more children implanted below the age of five achieve these categories four years after implantation than those implanted over

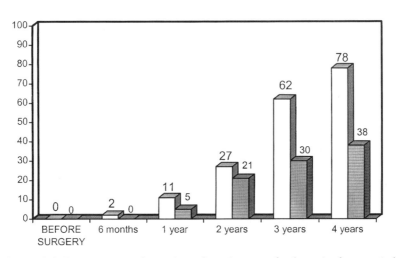

Figure 1.1. Percentages and actual numbers (on top of columns) of congenitally deaf children achieving the category of 'understanding conversation without lip-reading' or 'use of telephone with a known speaker' using Categories of Auditory Performance (CAP), comparing those implanted under five years of age with those implanted at five years of age and over.

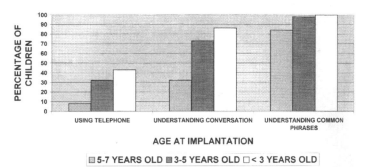

SPEECH PERCEPTION IN IMPLANTED
PRELINGUALLY DEAF CHILDREN 4 YEARS
AFTER IMPLANTATION

Figure 1.2. Pre-lingually deaf children achieving understanding of common phrases without lipreading, understanding conversation without lipreading and using the telephone, four years after implantation, comparing implantation at different ages.

five years of age. Figure 1.2 breaks this down further: it shows children born deaf or pre-lingually deafened, four years after implantation, and their attainments as rated by Categories of Auditory Perfomance on using the telephone, understanding conversation without lipreading and understanding common phrases without lipreading, comparing those implanted below the age of three, with those implanted between three and five, and those implanted over five. While there is little difference in outcomes on closed-set measures, such as understanding common phrases, there is a significant difference due to age at implantation in those achieving the understanding of conversation and the use of the telephone. A similar result is achieved using the Speech Intelligibility Rating, and shown in Chapter 10.

A consensus is now being established on the importance of early implantation, summarized by Miyamoto (2002) who considered that six months of age is now the youngest age to consider implantation. Other studies have supported the idea of implanting deaf children younger than two years of age (Lenarz in Honjo and Takahashi, 1997; Waltzman and Cohen, 1998), but there is, as yet, no strong evidence that a child implanted at one year of age will outperform a similar child implanted at two years of age. On the other hand, certain concerns have been raised with regard to implantation of very young children including:

- the relatively small size of the skull and its growth in young children with potential surgical difficulties of access and

possible increase in surgical risk (later complications of electrode displacement);
- the high prevalence of otitis media in this age group and
subsequent related complications; and
- difficulties in tuning, rehabilitation and identification of other
difficulties.

These issues are discussed more fully in Chapter 3, but the data
so far have not supported these concerns and implantation in
very young age is feasible and relatively safe (Waltzman and
Cohen, 1998; Miyamoto, 2002).

Other issues, such as post-meningitic ossification, may expe-
dite the decision to proceed, irrespective of the child's very young
age. On the other hand, adequate time is needed for parents to
realize the existence of, and adjust to, their child's deafness and
for audiologists to establish true hearing thresholds and to assess
the potential benefits of conventional hearing aids.

In conclusion, the current trend in paediatric cochlear
implantation is to implant younger children, and this is likely to
continue with the introduction of Newborn Hearing Screening.

Trends in educational management

The educational management of children following implantation has become a major issue.

Educational placement is an important outcome measure from
paediatric cochlear implantation as it is likely to have educational
implications (Archbold et al., 1998). Comparisons of the educational settings of profoundly deaf children implanted in the
Nottingham programme with those of profoundly deaf children in
the UK revealed that profoundly deaf children implanted early
(when they are still at the pre-school stage) are three times more
likely to attend mainstream school three years following implantation than profoundly deaf children of the same age using hearing
aids (Archbold et al., 2002). The educational settings of implanted
children with three years experience with their devices were: 41%
in mainstream schools, 52% in units in mainstream schools and
only 7% in schools for the deaf. The respective percentages for age-
matched profoundly deaf children with hearing aids were: 13% in
mainstream schools, 62% in units of mainstream schools, and 25%
are placed in schools for the deaf (Figure 1.3).

Data from the Nottingham programme also revealed that children implanted at an age younger than five years old are three

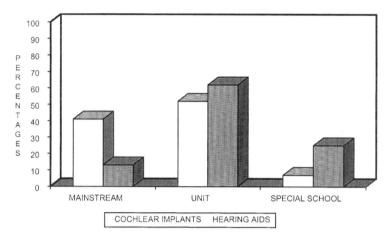

Figure 1.3. Educational placement of profoundly deaf children of the same age, comparing those with hearing aids and those with cochlear implants. Cochear implant children are at the three-year interval following implantation. All implanted children were implanted before five years of age.

times more likely to be placed in mainstream schools and five times less likely to be placed in schools for the deaf in comparison with children implanted above the age of five (Figure 1.4). However, educational placement continues to be monitored; with the challenges of secondary education, will this trend continue in the long term? Chapter 3 gives a fuller discussion of the educational issues, with its complexities.

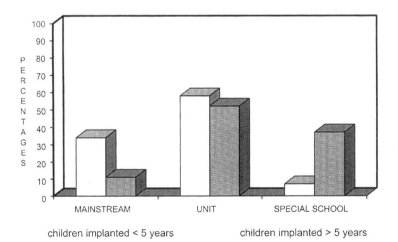

Figure 1.4. Educational placement of implanted children three years after implantation. Comparisons of those children implanted under five years of age with those implanted over five years of age.

A debate also exists with regard to the most appropriate mode of communication for deaf children. We explored the relationship between the approach to communication and measures of speech perception and production three, four, and five years following cochlear implantation in young pre-lingually deaf children (Archbold et al., 2000). The communication approach used by each child was classified by his/her teacher of the deaf at each interval into one of two categories: oral communication and signed communication. The results revealed that, at all intervals, those children classified as using oral communication significantly exceeded those using signed communication on measures of speech perception and intelligibility ($p < 0.05$). However, when those children who had changed from using signed to oral communication during the three years after implantation were compared at the three-year interval with those who used oral communication throughout, there was no significant difference in their results. It remains to be explored whether children use oral communication after implantation because they are doing well, or whether they do well because they are using oral communication.

Trends in patient-oriented healthcare

Parents' perspectives are very important and therefore there is a compelling need to involve them fully in assessment of outcomes. It is now becoming more broadly accepted that any new method of treatment should engage the wider public in discussion about what a national health service should provide and who should decide it (Chisholm, 1999). Moreover, it has also been suggested that repeated evaluation of patients' (or parental) views should become an integral part of routine healthcare (Richards, 1999).

However, the methods of assessment of quality of life issues with regard to both children and parents following paediatric cochlear implantation are extremely limited; as described in Chapter 11, parents at the Nottingham programme are asked to complete a questionnaire prior to implantation, and annually following implantation. The results show that their expectations were met, or surpassed, following implantation (Nikolopoulos et al., 2001; and see Chapter 11 for fuller discussion). A further questionnaire has been developed, based on open parental responses three years after implantation, which has been found to be robust and repeatable (Archbold et al., 2002). Content analysis of the open responses revealed the three most common constructs mentioned by parents to be the positive changes in confidence (linked to communication) seen in their children, the need for continuing links with the implant centre, particularly for long-term technical support, and the importance of liaison between the cochlear implant centre and the local educational service. Clearly, paediatric cochlear implantation is a service that necessarily closely interacts with parents and the local professionals providing long-term support to the child, and ways in which this can be organized are discussed in Chapter 3.

Trends in measures of effectiveness

It is no longer sufficient to provide information on safety or efficacy of healthcare services; we are now required to demonstrate cost effectiveness (Niparko in Niparko et al., 2000). This obliges services to produce information both on accurate costings and on outcomes, requiring careful data collection over time. Several measures, including Categories of Auditory Performance, and Speech Intelligibility Rating (Allen, Nikolopoulos and O'Donoghue, 1998) have been developed by the Nottingham programme to be accessible to the non-specialist, including purchasers of services, and to demonstrate outcomes over a long time-frame from different patient groups. Chapters 3 and 10 give further details. In addition, a major indication of effectiveness is the usage rate of the device. Unlike other implantable devices, the child can choose not to wear the external equipment, and thus continued high usage rates are an indication of patient satisfaction and an effective use of the financial investment. The Nottingham programme constantly monitors the usage rates via parents and teacher reports. Five years after implantation, 99% of our children are wearing their devices all or most of the time, according to parents, and only 1% are non-users at this stage of the programme. We have a few children who have later chosen to wear their devices only for some of the time, and 1% who are now choosing not to wear their devices at all. Maintaining this high usage rate relies on careful assessment of candidatures, appropriate tuning of devices, careful monitoring of functioning, and liaison with parents and local services.

Over the 10 years since the establishment of the programme, the necessary infrastructure to support this long-term effective use has become more evident, and the various chapters in this book describe the developing service provision, as the numbers grow. Dramatic changes have been seen in candidature, expectations and outcomes. Inevitably, practice has changed too, and those of us working in this challenging and ever-changing field have a responsibility to ensure that our children have the best possible lifelong care.

References

Allen C, Nikolopoulos T, O'Donoghue GM (1998) Speech intelligibility in children after cochlear implantation. The American Journal of Otology 19: 742–6.

Archbold SM, Nikolopoulos TP, Lutman ME, O'Donoghue GM (2002) The educational settings of profoundly deaf children with cochlear implants compared with age-matched peers with hearing aids: implications for management. International Journal of Audiology 41(3): pp. 157–161.

Archbold SM, Lutman ME, Gregory S, O'Neill C, Nikolopoulos TP (2002) Parents and their deaf child: their perceptions three years after cochlear implantation. Deafness and Education International 4(1): pp.12–40.

Archbold S, Nikolopoulos T, Tait M, O' Donoghue G, Lutman M, Gregory S (2000) Approach to communication and speech perception and intelligibility following paediatric cochlear implantation. British Journal of Audiology 34: 257–64.

Archbold S, Nikolopoulos T, O' Donoghue G, Lutman M (1998) Educational placement of deaf children following cochlear implantation. British Journal of Audiology 32: 295–300.

Archbold S, Lutman M, Nikolopoulos T (1998) Categories of auditory performance: inter-user reliability. British Journal of Audiology 32: 295–300.

Chisholm J (1999) Viagra: a botched test case for rationing. British Medical Journal 318: 273–4.

DeCasper AJ, Prescott PA (1984) Human newborns' perception of male voices: preference, discrimination and reinforcing value. Dev Psychol 17: 481–91.

Lenarz T (1997) Cochlear implantation in children under the age of two years. In Honjo I, Takahashi H (eds) Cochlear Implant and Related Sciences Update. Advances in Otorhinolaryngology. Basel: Karger, pp. 204–10.

Miyamoto RT (2002) Early Cochlear Implantation in Congenitally Deaf Children. Paper presented at 2nd International Conference on Newborn Hearing Screening Diagnosis and Intervention. Como May 30–Jun 1 2002.

Niparko JK, Cheng AK, Francis HW (2000) Outcomes of cochlear implantation: assessment of quality of life impact and economic evaluation of the benefits of the cochlear implant in relation to costs. In Niparko JK, Iler Kirk K, Mellon NK, McConkey Robbins A, Tucci DL, Wilson BS (eds) Cochlear Implants: Principles and Practices. Philadelphia, PA: Lippincott Williams & Wilkins, pp. 269–88.

Nikolopoulos TP, Lloyd H, Archbold S, O'Donoghue GM (2001) Pediatric Cochlear Implantation: The Parents' Perspective. Archives of Otolaryngology Head Neck Surgery 127: 363–7.

Nikolopoulos TP, O'Donoghue GM, Archbold S (1999) Age at implantation: its importance in pediatric cochlear implantations. Laryngoscope 109: 595–99.

Richards T (1999) Patients' priorities need to be assessed properly and taken into account. British Medical Journal 318: 277.

Ruben RJ (1997) A time frame of critical/sensitive periods of language development. Acta Otolaryngologica (Stockh) 117: 202–5.

Shea JJ, Domico EH, Lupfer M (1994) Speech perception after multichannel cochlear implantation in the pediatric patient. American Journal of Otology 15(1): 66–70.

Sininger YS, Doyle KJ, Moore JK (1999) The case for early identification of hearing loss in children. Pediatric Clinics of North America 46(1): 1–11.

Waltzman SB, Cohen NI (1998) Cochlear implantation in children younger than 2 years old. American Journal of Otology 19: 158–62.

Chapter 2
Cochlear implant systems

SARAH FLYNN

Introduction

Hearing impairment arises from dysfunction of any part of the auditory pathway. Medical or surgical treatment can alleviate some specific types of hearing loss. It is possible to compensate for the dysfunction of the inner ear (cochlea) by amplifying sound with conventional hearing aids or, in the case of minimal cochlear function, by stimulating remaining nerve tissue in the cochlea electrically with a cochlear implant. Partial hearing can be restored to profoundly deaf people with cochlear implants that attempt to bypass dysfunction in the cochlea.

Sound undergoes transformation in the ear. The outer ear picks up acoustic pressure waves that are transformed into mechanical vibrations by the tympanic membrane and small bones in the middle ear. In the cochlea or inner ear the mechanical vibrations are converted into fluid vibrations, which cause the basillar membrane inside the cochlea to move. On the basillar membrane are thousands of hair cells that bend where the membrane moves and release an electrochemical substance causing excitation of adjacent neurones. From these nerve endings the signal is sent through the auditory nerve to the brain where it is perceived as hearing. More hair cells are bent at the location of maximum displacement of the basillar membrane. This location varies with frequency and, thus, each place in the cochlea responds best to specific frequencies. Low frequencies result in the largest movement of the basillar membrane at the apex of the cochlea whereas high frequencies give the largest displacement at the base of the cochlea. The rate that neurones fire at may also play a role in the analysis of sound in the cochlea (Shannon et al., 1995; Langer, 1997; Pijl, 1997). When the hair cells in the cochlea are damaged or absent there is a break in the auditory pathway resulting in a sensory hearing loss. There may also be some accompanying degeneration of adjacent neurones giving a neural component and, therefore, a sensorineural hearing loss. Research suggests that cochlear implants can give benefit even if there is degeneration of some spiral ganglion cells in the auditory system (Nadol, Young and Glynn, 1989; Hinjosa, Douglas Green and Marion, 1991; Fayad et al., 1991; Blamey, 1997; Kawano et al., 1998). Cochlear implants induce a sensation

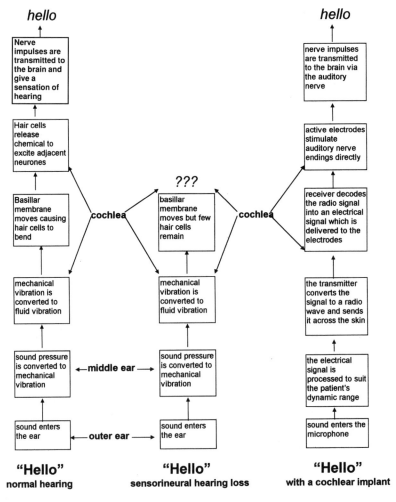

Figure 2.1. Flow diagram of how a cochlear implant works showing how sound is processed in a normally hearing ear, in an ear with sensorineural hearing loss and in an implanted ear.

of hearing to people with sensorineural hearing loss by directly stimulating the remaining auditory nerve tissue thus bridging the break in transmission of sound caused by lost or damaged hair cells in the cochlea.

Adults and older children with acquired hearing losses have gained better speech perception and psychological benefits from cochlear implantation although the degree of benefit varies considerably between individuals (Cohen, Waltzman and Fisher, 1993; Summerfield and Marshall, 1995; Tyler and Summerfield, 1996; Knutson et al., 1998; Maillet, Tyler and Jordan, 1995). Profoundly deaf children implanted at a young age have been able to develop auditory/verbal means of communication with the aid of cochlear implants even though they have had little or no experience of hearing (Osberger et al., 1996; Tait and Lutman, 1994; Waltzman et al., 1994; Gantz et al., 1994; Miyamoto et al., 1993; Miyamoto et al., 1995; Cohen and Waltzman, 1996; Miyamoto, Svirsky and Robbins, 1997; Snik et al., 1997; Parkinson, El-Kholy and Tyler, 1998; Spencer, Tye-Murray and Tomblin, 1998; O'Donoghue et al., 1999; Miyamoto et al., 1999). This chapter looks at the development of cochlear implants and reviews the most widely used systems with particular reference to the choice of suitable implants for children.

Development of cochlear implants

Early development of cochlear implants

Interest in the electrical stimulation of the cochlea has a long history, beginning with Volta's experiment in 1800 in which he stimulated his own ears electrically producing an unpleasant sound-like sensation.

Considerably later, in 1930, Weaver and Bray discovered that the cochlea acts as a transducer of mechanical energy into electrical energy, which is then transmitted via the auditory nerve to the brain. Dijourno and Eyries (1957) carried out direct electrical stimulation of the auditory nerve. The subject described some auditory sensation that helped with lipreading and made him aware of background noise. At this time there were doubts about safety and the long-term feasibility of electrical stimulation of auditory nerve cells. In the 1960s, however, the first clinical cochlear implant, developed by House and Urban, became available (House et al., 1976; House and Berliner, 1986; House and Berliner, 1991). This first system, the 3M/House device, was

a relatively simple single channel device with one active electrode and gave benefit mostly as an aid to lip-reading. Another
widely used single channel implant was the 3M/Vienna cochlear
implant. This device preserved more of the temporal features of
speech than the 3M/House device by applying frequency equal-
ization to the incoming signal and improving the compression of
the signal to better suit patients' dynamic ranges (Burian,
Hochmair-Desoyer and Eisenwort, 1986; Tyler 1988). The early
development of cochlear implants is reviewed by Simmons
(1966).

Single and multi-channel implants

Single channel implants deliver auditory information through
one channel. Multi-channel implants convey different parts of
the signal via several distinct channels that stimulate different
regions of the cochlea. The terms single and multi-channel are
used to describe the number of active electrodes through which
different information is sent; whereas single or multi-electrode
refers to the number of electrodes that the implant has. Thus, in
a single channel system the same information may be duplicated
on several electrodes or just conveyed via a single electrode.
Cochlear implants have been developed with active electrodes
placed inside the cochlea (intra-cochlear) and outside the
cochlea (extracochlear). Extracochlear devices are less invasive
because there is no damage to the cochlea but higher current
levels are required to give stimulation because the active electrodes are further away from nerve endings. Implantees' speech
perception is not as good with extracochlear systems (Hortman
et al., 1989; Kasper, Pelizzone and Montandon, 1991).

  Following the success of single channel implants in giving
auditory stimulation safely (Bilger, 1977) multi-channel intra-
cochlear devices were developed. The first commercially available multi-channel cochlear implants were the Symbion or Utah
device, later known as the Ineraid implant, developed by
Eddington et al. (1978) and the Nucleus Melbourne cochlear
implant developed by Clark et al. (1987). Several other cochlear
implants were developed for research and clinical use and are
discussed in more detail by Mecklenberg and Lehnhardt (1991)
and Lance de Foa and Loeb (1991).

  Intra-cochlear multi-channel cochlear implants give rise to
larger improvements in speech discrimination over a wide range
of tests compared with single channel or extracochlear devices

(Gantz et al., 1988; Cohen, Waltzman and Fisher, 1993; Weston and Waltzman, 1995). Most patients who have had single channel implants replaced with multi-channel implants have shown varying degrees of improvement in speech and environmental sound recognition (Doyle, Pilj and Noel, 1991; Pijl, 1991; Eyles, Aleksy and Boyle,1995). Children using multi-channel implants have shown greater improvements in speech production than those using single channel devices (Osberger et al., 1991). Most studies reporting the differences in benefit between multi-channel and single channel implants demonstrate considerable variation in results between different individuals. Many other factors than the implant itself can influence implantees' performance such as the patient's age, duration of deafness, auditory neurone survival and length of time of implant use. Given the body of evidence, however, implant programmes now choose to use multi-channel, intra-cochlear implants because they generally give superior patient performance.

Cochlear implants for children

All the early work with cochlear implants was with adults. There was a reluctance to implant children, especially those who were born deaf or had lost their hearing in the early stages of language development. The deaf community worldwide is generally resistant to implantation and believe that the hearing people are trying to 'cure' deafness (House, 1986; Tyler, 1993; Cohen, 1994; Lane, 1995). Cochlear implants do not cure deafness and should be regarded as sophisticated hearing aids that offer alternative help with communication. The benefits of implantation for adults had exceeded initial expectations and there were few adverse effects. House, therefore, began implanting children with single channel implants and most received benefit (House, Berliner and Eisenberg, 1983). Multi-channel implants were used in children when their increased benefit over single channel devices had been demonstrated in adults. Initially, only children with post-lingually acquired hearing losses were implanted but it became clear that young congenitally deafened children could also benefit from cochlear implantation (McCormick, 1991; Osberger et al., 1996; Miyamoto et al., 1995). Nearly 800 children had received cochlear implants in the UK by the end of 1997 (Summerfield and Marshall, 1999).

Children are now being implanted at younger ages (Lenarz, Battmer and Bertram, 2000; Cohen and Waltzman, 1996; Waltzman et al., 1994; Miyamoto, Svirsky and Robbins, 1997; Miyamoto et al., 1999) and those with more residual hearing are likely to gain from implantation (Kiefer et al., 1998; Rubenstein et al., 1999). Cochlear deformity (Bent, Chute and Parisier, 1999), ossification in the cochlea (Balkany, Gantz and Nadol, 1988; Bredberg et al., 1997; Ramsden et al., 1997; Kirk, Sehgal and Miyamoto, 1997; Richardson et al., 1999) and other medical conditions no longer necessarily preclude implantation (Gibbin, O'Donoghue and Murty, 1993; Axon et al., 1997; Szilvassy et al., 1998; Cinamon et al., 1997; Camilleri et al., 1999).

Evolving speech processing for multi-channel implants

The first two widely used multi-channel devices used different speech processing philosophies. The Ineraid device used the compressed analogue (CA) strategy in which the raw signal is filtered and compressed and then split into different frequency bands, which are delivered to each of four separate channels simultaneously and continuously (Eddington et al., 1978; Parkin and Stewart, 1988). The early Nucleus devices delivered stimulation as a series of pulses sampled from the incoming sound. Formant features of speech, which are important for speech recognition, were extracted and delivered to different channels depending on their frequency (Clark et al., 1987). The original F0F2 strategy was improved by including additional formant information to give strategies such as F0F1F2 (Tye-Murray, Lowder and Tyler, 1990). The MPEAK strategy was then developed, which extracted higher frequency information as well as the formants and delivered this to other channels depending on the frequency of the input signal. This improved implantees' performance further (Koch et al., 1990; Patrick and Clark, 1991; Von Wallenberg and Battmer, 1991).

Many implanted patients did remarkably well with both the MPEAK and CA strategies despite their different approaches to speech processing (Teig et al., 1992; Tye-Murray et al., 1992). There was, however, more inter-subject variation with the same device than variation between devices. With the simultaneous stimulation of the Ineraid device some patients were unable to benefit from different information being delivered to different parts of the cochlea (Dorman et al., 1990). This is caused by current spreading and giving rise to channel interactions that resulted in some neurones being stimulated by two channels at the same time (Favre and Pelizzone, 1993). The Nucleus device delivered stimulus pulses to different channels sequentially so that channel interaction was minimized. Performance with the feature extraction strategies of the Nucleus implant was, however, limited by the feature extraction algorithms, which tended to make errors in formant extraction especially when the speech was embedded in noise (Dillier et al., 1995; Skinner et al., 1994).

A new signal processing method was developed for the Nucleus implant, which analyses the incoming waveform and extracts a given number of peaks from the signal. The loudest frequencies, or spectral maxima, in the incoming signal are extracted, processed and delivered to different electrodes depending on their frequency. No attempt is made in this strategy to extract specific features of speech. This strategy is known as the SPEAK strategy (Skinner et al., 1994) and is still widely and successfully used with patients who have the Nucleus 22 implant. The majority of both adults and children have been shown to achieve better speech recognition with the SPEAK strategy compared with older Nucleus strategies (Shallop and McGinn-Brunelli, 1995; Cowan et al., 1995; Lenarz and Battmer, 1995; Sehgal et al., 1998).

A significant number of Ineraid patients have had access to the newer continuous interleaved sampling (CIS) speech processing strategy (Wilson et al., 1991; Wilson et al., 1995) with alternative speech processors adapted for use with the Ineraid implant. All Ineraid patients improved their speech perception scores in quiet, but not always in noise, with the new CIS processors after a period of adjustment (Wilson, 1993; Pelizzone, Cosendai and Tinembart, 1999; Kompis, Vischer and Hausler, 1999).

The success of cochlear implantation does not, however, consist only of the implant system itself; implantees need help in learning how to use the new sound sensation. In a survey by Tucci, Lambert and Ruth (1990) all clinicians who were polled agreed that rehabilitation was of great importance and required considerable time, especially for children, to promote the successful use of the implant. Improvements in cochlear implant technology are likely to continue to lead to better speech recognition at an earlier stage, thus encouraging patients in the use of their implants and having a synergistic effect with rehabilitation.

Components of cochlear implant systems

Cochlear implant systems are made up of several components and all require the patient to wear equipment externally as well as having the internal, surgically implanted electrode array. The external equipment comprises the microphone, the speech processor and a means of transferring the signal to the implanted electrodes. More than one component may be housed in the same casing in some systems.

Microphone

The microphone collects sound from the environment and converts it into an electrical signal. For most body-worn systems the microphone is housed in its own case which is similar in appearance to a small post-aural hearing aid. The microphone for the Clarion S series device is on the transmitter. The signal is transferred from the microphone to the body-worn speech processor via a lead. The Nucleus CI24M, Medel Combi 40+ and Clarion CII systems have the option of behind the ear processors which have integral microphones.

Speech processors

The speech processor converts the raw signal from the microphone into a form that can be delivered to the implanted electrodes and produces an audible yet comfortable sensation of hearing. The parameters of the various speech processing strategies used in different implants are discussed in a later section. The speech

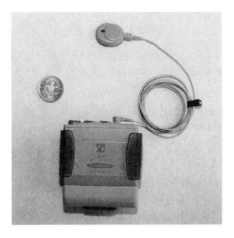

Figure 2.2. Clarion S series speech processor and integral transmitter coil and microphone.

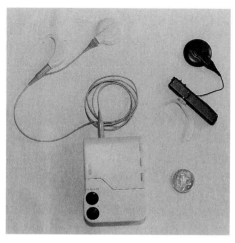

Figure 2.3. Medel Combi 40+ speech processors; the Cispro+ body-worn processor, microphone and transmitter coil (left) and the Tempo+ post-aural speech processor with integral microphone and transmitter coil (right).

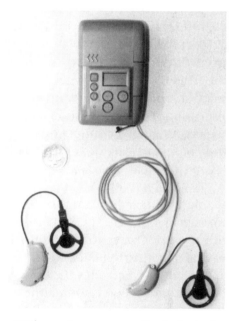

Figure 2.4. Nucleus C124 speech processors; the Sprint body-worn processor, microphone and transmitter coil (left) and the Esprit post-aural speech processor with integral microphone and transmitter coil (right).

processor has programmable electronics that are set individually to suit each patient by an audiologist with the aid of a computer and a device-specific interface. Implant programming is discussed in detail in Chapter 7. Speech processors have on/off switches and adjustable sensitivity controls. They may also have volume controls and programme selection buttons if the processor can store more than one programme. Most new-generation processors have warning lights or sounds to indicate faults; a particularly useful feature for children. Speech processors may be body-worn or post-aural but at the present time most children are still using body-worn processors. The Nucleus Esprit and Esprit 22 post-aural processors support the SPEAK strategy only. The Nucleus 3G post-aural processor can support SPEAK and other faster rate speech processing strategies. The Medel Tempo+ post-aural speech processor supports the CIS processing strategy. The Clarion CII post-aural processor supports a range of speech processing options. This processor uses its own rechargeable batteries that generally need to be changed more than once a day.

Signal transfer to the implanted electrodes

The signal and power from the speech processor needs to be delivered to the internal electrode array. The simplest method of doing this is a direct hardware connection through the skin via a plug or pedestal fixed surgically to the skull as used in the Ineraid implant. This method of connection is known as percutaneous connection and has the advantage that it is easier to apply new processing strategies without replacing the internal electrode array. Percutaneous connections are, however, prone to damage and infection can develop around the pedestal, which in the worst case can necessitate reimplantation (Cohen and Hoffman, 1991; Eyles et al., 2000). For this reason all currently available cochlear implants use transcutaneous links where the skin remains intact. The signal is transmitted across the skin via an FM carrier wave to the internal receiver stimulator; here the signal is converted back to an electrical signal and stimulates the implanted electrodes. In most systems the transmitter and the internal receiver stimulator are magnetized to keep the transmitter and receiver correctly aligned and thus maintain good contact across the skin.

Implanted electrode array

The electrode array is connected to the internal receiver stimulator. The intra-cochlear electrodes are housed in flexible casing and have contacts at points spaced along the electrode array. At the contacts, which may be rings, discs or rectangles, the electric current coded by the speech processor excites remaining nerve cells in the cochlea. The signal is then transmitted up the auditory neural pathway to the brain and gives a sensation of hearing. The implant must be constructed to a very high standard and under clean conditions so that it is safe and maintenance free over a long period of time. The internal implant package is sealed within a biocompatible material, such as silastic, to isolate it from body tissue and fluids and to avoid any undesired non-auditory stimulation or tissue changes (Shepherd, Franz and Clark, 1990).

Different systems have varying numbers of intra-cochlear electrodes. The electrode contacts, spacing of electrodes and the overall length of the electrode array also vary with different implants. The position and number of electrodes affects how current is delivered to remaining nerve endings in the cochlea. Electrode arrays are not inserted the whole depth of the cochlea and there is, therefore, a frequency mismatch between the normal tonotopic organization in the cochlea and the frequency of the signal from the implant in a given region of the cochlea. Deeper insertion might be expected to result in better patient performance but some implantees with shallow insertions perform as well as those with deeper insertions possibly because of the many other factors that also influence performance with an implant (Loizou, 1998). The Medel Combi 40+ implant currently allows the deepest insertion (Gstoellner et al., 1997). Electrode spacing can influence implantees ability to discriminate between different stimuli on different channels; if electrodes are too closely spaced true channel separation may not be possible (Fu and Shannon, 1999a; Fu and Shannon, 1999b). There may be some advantage to having more electrodes than channels so that the 'best' electrodes can be selected for stimulation in each individual implantee (Lawson et al., 1996).

Until recently most patients were implanted with straight but flexible electrode arrays. Clarion and Nucleus now have curved arrays. Clarion previously used a coiled array that required separate mirror image electrode arrays for left and right ears (Balkany, Cohen and Gantz, 1999; Filipo et al., 1999). The rationale for having a curved array is to position the electrodes closer to remaining nerve tissue in the modiolus or central axis of the cochlea, thus reducing the level of stimulation required and increasing the specificity of stimulation. The design of electrode arrays that 'hug' the modiolus is currently an area of intense research activity.

Cochlear implant manufacturers may offer a choice of electrode arrays. Medel and MXM have split electrode arrays and Nucleus has the option of a double array that may be more suited to cochleae where there is ossification. Different parts of the cochlea are drilled out and then two or more sections of the split array are placed in different regions of the cochlea thus maximizing the possibility of making use of the tonotopic organization of the cochlea (Bredberg et al., 1997; Richardson et al., 1999). Medel also has a short electrode array, which still has the twelve electrodes of the standard array but they are closer together. This array is designed for patients with deformed cochleae when it may not be possible to insert the standard length Medel array.

Stimulation mode

To induce an electrical field current must flow from an active electrode or positive pole to a reference or ground electrode or negative pole. The relative positions of the active and reference electrodes can affect the level of current required for stimulation and the degree of current spread. For monopolar stimulation the active and reference electrodes are positioned remotely; the active electrode is inside the cochlea and the reference electrode is on the receiver stimulator case or embedded in muscle outside the cochlea. If the active and reference electrodes are adjacent to each other inside the cochlea stimulation is bipolar. Current spreads over a wider area with monopolar stimulation than bipolar configurations that activate more discrete groups of neurones. Bipolar stimulation gives more specific stimulation but because fewer neurones are stimulated a higher current level is required to produce the same loudness sensation as monopolar stimulation. All the current generation of implants can use monopolar stimulation and some have the option of bipolar stimulation as well. The Nucleus implant can also use common ground stimulation where all non-active electrodes at a given moment of stimulation form the reference or ground electrode. Pseudo-monopolar stimulation can be used with older versions of the Nucleus 22 implant, which does not have an extracochlear reference electrode, where the first or second electrode inside the cochlea is designated the reference electrode. The modified 20+2 Nucleus implant has extracochlea electrodes for monopolar stimulation (von Wallenberg et al., 1993). The main features of the most commonly used cochlear implants are shown in Table 2.1.

Table 2.1. Features of the most widely used cochlear implant systems including electrode and speech processor characteristics and the stimulus modes and speech processing strategies supported by each device

Implant	Number of electrodes	Spacing of electrodes	Stimulation modes available	Speech processors	Speech processing strategies
Nucleus 22	22	0.75mm	BP CG (MP with newer 22+2 version)	Spectra *Esprit 22	SPEAK SPEAK
Nucleus 24	22	0.75mm	BP MP CG	Sprint *Esprit *3G	SPEAK, ACE, CIS SPEAK SPEAK, ACE, CIS
Clarion	8 pairs	2.0mm	BP MP	S Series *Clarion CII	CIS, SAS, PPS and others CIS, SAS, PPS and others
Medel Combi 40 +	12	2.4mm	MP	CIS pro + *Tempo +	CIS, n of m CIS
Ineraid	6	4.0mm	MP	Ineraid processor CISlink	CA CIS

* indicates post-aural speech processor.
SPEAK - spectral peak strategy.
ACE - advanced combination encoder.
CIS - continuous interleaved sampling strategy.
SAS - simultaneous analogue strategy.
PPS - paired pulsatile strategy.
n of m - n spectral peaks of m channels.
CA - compressed analogue strategy.
MP - monopolar
BP - bipolar
CG - common ground

Speech processing strategies

What is speech processing?

A normally hearing ear can discriminate speech and other sounds by detecting changes in the pitch or frequency and loudness or intensity of the sound with time. The electrical signal of the implant must represent the changes in the sound input to the speech processor so that the implantee can detect pitch and loudness variations and thus have some ability to discriminate speech auditorily.

A normally hearing human ear can detect sound at 0 dB and sound does not cause discomfort until it reaches about 120 dB. This gives a wide dynamic range of 120 dB. The dynamic range for electrical stimulation is between 5 and 20 dB, thus there is only a narrow range between sound being just audible to the level where sound is uncomfortable. Compression of the signal is therefore essential to include a reasonable range of quiet to loud sound. The loudness changes as current density changes in all implant systems. For pulsatile systems the current density can be increased by increasing both current amplitude and pulse duration. Loudness growth functions are usually steeper for quieter sounds, but level off as sound becomes loud, to better represent conversational speech (Zeng and Shannon, 1993; Skinner et al., 1997; Brill, Stobich and Hochmair, 2000). Different implants vary in their implementation of loudness growth (for example, logarithmic type function for Clarion, map law for Medel, Q value for Nucleus) but aspects of loudness growth can be varied to suit individual implantees. Optimum representation of different loudness levels can aid implantees' ability to discriminate phonemes (Zeng and Galvin, 1999). Stobich, Zierhofer and Hochmair (1999) have looked at the possibility of using two-stage compression to improve patient performance in variable noise conditions.

Multi-channel cochlear implants make use of the tonotopic organization of the cochlea by dividing incoming sound into separate frequency bands and delivering different spectral information to the most appropriate places in the cochlea. The range of frequencies delivered via the implant can affect speech perception ability; Lawson et al. (1996) found that eight out of 10 implantees achieved better results with an extended frequency range of 350 Hz to 9,500 Hz. The allocation of frequencies to different channels can also affect speech perception with cochlear implants (Fu and Shannon, 1999b; Skinner, Holden and Holden, 1995).

A variety of different strategies are available and many of the newest implant systems can support a choice of different strategies. Within strategies parameters can be adjusted to suit individual patients. Shannon (1996), Wilson (1997) and Loizou (1998) have reviewed developments in speech processing for cochlear implants.

Waveform options

Sound may be delivered as an analogue waveform where there is continuous and simultaneous stimulation of the implanted electrodes. Alternatively, pulsatile waveforms that comprise a series of pulses generated from sampling the incoming sound signal can be used.

Analogue waveform

An analogue waveform was used in the compressed analogue (CA) strategy of the Ineraid cochlear implant and gave varying degrees of benefit to many implantees (Eddington et al., 1978; Parkin and Stewart, 1988). The Clarion device is the only currently available cochlear implant that uses an analogue waveform with its Simultaneous Analogue Stimulation (SAS) strategy. The SAS strategy emphasizes the temporal information in the sound signal. The Clarion has a transcutaneous rather than percutaneous link across the skin and it also differs from the Ineraid implant in that the SAS strategy of the Clarion implant has eight channels and the stimulation mode is bipolar rather than monopolar. There are 16 electrodes in the Clarion device which form eight pairs of one active and one reference electrode for bipolar stimulation. The use of bipolar stimulation aims to reduce current spread and minimize the channel interaction characteristic of the monopolar CA strategy although the electrodes of the Clarion device are closer together than the Ineraid electrodes (Dorman et al., 1990; Favre and Pelizzone, 1993). Some patients achieve good speech recognition with SAS and prefer the quality of sound over the CIS strategy as implemented in the Clarion implant (Battmer et al., 1999).

Pulsatile waveform

A pulsatile waveform comprises series of pulses extracted from the incoming signal and delivered to different channels, according to their frequency. Each pulse is presented to each channel sequentially which minimizes the possibility of channel interactions and maximizes spectral information. Pulsatile strategies do not, therefore, convey the whole waveform but rapidly updated samples of the sound signal. Rapid updating of the incoming signal is required so that changes in the signal with time are adequately represented. The amplitude of each pulse is derived by extracting the envelope of bandpassed waveform. There are variations in how the pulse trains are extracted between different devices and strategies (Loizou, 1998; Wilson, 1997; Lawson et al., 1996). The order in which pulses are delivered to different channels may be varied such as apex to base of the cochlea; channels 1,2,3,4,5,6, or in a staggered order; channels 1,4,2,5,3,6, in a hypothetical six channel device.

Most pulsatile strategies available in the current generation of cochlear implants use sequential stimulation and fall into two broad categories, the n of m or spectral maxima type of strategy and Continuous Interleaved Sampling (CIS) strategy.

Spectral maxima or 'n of m' strategies

The spectral maxima strategies sample peaks from the incoming sound signal and these are delivered to different electrodes according to their frequency. Thus, the most dominant features of the incoming waveform are used for stimulation, not samples of the whole waveform. Active intra-cochlear electrodes are each allocated a frequency band but only those electrodes that correspond to the frequency peaks extracted will be stimulated in each cycle of pulses. Stimulation roves between electrodes according to the frequency of the spectral peaks extracted in the speech processor. The 'n' of 'n of m' refers to the number of peaks extracted from the sound signal and the 'm' is the maximum number of electrodes of the implant available for stimulation. Examples of spectral maxima type strategies are the Nucleus SPEAK and ACE strategies and the Medel n of m strategy.

SPEAK Strategy

SPEAK is a slow-rate (180–300 pps) spectral maxima strategy. The speech processor extracts up to nine maxima from the incoming signal and presents these maxima to different electrodes of 20 active electrodes inside the cochlea according to their frequency. The average number of maxima is six but varies according to the incoming signal. For a broad band signal there would be more maxima but the stimulation rate is slower but if there is limited spectral content to the signal there will be fewer maxima and the rate will be faster. Frequency bands are typically allocated within the range 187–7,937 Hz although alternative frequency allocations can be set. The SPEAK strategy is available with all the Nucleus processors for both the Nucleus 22 and the Nucleus 24 implants.

ACE

The Advanced Combination Encoder (ACE) is a fast rate, flexible spectral maxima strategy. Up to 22 channels can be used and up to 20 maxima although eight to 12 maxima are most commonly used. The frequency band allocation is variable but typically 187–7,937 Hz. Stimulation rates up to 2,400 pulses per second (pps) per channel are available with a maximum overall rate of 14,400 pps. The more maxima are used the slower the overall stimulation rate will be, for example if 12 channels are used the maximum rate per channel will be 14,400 divided by 12 which equals 1,200pps; if only six channels are used the maximum rate per channel will be 14,400/6 = 2,400pps. ACE is available with the 3G and Sprint processors of the Nucleus 24 implant.

Medel 'n of m'

Medel n of m strategy extracts up to 11 spectral peaks from the signal to be delivered to a maximum of 12 electrodes. Fast rates up to a maximum overall rate of 18,000 pps can be used. The fewer channels that are used the faster the rate of stimulation. More spectral information is delivered if more spectral peaks are extracted but more temporal information is delivered if the sampling rate is faster. The spectral peaks are extracted up to 7.5 KHz frequency. This strategy can be used in the CIS pro+ processor only.

CIS strategy

The continuous interleaved sampling (CIS) strategy was first developed by Wilson et al. (1991) and was the first fast rate strategy. The waveform is sampled and split into frequency bands from which pulses are generated and delivered sequentially to different electrodes according to their frequency, thus giving good spectral information. Every active intra-cochlear electrode is available for stimulation in each cycle of pulses. The fast stimulation rate allows for more frequent sampling of the incoming signal and therefore better temporal resolution than slower rate strategies. The CIS strategy showed the potential for better performance than speech feature extraction, the SPEAK strategy of the Nucleus 22 implant (Kiefer et al., 1996) and CA strategy of the Ineraid implant (Wilson et al., 1995). All the currently available cochlear implants can be programmed with the CIS strategy but the implementation of the strategy is not identical in different implants; parameters such as filtering, envelope extraction, the number of channels, the pulse rate and the update rate vary.

Other strategies

Partially simultaneous, pulsatile strategies are available in the Clarion implant. The Paired Pulsatile Strategy (PPS) comprises pairs of pulses that are delivered to two channels at a time thereby increasing the pulse rate per channel (Zimmerman-Phillips and Murad, 1999). Hybrid strategies that combine simultaneous analogue and non-simultaneous pulsatile stimulation are possible with the Clarion implant but have not yet been widely used.

Parameters affecting speech processing strategies

New cochlear implant devices are very flexible but we know little of how to best match the processor parameters to the residual capabilities of the individual cochlear implant listener. Two of the main areas of research are addressing the issues of the optimum number of channels and the best stimulation rate.

Number of channels

Dorman, Loisou and Rainey (1997) looked at the effect of channel number with normally hearing subjects listening to processed speech. They found that eight channels were required for vowel recognition but only five channels were required for sentence recognition. In a further study some implantees were able to achieve similar speech discrimination scores to normally hearing subjects listening to speech processed through six channels (Dorman and Loizou, 1998). The implantees' ability to achieve these good levels of speech recognition was thought to be related to a larger electrical dynamic range.

To benefit from multiple channels implantees need to be able to perceive differences in pitch between different channels. Local variations in channel discrimination can be significant for some implant users (Eddington et al., 1994; Nelson et al., 1995). Nucleus 22 implants were modified to use CIS with varying numbers of channels and the same number of channels but with different electrodes selected to be active. Speech discrimination results showed that in no case were eight, 11 or 21 channels better than the six best channels but selecting the electrodes to give the six 'best' channels did influence speech recognition. Significant increases in consonant recognition were found to be unlikely above four channels when electrodes were optimally selected with only one out of five subjects doing better with more than eight channels (Lawson et al., 1996; Wilson, 1997). Fishman, Shannon and Slattery (1997) altered the number of channels available with the SPEAK strategy. As the number of channels was reduced the pulse rate was increased to improve temporal features. A few individuals reached their peak performance by four channels but implantees more commonly performed best with seven channels and a few implantees needed 10 channels for optimum performance. Above 10 channels performance did not improve significantly. Some subjects commented that the 10-channel strategy gave a pleasanter voice quality than the 20-channel strategy. There may be a trade-off between the number of channels and rate of stimulation because more channels result in slower rates of stimulation possibly making more channels less beneficial above a certain number. Physiological limitations in some patients may mean than they cannot benefit from a lot of channels, rather like having a washing machine with 20 programmes but you can get all your clothes clean using four different programmes. With the CIS strategy Brill et al. (1997) and Kiefer et al. (2000) found that it may be better to select the six to eight 'best' channels, so that a higher pulse rates of 1,500–1,600 pps per channel can be used. Current implants have some channel redundancy in that they have the potential to use more channels than are currently needed. New electrode designs may, however, give more selective stimulation that may enable at least some implantees to obtain increased benefit from many more channels.

Stimulation rate

The understanding of speech relies on the interpretation of frequency differences, and changes in the signal amplitude or temporal features. Although more channels allow more detailed frequency representation, on different channels of the implant, the sampling rate of the signal is slower because it takes longer to deliver pulses to more channels sequentially. At higher stimulation rates the incoming sound can be sampled more often so that rapid variations in the original signal can be delivered. At lower stimulation rates the incoming signal cannot be sampled so often and some of the changes of the signal with time will be missed. It is possible to speed up the pulse rate by delivering the same pulse more than once but the most accurate representation of the incoming signal is achieved when the sampling rate matches the stimulation rate such that each pulse provides different, updated information. Pulse rates can be expressed as the rate of pulses stimulating each channel in a second (pps per channel) or the overall rate at which all pulses are delivered on all channels in a second (pps). The maximum overall pulse rate cannot be exceeded and each channel is stimulated in turn; for example, for the Combi 40+ implant the overall pulse rate is 18,000 pps and if 12 channels are used the rate per channel will be 18,000/12 = 1,500 pps per channel whereas if four channels are used in the same device there will be 18,000/4 = 4,500 pps per channel. There may be a maximum channel rate such that reducing the channel number does not increase the overall rate – for example, the Nucleus CI24M implant can support channel rates up to 2,400 pps per channel and an overall rate of 14,400 pps so that four channels cannot be used at a faster channel rate than six channels because 14,000/4 = 3,500pps per channel which is greater than the maximum possible of 2,400 pps per channel.

Fast pulse rates tend to represent temporal features better. Lawson et al. (1996) found that reducing the stimulation rate from 833 pps per channel to 250 pps per channel with six channels gave a 70% likelihood of reducing speech discrimination performance. In the same study, 'n of m' and CIS strategies were compared; two subjects did better with CIS, one did better with 'n of m' and two found CIS better for male voices and 'n of m' better for female voices but all did better than with their usual SPEAK strategy probably because of the higher stimulation rate and extended high frequency range. Studies with the CIS strategy and Combi 40+ implant found that for four or more channels a reduction in stimulation rates to less than 1,500 pps per channel led to a reduction in word understanding and some implant users gained more benefit with even higher rates (Brill et al., 1997; Kiefer et al., 2000). There may, however, be a level above which increasing pulse rate does not continue to improve speech discrimination. Even with sequential stimulation residual current could cause channel interactions at very high pulse rates because there is insufficient interval between each pulse for the neurone to go back to its resting state thus reducing the clarity of the signal (Abbas, 1993).

Comparative studies of different implant systems and strategies

Comparisons between different devices and processing strategies are problematic because of the many other variables involved. These include the wide variation in individual performance with implants seen with all devices and strategies, changes in criteria for suitability for implantation and the desire of clinics to give patients the most advanced devices. Nevertheless some comparative studies have been attempted. Wilson et al. (1995) and Lawson et al. (1996) have compared the Nucleus roving spectral maxima (SPEAK type) of strategy with CIS strategies but found no clear difference when stimulus rate and frequency ranges are similar. The CIS strategy is, however, typically implemented in commercially available processors at higher stimulus rates and with extended high frequency range. Some studies show improved speech perception performance with the Clarion CIS/SAS strategies than the Nucleus 22 SPEAK or Ineraid CA strategies (Tyler et al., 1996; Battmer, Reid and Lenarz, 1997). The Combi 40 Medel implant with CIS strategy tends to show better patient performance than the Nucleus 22 SPEAK strategy (Helms et al., 1997; Kiefer et al., 1996). Arndt et al. (2000) have reported encouraging three- and six-month post-implant results with the Nucleus CI24M implant in children but did not give details of the strategies used. Most of the data currently available compares patient performance with newer devices and strategies with older devices and strategies. As clinical experience with the latest and most widely used devices with fast rate strategies grows, more rigorous comparisons between more 'equivalent' devices will be possible. Future research could show that different implant candidates may suit certain strategies or implants better than others.

Choice of a cochlear implant for children

Children are implanted early in their lives and are likely to need to use their implants for considerably longer than many adults. Device safety over long time periods is therefore essential. Young children being considered for implantation often have little or no memory of spoken language but they do have more neural plasticity than older children and adults. The best possible speech processing strategy will be required because the

signal will be used to develop speech and language auditorily
and it is possible that the electrical signal could influence neural
connections in the developing brain in the very young (Leake et
al., 2000). Ideally cochlear implants should not introduce too
many restrictions to young children's active lifestyle. It is important that parents are made aware of any restrictions that an
implant may confer such as avoiding some contact sports, mini-
mizing exposure to static discharge, or post-implantation use of
magnetic resonance imaging (MRI), before the child is
implanted. Several factors affect the choice of cochlear implants
for children but the three most essential requirements will be
considered first and these are:

- the safety of the device;
- the benefit it can afford;
- the long-term availability of spares and backup.

Device safety and longevity

The safety and longevity of cochlear implants are dependent on
the design of the implant, the quality of the components used
and the quality and cleanliness of the manufacturing process.
The desire to use the most advanced components for implants
is confounded by the unprecedented challenge of service-free
use for a child's lifetime. Most implant teams select devices that
have been widely and successfully used in adults before considering them for children. In the US the Food and Drug Administration (FDA) regulates trials of new cochlear implants and
devices must have FDA approval before they can be used other
than in a controlled research setting. In Europe regulation is by
the CE mark. Issues of safety and biocompatibility have been
discussed in detail by House and Berliner (1986) and Shepherd,
Franz and Clark (1990). Safety features such as capacitors are
incorporated into some implants to guard against the effects of
DC current leakage (McCreery et al., 1990; Brummer, Roblee
and Hambrecht, 1983). Terr, Sfogliano and Riley (1989) and
Waltzman, Cohen and Shapiro (1991) have found no deleteri-
ous effects from electrical stimulation in patients implanted for
several years. Device failure rates and surgical complications
have been reported (Cohen and Hoffman, 1991; Parisier et al.,
1991; Parisier, Chute and Popp, 1996; von Wallenberg and
Brinch, 1995; Balkany et al., 1999, Lehnhardt, von Wallenberg
and Brinch, 2000). The definition of a device failure varies in

the scientific literature and in implant companies' information. Device failure can be a complete failure with no sound signal being delivered or, if several electrodes malfunction this may effectively constitute a device failure. Von Wallenberg and Brinch (1995) expressed Nucleus implant reliability on the basis of failures per cumulative years of use. Newer devices may appear to have lower failure rates because problems have not yet been identified and reported. Overall numbers of failures will be lower if fewer patients have been implanted with a particular device. Should implant failure occur, reimplantation is possible and gives similar levels of patient performance in most cases (Gantz, Lowder and McCabe, 1989; Jackler, Leake and McKerrow, 1989; Cohen and Hoffman, 1991; Ray, Gray and Court, 1998; Balkany et al., 1999).

Proven benefit

Cochlear implantation involves surgery and the usual risks that accompany general anaesthesia. Implantation also damages residual hearing (Boggess, Baker and Balkany, 1989). Ethically clinicians need to be confident that an individual will benefit more from implantation with a particular device than from using conventional hearing aids. Implant candidacy issues concerning children are discussed in detail in Chapter 4. There is a large body of evidence that shows that multi-channel cochlear implants provide significant gains in speech perception and production to suitable children although the benefits appear over long time periods (Osberger et al., 1991; Staller et al., 1991; Gibbin, 1992; Gantz et al., 1994; Miyamoto et al., 1995; Summerfield and Marshall, 1995; Osberger et al., 1996; Cohen and Waltzman, 1996; Miyamoto, Svirsky and Robbins, 1997; Tait and Lutman, 1994; Parkinson, El-Kholy and Tyler, 1998; Miyamoto et al., 1999; O'Donoghue et al., 1999). The performance of adults can be used as a guide as to whether a new implant or processing strategy gives better speech recognition. As the benefits of implantation increase with better implants and better speech processing children with more residual hearing may get more benefit from implantation (see Chapter 4 and also Kiefer et al., 1998; Rubenstein et al., 1999). Evaluation of the benefit afforded by the latest generation of implants is confounded by changes in candidature for implantation over time and the subjects in different studies having different histories of hearing loss e.g. different durations of deafness or levels of residual hearing.

Availability of spares and backup

A cochlear implant can only be successful with consistent use for the lifetime of the implanted patient. Replacement external equipment compatible with the implanted components and the means to programme the processor should be available for the lifetime of the implanted device. The external equipment of different cochlear implant systems is not interchangeable. It is, therefore, essential that the implant company has a secure financial basis and is committed to providing replacement external components to existing patients. In addition to maintaining the external equipment for existing patients, it is advantageous if new processors or processing strategies are designed so that existing implantees, as well as new implantees, can benefit from them. The flexibility of the currently available implant systems goes some way to enabling new developments in speech processing to be adopted by patients implanted now. A post-aural processor has been developed for the Nucleus 22 device but it will not be able to use the newest fast rate processing strategies. Clarion have developed a post-aural processor that is compatible with their previous and current electrode arrays.

Telemetry

Telemetry enables the clinician to detect electrode short circuits easily and quickly from information sent back from the internal implant. Telemetry testing can be carried out in the operating theatre during implantation. It is useful for the clinician to know which electrodes are functioning correctly and are likely to give a good response for young children when tuning the processor may be difficult. Telemetry at routine appointments can also be helpful to identify electrode shorts early rather than by relying on observation of changes in the child's auditory responsiveness or behaviour. Should a problem arise with an implant system a check of the internal electrodes is reassuring and can lead to a quicker identification of the source of a problem. In a few seconds it is now possible to test for electrode shorts that, on older implants without telemetry, would require lengthy threshold and comfort level testing and/or integrity tests. With the Nucleus CI24M implant a new measurement of neural response telemetry (NRT) is available which detects neural responses with electrically evoked compound action potentials. NRT measurements have potential in helping with device tuning and selection of the electrodes with the 'best' neural responses (see Chapter 6 and also Abbas et al., 1999; Shallop, Facer and Peterson, 1999).

Objective tests

With young children the possibility of doing objective measurements together with telemetry measurements is a great help with tuning the device especially in the early stages of tuning when the child may not fully understand the tasks required and may not have formed a concept of loudness. Intra-operative objective measurements also give reassurance of an auditory response being elicited by stimulation through the implant immediately after surgery before initial stimulation. The electrical stapedial reflex is caused by the stapedius muscle contracting in response to loud sound conveyed through the implant (Stephan, Welzl-Muller and Stiglbrumer, 1991; Battmer, Laszig and Lehnhardt, 1990; Hodges et al., 1999). Electrical auditory brainstem responses can be recorded which fall between the behavioural threshold and comfort level (Shallop et al., 1990; Mason et al., 1993). Objective measurements are discussed in detail in Chapter 6.

Ergonomics

Ergonomic features of the cochlear implant system can facilitate or hinder the child's use of the implant system. Transcutaneous signal transmission is now used universally because of the problems of infection and risk of damage with percutaneous systems that were used with a few children (Montandon, Kasper and Pelizzone, 1991). The size of the external equipment should be small enough to be worn by very young children and discrete enough to suit teenagers. Many young children are happy with body-worn processors but as they become older and more self-conscious they may prefer a less noticeable processor. Post-aural processors may be less prone to damage than body-worn processors because there are fewer connections and the processor is out of the way of most of the child's activities but they should not be small enough to present a choking hazard. Battery compartments need to be tamper-proof for very young children to avoid batteries being swallowed. Tamper-proof switches are important to avoid accidentally changing the processor settings. External equipment should have no sharp components. Any leads should be unpluggable so that they can easily be replaced.

Durability

The whole implant system should be durable enough to cope with a young child's active lifestyle without imposing too many restrictions. Breakdowns of external equipment can be rectified but may require the child being without his or her implant for up to 24 hours, while equipment is sent out or collected. Frequent processor or microphone breakdowns result in inconsistent use of the implant and poorer outcomes. Frequent breakdowns also place heavy demands on equipment spares and staff time.

Batteries

Implant systems are powered by batteries in the speech processor. Advances in battery technology are allowing speech processors to get smaller and not require such frequent battery changes. Rechargeable batteries would be ideal from cost and environmental viewpoints, but unfortunately in some processors these batteries may not last all day. Young children will not always indicate immediately when a battery needs changing and in the school environment it is not always convenient for teachers to change batteries in the middle of the day. In most circumstances young children should use a system that has a battery that lasts at least one whole waking day even if disposable rather than rechargeable batteries have to be used to maintain continuity of sound. The batteries for the implant system should be easily and locally available for the implanted child.

Indicators of processor function

Most speech processors have some form of indicator lights on the processor that indicate that the processor is working normally or show a fault. With young children, especially, an indicator light that shows normal function reassures parents and teachers that the child is receiving a signal. Indicator lights or sounds audible to the parent or teacher are beneficial for the early identification of faults or flat batteries, thus reducing the time that children are without a signal from their implants. In the newer devices different signals can indicate different faults thus helping the audiologist identify the fault and issue replacement equipment quickly. All of the commonly used body-worn processors have integral visual or auditory indicators of processor function. Of the postaural speech processors currently available the Medel Tempo+ is the only one with integral indicator lights. A signal check and listening earphones are available for checking the function of all

Nucleus post-aural processors and the Tempo+. The lack of any indicator system for checking processor function could present difficulties in achieving consistent processor use with young or newly implanted children. It is possible, of course, for young children to be fitted with a body-worn processor and later, when they are able to report about sound quality themselves, change to an appropriate behind the ear processor.

Possibility of using an FM radio aid and accessories

Once fitted with an implant the aim is for the implantee to use the device as much as possible. In educational settings implanted children experience the same problems with background noise that occur for those with conventional hearing aids. In certain circumstances it is useful to interface the implant with an FM radio aid. This is possible for the most widely used modern implant systems in the UK with a specially shielded lead to connect the speech processor to the radio aid. Different leads are required for use with different radio aids and each of the implant manufacturers supply their own sets of leads. It is important even with the proper equipment and leads to be vigilant against interference from external sources (Hocking, Joyner and Fleming, 1991). If a child reports unusual noises, such as hissing, the possibility of interference should be investigated and other carrier frequencies can be tried. Separating the leads from a body-worn processor to the headset and the radio aid and preventing them from touching can help to reduce interference.

Cochlear implant users may benefit from loop systems in public places such as theatres and churches. Specialized leads may give a better signal from the television or for listening to music. Varying sets of accessories are available with some cochlear implants for specific listening conditions. The use of accessories will depend on the age and lifestyle of the child.

Other types of accessories available with implant systems are harnesses, pouches, bags and belt clips that give the child different options for wearing the external equipment depending on their age, lifestyle and preference.

Magnetic resonance imaging compatibility

Medical investigations using magnetic resonance imaging (MRI) are becoming more common but are problematic with cochlear implants because of the torsion resulting from the strong magnetic fields required for the technique (Portnoy and Mattucci, 1991). The implant would also cause a shadow on the MRI scan. Newer implant designs such as the removable magnet in the Nucleus 24 implant (Heller et al., 1996) or the magnetless Clarion device do permit the use of MRI. The latter would be useful if the implant candidate was known to have a medical condition that may require regular MRI investigation (Weber et al., 1999; Graham et al., 1999). Whilst the magnet of the Nucleus device is removable it requires minor surgery and a local anaesthetic. Studies with the Medel Combi 40+ implant have shown that MRI is possible with the implant in situ under certain controlled conditions and with certain strengths of magnetic field (Teissl et al., 1998). Medical aspects of cochlear implantation are discussed further in Chapter 5.

Conclusion

Cochlear implants now offer choices of processing strategy, several programmes within one processor, post-aural multi-channel processors and choices of electrode array. Average speech perception performance has improved considerably but there is still wide variation in individual outcomes from implantation. More knowledge about basic implant function and the effects of changing processing parameters is needed to make full use of the flexibility offered by the latest generation of cochlear implants. Improved assessment of residual nerve function could also help customizing implants for individuals and thus improve performance for all implantees. Animal research into regeneration of auditory neural tissue may have applications in further development of cochlear implants (Salvi et al., 1998; Staecker and van de Water, 2000).

Technological advances will allow cochlear implants to become even smaller and possibly wholly implanted. Remote control adjustment of the processor to suit different listening situations may become possible. Further development of telemetry and objective measures may lead to partially automated tuning of devices which would benefit the very young in ensuring good processor settings and, therefore, good sound quality earlier.

Implant and hearing aid users find listening in background noise particularly difficult (Agelfors, 1998). The possibility of using beamforming (Margo, Schweitzer and Feinman, 1997), binaural microphones (Pedley, 1998) and binaural implants (Van Hoesel and Clark, 1999) is under investigation. Further improvements in speech processing may also help cochlear implant users with speech recognition in noise.

There have been rapid advances in the field of cochlear implantation in which the benefits of implantation have exceeded expectations. Over the next few years there will no doubt be further advances in the design of cochlear implants and the application of speech processing strategies to further increase the benefit that cochlear implants can give to severely to profoundly deaf children.

References

Abbas PJ (1993) Electrophysiology. In Tyler RS (ed.) Cochlear Implants: Audiological Foundations. San Diego, CA: Singular, pp 317–56.

Abbas PJ, Brown CJ, Shallop JK, Firszt JB, Hughes ML, Hong SH, Staller SJ (1999) Summary of results using the Nucleus CI24M implant to record the electrically evoked compound action potential. Ear and Hearing 20: 45–59.

Agelfors E (1998) A comparison of speech performance in quiet and noise between persons using cochlear implants and hearing aids. Speech, Music and Hearing Quarterly Progress and Status Report. TMH-QPSR 1-2/1998: 81–8.

Arndt P, Staller SJ, Beiter AL, LeMay M (2000) Initial paediatric results with the Nucleus 24 cochlear implant system. In Waltzman SB, Cohen NL (eds) Cochlear Implants. New York: Thieme, pp 207–9.

Axon PR, Mawman DJ, Upile T, Ramsden RT (1997) Cochlear implantation in the presence of chronic suppurative otitis media. The Journal of Laryngology and Otology 111: 228–32.

Balkany T, Gantz B, Nadol JB (1988) Multichannel cochlear implants in partially ossified cochleas. Annals of Otology, Rhinology and Laryngology 97: 3–7.

Balkany TJ, Cohen NL, Gantz BJ (1999) Surgical technique for the Clarion cochlear implant. Annals of Otology, Rhinology and Laryngology 108: 27–30.

Balkany TJ, Hodges AV, Gomez-Marin O, Bird PA, Dolan-Ash S, Butts S, Telischi FF, Lee D (1999) Cochlear reimplantation. The Laryngoscope 109: 351–5.

Battmer RD, Laszig R, Lehnhardt E (1990) Electrically elicited stapedius reflex in cochlear implant patients. Ear and Hearing 11: 370–4.

Battmer RD, Reid JM, Lenarz T (1997) Performance in quiet and noise with the Nucleus Spectra 22 and the Clarion CIS/CA cochlear implant devices. Scandinavian Audiology 26: 240–6.

Battmer RD, Zilberman Y, Haake P, Lenarz T (1999) Simultaneous analog stimulation (SAS) – continuous interleaved sampler (CIS) pilot study in Europe. Annals of Otology, Rhinology and Laryngology 108: 69–73.

Bent JP, Chute P, Parisier SC (1999) Cochlear implantation in children with large vestibular aqueducts. The Laryngoscope 109: 1019–22.

Bilger RC (1977) Evaluation of subjects presently fitted with auditory prostheses. Annals of Otology, Rhinology and Laryngology 86 (suppl 38) 1–140.

Blamey P (1997) Are spiral ganglion cell numbers important for speech perception with a cochlear implant? The American Journal of Otology 18 (suppl): S11–S12.

Boggess WJ, Baker JE, Balkany TJ (1989) Loss of residual hearing after cochlear implantation. The Laryngoscope 99: 1002–5.

Bredberg G, Lindstrom B, Lopponen H, Skarzynski H, Hyodo M, Sato H (1997) Electrodes for ossified cochleas. The American Journal of Otology 18 (suppl): S42–S43.

Brill SM, Gstottner W, Helms J, Ilberg C, Baumgartner W, Muller J, Kiefer J (1997) Optimization of channel number and stimulation rate for the fast continuous interleaved sampling strategy in the Combi 40+. The American Journal of Otology 18 (suppl): S104–S106.

Brill SM, Stobich B, Hochmair ES (2000) Influence of sound pressure level on speech understanding with the continuous interleaved sampling strategy in the Combi 40/Combi 40+. In Waltzman SB, Cohen NL (eds) Cochlear Implants. New York: Thieme, pp. 333–4.

Brummer SB, Robblee LS, Hambrecht FT (1983) Criteria for selecting electrodes for electrical stimulation: theoretical and practical implications. Annals of the New York Academy of Sciences 405: 159–71.

Burian K, Hochmair-Desoyer IJ, Eisenwort B (1986) The Vienna cochlear implant programme. Otolaryngology Clinics of North America 19: 313–28.

Camilleri AE, Toner JG, Howarth KL, Hampton S, Ramsden RT (1999) Cochlear implantation following temporal bone fracture. The Journal of Laryngology and Otology 113: 454–7.

Cinamon U, Kronenberg J, Hildesheimer M, Taitelbaum T (1997) Cochlear implantation in patients suffering from Cogan's syndrome. The Journal of Laryngology and Otology 111: 928–30.

Clark GM, Blamey PT, Brown AM, Gusby PA, Dowell RC, Franz BK-H, Pyman BC, Shepherd RK, Tong YC, Webb RL, Hirshorn MS, Kuzuma J, Mecklenberg DJ, Money DK, Patrick JF, Seligman PM (1987) The University of Melbourne – Nucleus multi-electrode cochlear implant. In Pfaltz CR (ed.) Advances in Otology, Rhinology and Laryngology, vol. 38. Basel: Karger.

Cohen NL (1994) The ethics of cochlear implants in young children. The American Journal of Otology 15 (suppl): 1–2.

Cohen NL, Hoffman RA (1991) Complications of cochlear implant surgery in adults and children. Annals of Otology, Rhinology and Laryngology 100: 708–11.

Cohen NL, Waltzman SB, Fisher SG (1993) A prospective randomized study of cochlear implants. New England Journal of Medicine 328: 233–7.

Cohen NL, Waltzman SB (1996) Cochlear implants in infants and young children. Seminars in Hearing 17: 215–21.

Cowan RSC, Brown C, Whitford LA., Galvin KL, Sarant JZ, Barker EJ, Shaw S, King A, Skok M, Seligman PM, Dowell RC, Everingham C, Gibson WPR, Clark GM (1995) Speech perception in children using the advanced (SPEAK) speech processing strategy. Annals of Otology, Rhinology and Laryngology 104 (suppl 166): 318–21.

Dijourno A, Eyries C (1957) Prosthese auditive par excitation electrique a distance du nerf sensoriel a l'aide d'un bobinage inclus a demeure. Presse Medicale 35: 14–17.

Dillier N, Battmer RD, Doring WH, Muller-Deile J (1995) Multicentric field evaluation of a spectral peak (SPEAK) cochlear implant speech coding strategy. Audiology 34: 145–59.

Dorman MF, Smith L, McCandless G, Dunnavant G, Parkin J, Dankonski K (1990) Pitch scaling and speech understanding by patients who use the Ineraid cochlear implant. Ear and Hearing 11: 310–15.

Dorman M, Loizou P, Rainey D (1997) Speech intelligibilty as a function of the number of channels of stimulation for signal processors using sine-wave and noise band outputs. Journal of the Acoustical Society of America 102: 2403–11.

Dorman MF, Loizou PC (1998) The identification of consonants and vowels by cochlear implant patients using a 6 channel CIS processor and normally hearing subjects using simulations of processors with 2 to 9 channels. Ear and Hearing 19: 162–6.

Doyle PJ, Pijl S, Noel FJ (1991) The cochlear implant: a comparison of single and multi-channel results. The Journal of Laryngology and Otology 20: 204–8.

Eddington DK, Dobelle WH, Brackmann EE, Mladejovsky MG, Parkin JL (1978) Auditory prosthesis research with multiple channel intracochlear stimulation in man. Annals of Otology, Rhinology and Laryngology 87 (suppl 53): 1–39.

Eddington DK, Noel VA, Rabinowitz WM, Svirsky MA, Tierney J, Zissman MA (1994) Speech Processors for Auditory Prostheses. Ninth quarterly progress report, NIH project NO1-DC-2-2402, Massachusetts Institute of Technology, Research Laboratory of Electronics, Cambridge, MA.

Eyles JE, Aleksy WL, Boyle PJ (1995) Performance changes in University College Hospital/ Royal National Institute for the Deaf single-channel cochlear implant users upgraded to the Nucleus 22 channel cochlear implant system. Annals of Otology, Rhinology and Laryngology 104 (suppl 166): 263–5.

Eyles JE, Pringle MB, Flynn SL, French ML (2000) Implantation with a Nucleus 22, and Ineraid Mk2, and Med-el Combi 40+: a clinical case study. poster presentation at the 6th International Cochlear Implant Conference, Miami Beach, FL, 3–5 February.

Favre E, Pelizzone M (1993) Channel interactions in patients using the Ineraid multi-channel cochlear implant. Hearing Research 66: 150–6.

Fayad J, Linthicium FH, Otto SR, Galey FR, House WF (1991) Cochlear implants: histopathological findings related to performance in 16 human temporal bones. Annals of Otology, Rhinology and Laryngology 100: 807–11.

Filipo R, Barbara M, Monini S, Mancini P (1999) Clarion cochlear implants: surgical implications. The Journal of Laryngology and Otology 113: 321–5.

Fishman KE, Shannon RV, Slattery WH (1997) Speech recognition as a function of the number of electrodes used in the SPEAK cochlear implant speech processor. Journal of Speech, Language and Hearing Research 40: 1201–15.

Fu G-J, Shannon RV (1999a) Effects of electrode location and spacing on phoneme recognition with the Nucleus 22 cochlear implant. Ear and Hearing 20: 321–31.

Fu G-J, Shannon RV (1999b) Effects of electrode configuration and frequency allocation on vowel recognition with the Nucleus 22 cochlear implant. Ear and Hearing 20: 332–44.

Gantz BJ, Tyler RS, Knutson JF, Woodworth GG, Abbas P, McCabe BF, Hinrichs J, Tye-Murray N, Lansing C, Kirk F, Brown C (1988) Evaluation of 5 different cochlear implant designs: audiological assessment and predictors of performance. The Laryngoscope 98: 1100–6.

Gantz BJ, Lowder MW, McCabe BF (1989) Audiological results following reimplantation of cochlear implants. Annals of Otology, Rhinology and Laryngology 98: 12–16.

Gantz BJ, Tyler RS, Woodworth GG, Tye-Murray N, Fryauf-Bertschy H (1994) Results of multi-channel cochlear implants in congenitally deaf and prelingually deafened children. The American Journal of Otology 15 (suppl 2): 1–8.

Gibbin KP (1992) Paediatric cochlear implantation. Archives of Diseases in Childhood 67: 669–71.

Gibbin KP, O'Donoghue GM, Murty GE (1993) Paediatric cochlear implantation: the Nottingham surgical experience. In Hochmair-Desoyer IJ, Hochmair ES (eds) Advances in Cochlear Implants. Vienna: Manz, pp 230–2.

Graham J, Lynch C, Weber L, Stollwerck L, Wei J, Brookes G (1999) The magnetless Clarion cochlear implant in a patient with neurofibromatosis 2. Journal of Laryngology and Otology 113: 458–63.

Gstoettner W, Plenk H, Franz P, Hamzavi J, Baumgartner W, Czerny C, Ehrenberger K (1997) Cochlear implant deep electrode insertion: extent of insertional trauma. Acta Otolaryngology (Stockh) 117: 274–7.

Heller J, Brackmann D, Tucci D, Nyenhuis J, Chou C (1996) Evaluation of MRI compatibility of the modified Nucleus cochlear implants. The American Journal of Otology 17: 724-9.

Helms J, Muller J, Schon F, Moser L, Arnold W, Janssen T, Ramsden R, Schon F, von Ilberg C, Kiefer J, Pfennigdorff T, Gstottner W, Baumgartner W, Ehrenberger K, Sharzyinski H, Ribari O, Thumfart W, Stephan K, Mann W, Heinmann M, Zorowka P, Lippert KL, Zenner HJ, Bohndorf M, Huttenbrink K, Muller-Aschoff E, Hofmann G, Fiegang B, Begall K, Ziese M, Frogbert O, Hausler R, Vischer M, Schlatter T, Schlodorff G, Korves B, Doring H, Gerhardt HJ, Wagner H, Schorn K, Schilling V, Baumann U, Kastenbauer E, Albegger K, Mair A, Gammert CH, Mathis A, Streitberger CH, Hochmair-Desoyer I (1997) Evaluation of performance with the Combi 40 cochlear implant in adults: a multicentric clinical study. Otology, Rhinology and Laryngology 59: 23-35.

Hinjosa R, Douglas Green Jr.J, Marion MS (1991) Ganglion cell populations in labyrinthitis ossificans. The American Journal of Otology 12(suppl): 3-7.

Hocking B, Joyner KH, Flemming AHJ (1991) Implanted medical devices in workers exposed to radio-frequency radiation. Scandinavian Journal of Work and Environmental Health 17: 1-6.

Hodges AV, Balkany TJ, Ruth RA, Lambert PR, Dolan-Ash S, Schloffman JJ (1999) Electrical middle ear muscle reflex: use in cochlear implant programming. Otolaryngology, Head and Neck Surgery 117: 255-61.

Hortman G, Pulec JL, Causse JB, Causse JR, Briand C, Fontaine JP, Tetu F, Azema B (1989) Experience with the extracochlear multi-channel implex system. In Fraysse B (ed.) Cochlear Implant Acquisitions and Controversies. Basel: Cochlear, pp 307-317.

House WF (1986) Opposition to the cochlear implant in deaf children. The American Journal of Otology 7: 89-92.

House WF, Berliner K, Crary W, Graham M, Luckey R, Norton N, Selters W, Tobin H, Urban J, Wexler M (1976) Cochlear implants. Annals of Otology, Rhinology and Laryngology 85 (suppl 27): 1-93.

House WF, Berliner KI, Eisenberg LS (1983) Experiences with the cochlear implant in preschool children. Annals of Otology, Rhinology and Laryngology 92: 587-92.

House WF, Berliner KI (1986) Safety and efficacy of the House/3M cochlear implant in profoundly deaf adults. Otolaryngology Clinics of North America 19: 275-86.

House WF, Berliner KI (1991) Cochlear implants: from idea to clinical practice. In Cooper H (ed.) Cochlear Implants: A Practical Guide. London: Whurr, pp 9-33.

Jackler RK, Leake PA, McKerrow WS (1989) Cochlear implant revision: effects of reimplantation on the cochlea. Annals of Otology, Rhinology and Laryngology 98: 813-20.

Kasper A, Pelizzone M, Montandon P (1991) Intracochlear potential distribution with intracochlear and extracochlear electrical stimulation in humans. Annals of Otology, Rhinology and Laryngology 100: 812-16.

Kawano A, Seldon HL, Clark GM, Ramsden RT, Raine CH (1998) Intracochlear factors contributing to psychophysical percepts following cochlear implantation. Acta Otolaryngology (Stockholm) 118: 313-26.

Kessler D (1999) The Clarion multi-strategy cochlear implant. Annals of Otology, Rhinology and Laryngology 108: 8-16.

Kiefer J, Muller J, Pfennigdorff T, Schon F, Helms J, Von Ilberg C, Baumgartner W, Gstottner W, Ehrenberger K, Arnold W, Stephan K, Thumfart W (1996) Speech understanding in quiet and noise with the CIS speech coding strategy (Medel

Combi 40) compared to the multipeak and spectral peak strategies (Nucleus). Otology, Rhinology and Laryngology 58: 127–35.

Kiefer J, Von Ilberg C, Reimer B, Knecht R, Diller G, Sturzebecher E, Pfennigdorff T, Spelsberg A (1998) Results of cochlear implantation in patients with severe to profound hearing loss – implications for patient selection. Audiology 37: 382–95.

Kiefer J, Von Ilberg C, Rupprecht V, Huber-Egener J, Baumgartner W, Gstottner W, Forgasi K, Stephan K (2000) Optimized speech understanding with the speech coding strategy in cochlear implants: the effect of variations in stimulus rate and number of channels. In Waltzman SB, Cohen NL (eds) Cochlear Implants. New York: Thieme, pp. 339–40.

Kirk KI, Sehgal M, Miyamoto RT (1997) Speech perception performance of Nucleus multi-channel cochlear implant users with partial electrode insertions. Ear and Hearing 18: 456–71.

Knutson JF, Murray KT, Husarek S, Westerhouse K, Woodworth G, Gantz BJ, Tyler RS (1998) Psychological change over 54 months of cochlear implant use. Ear and Hearing 19: 191–201.

Koch DB, Seligman PM, Daly C, Whitford LA (1990) A mulitpeak feature extraction coding strategy for a multi-channel cochlear implant. Hearing Instruments 41: 28–30.

Kompis M, Vischer MW, Hausler R (1999) Performance of compressed analogue (CA) and continuous interleaved sampling (CIS) coding strategies for cochlear implants in quiet and noise. Acta Otolaryngology (Stockh) 119: 659–64.

Lance de Foa J, Loeb GE (1991) Issues in cochlear prosthetics from an international survey of opinions. International Journal of Technology Assessment in Health Care 7: 403–10.

Lane H (1995) Letter to the editor. The American Journal of Otology 16: 1–6.

Langer G (1997) Neural processing and representation of periodicity pitch. Acta Otolaryngology (Stockh) 532 (suppl): 68–76.

Lawson DT, Wilson BS, Zerbi M, Finley CC (1996) Speech processors for auditory prostheses. Third quarterly progress report, NIH project NO1-DC-5-2103, Neural Prosthesis Program, National Institutes of Health, Bethesda, MD.

Leake PA, Synder RL, Rebscher SJ, Hradek GT, Moore CM, Vollmer M, Sato M (2000) Long term effects of deafness and chronic electrical stimulation of the cochlea. In Waltzman SB, Cohen NL (eds) Cochlear Implants. New York: Thieme, pp. 31–42.

Lehnhardt M, von Wallenberg EL, Brinch J (2000) Reliability of the Nucleus CI22 and CI24M cochlear implants. Annals of Otology, Rhinology and Laryngology 109 (suppl 185): 14–6.

Lenarz T, Battmer RD (1995) First results with the Spectra 22 speech processor at the Medizinsche Hochschule Hannover. Annals of Otology, Rhinology and Laryngology 104 (suppl 166): 285–7.

Lenarz T, Battmer RD, Bertram B (2000) Cochlear implants in children under 2 years of age. In Waltzman SB, Cohen NL (eds) Cochlear Implants. New York: Thieme, pp. 163–5.

Loizou P (1998) Mimicking the human ear. An overview of signal processing strategies for converting sound into electrical signals in cochlear implants. IEEE Signal Processing Magazine Sept 1053-5888/98/101–30.

Maillet CJ, Tyler RS, Jordan HN (1995) Change in the quality of life of adult cochlear implant patients. Annals of Otology, Rhinology and Laryngology 104 (suppl 165): 31–8.

Margo V, Schweitzer C, Feinman G (1997) Comparisons of Spectra 22 performance in noise with and without an additional noise reduction pre-processor. Seminars in Hearing 18: 405–15.

Mason S, Sheppard S, Garnham CW, Lutman M, O'Donoghue G, Gibbin K (1993) Improving the relationship of intraoperative EABR threshold to T-level in young children receiving the Nucleus cochlear implant in Hochmair-Desoyer IJ, Hochmair ES (eds) Advances in Cochlear Implants. Vienna: Manz, pp 44-9.

McCormick B (1991) Paediatric Cochlear Implantation in the United Kingdom – a delayed journey on a well marked route. British Journal of Audiology 25: 145-9.

McCreery DB, Agnew WF, Yuon TGH, Bullara L (1990) Charge density and charge per phase as cofactors in neural injury induced by electrical stimulation. IEEE Transactions on Biomedical Engineering BME-37: 996-1001.

Mecklenburg D, Lehnhardt E (1991) The development of cochlear implants in Europe Asia and Australia. In Cooper H (ed.) Cochlear Implants: A Practical Guide. London: Whurr, pp. 34-57.

Miyamoto RT, Osberger MJ, Todd SL, Robbins AM (1993) Speech perception skills of children with multi-channel cochlear implants. In Hochmair-Desoyer IJ, Hochmair ES (eds) Advances in Cochlear Implants. Vienna: Manz, pp. 498-502.

Miyamoto RT, Kirk KI, Todd SL, Robbins AM, Osberger MJ (1995) Speech perception skills of children with multi-channel cochlear implants or hearing aids. Annals of Otology, Rhinology and Laryngology 104 (suppl 166): 334-7.

Miyamoto RT, Svirsky MA, Robbins AM (1997) Enhancement of expressive language in prelingually deaf children with cochlear implants. Acta Otolaryngology (Stockh) 117: 154-7.

Miyamoto RT, Kirk KI, Svirsky MA, Sehgal ST (1999) Communication skills in pediatric cochlear implant recipients. Acta Otolaryngology (Stockh) 119: 219-24.

Montandon P, Kasper A, Pelizzone M (1991) A case study of a 4 year old prelingually deaf child implanted with an Ineraid multi-channel cochlear implant. Otorhinolaryngology 53: 315-18.

Nadol JB, Young Y-S, Glynn RJ (1989) Survival of spiral ganglion cells in profound sensorineural hearing loss: implications for cochlear implantation. Annals of Otology, Rhinology and Laryngology 98: 411-16.

Nelson DA, Van Tassel DJ, Schroeder AC, Soli S, Levine S (1995) Electrode ranking of 'place pitch' and speech recognition in electrical hearing. Journal of the Acoustic Society of America 98: 1987-99.

O'Donoghue GM, Nikolopoulos TP, Archbold SM, Tait M (1999) Cochlear implants in young children: the relationship between speech perception and speech intelligibilty. Ear and Hearing 20: 419-25.

Osberger MJ, Robbins AM, Berry SW, Todd SL, Hesketh LJ, Sedley A (1991) Spontaneous speech samples of children with cochlear implants or tactile aids. The American Journal of Otology 12 (suppl): 151-64.

Osberger MJ, Robbins AM, Todd S, Riley A, Kirk K, Carney A (1996) Cochlear implants and tactile aids for children with profound hearing impairment. In Bess F, Gravel J, Tharpe AM (eds) Amplification for Children with Auditory Deficits. Nashville, TN: Bill Wilkerson Centre Press, pp 283-308.

Parisier SC, Chute PM, Weiss MH, Hellman SA, Wang RC (1991) Results of cochlear implant reinsertion. The Laryngoscope 101: 1013-15.

Parisier SC, Chute PM, Popp AL (1996) Cochlear implantation mechanical failures. American Journal of Otology 17: 730-4.

Parkin J, Stewart BE (1988) Multichannel cochlear implantation: Utah – design. The Laryngoscope 98: 262-5.

Parkinson AJ, El-Kholy W, Tyler RS (1998) Vowel perception in prelingually deafened children with multichannel cochlear implants. Journal of the American Academy of Audiology 9: 179-90.

Patrick JF, Clark GM (1991) The Nucleus 22 channel cochlear implant system. Ear and Hearing 12: 3s-9s.

Pedley K (1998) Comparison of conventional and dual microphone cochlear implant headsets - a case study. The Australian Journal of Audiology 20: 17-20.

Pelizzone M, Cosendai G, Tinembart J (1999) Within-patient longitudinal speech reception measures with continuous interleaved sampling processors for Ineraid implanted subjects. Ear and Hearing 20: 228-37.

Pijl S (1991) Single channel versus bilateral multi-channel implant results: a case report. Ear and Hearing 12: 431-3.

Pijl S (1997) Pulse rate matching by cochlear implant patients: effects of loudness randomization and electrode position. Ear and Hearing 18: 316-25.

Portnoy WM, Mattucci K (1991) Cochlear implants as a contraindication to magnetic resonance imaging. Annals of Otology, Rhinology and Laryngology 100: 195-7.

Ramsden R, Bance M, Giles E, Mawman D (1997) Cochlear implantation in otosclerosis: a unique positioning and programming problem. The Journal of Laryngology and Otology 111: 262-5.

Ray J, Gray RF, Court I (1998) Surgical removal of 11 cochlear implants - lessons from the 11 year Cambridge programme. The Journal of Laryngology and Otology 112: 338-43.

Richardson HC, Beliaeff M, Clarke G, Hawthorne M (1999) A three array cochlear implant: a new approach for the ossified cochlea. The Journal of Laryngology and Otology 113: 811-14.

Rubenstein JT, Parkinson WS, Tyler RS, Gantz BJ (1999) Residual speech recognition and cochlear implant performance: effects of implantation criteria. The American Journal of Otology 20: 1-7.

Salvi RJ, Chen L, Trautwein P, Powers N, Shero M (1998) Hair cell regeneration and recovery of function in the avian auditory system. Scandinavian Audiology suppl. 48: 7-14.

Sehgal ST, Kirk KI, Svirsky M, Miyamoto RT (1998) The effects of speech processor strategy on the speech perception performance of pediatric Nucleus multichannel cochlear implant users. Ear and Hearing 19: 149-61.

Shallop JK, Beiter AL, Goin DW, Mischke RE (1990) Electrically evoked auditory brainstem responses (EABR) and middle latency responses (EMLR) obtained from patients with the Nucleus multi-channel cochlear implant. Ear and Hearing 11: 5-15.

Shallop JK, McGiun-Brunelli T (1995) Speech recognition performance over time with the Spectra 22 speech processor. Annals of Otology, Rhinology and Laryngology 104 (suppl 166): 306-7.

Shallop JK, Facer GW, Peterson A (1999) Neural response telemetry with the Nucleus CI24M cochlear implant. The Laryngoscope 109: 1755-9.

Shannon R, Zeng F-G, Kamath V, Wygonski J, Ekelid M (1995) Speech recognition with primarily temporal cues. Science 270: 303-4.

Shannon RV (1996) Cochlear implants: what have we learned and where are we going? Seminars in Hearing 17: 403-15.

Shepherd RK, Franz BK-HG, Clark G (1990) The biocompatibility and safety of cochlear prostheses. In Clark G, Tong YC, Patrick JF (eds) Cochlear Prostheses. London: Churchill Livingstone, pp. 69-98.

Simmons FB (1966) Electrical stimulation of the auditory nerve in man. Archives of Otolaryngology, Chicago, IL, 84: 2-54.

Skinner MW, Clark GM, Whitford LA, Seligman PM, Staller SJ, Shipp DB, Shallop JK, Everingham C, Menapace CM, Arndt PL, Antogenelli T, Brimacombe JA, Pijl S, Daniels P, George CR, McDermott HJ, Beiter AL (1994) Evaluation of the new spectral peak (SPEAK) coding strategy for the Nucleus 22 channel cochlear implant system. The American Journal of Otology 15 (suppl 2): 15-27.

Skinner MW, Holden LK, Holden TA (1995) Effect of frequency boundary assignment on speech recognition with the SPEAK speech coding strategy. Annals of Otology, Rhinology and Laryngology 104 (suppl 166): 307-9.

Skinner MW, Holden LK, Holden TA, Demorest ME, Fourakis MS (1997) Speech recognition at simulated soft, conversational, and raised-to-loud vocal efforts by adults with cochlear implants. Journal of the Acoustical Society of America 101: 3766-82.

Snik Ad FM, Vermeulen AM, Geelen CP, Brohx JPL, Van den Broek P (1997) Speech perception performance of children with a cochlear implant compared to that of children with conventional hearing aids II. Results of prelingually deaf children. Acta Otolaryngology (Stockh) 117: 755-9.

Spencer LJ, Tye-Murray N, Tomblin JB (1998) The production of English inflection morphology, speech production and listening performance in children with cochlear implants. Ear and Hearing 19: 310-18.

Staecker H, Van der Water TR (2000) Regeneration, repair and protection in the inner ear: implications for cochlear implantation. In Waltzman SB, Cohen NL (eds) Cochlear Implants. New York: Thieme, pp. 17-30.

Staller S, Beiter AL, Brimacombe JA, Mecklenburg DJ, Arndt P (1991) Paediatric performance with the Nucleus 22 channel cochlear implant system. The American Journal of Otology 12 (suppl): 126-36.

Stephan K, Welzl-Muller K, Stiglbrumer H (1991) Acoustic reflex in patients with cochlear implants (analog stimulation). The American Journal of Otology 12 (suppl): 48-51.

Stobich B, Zierhofer CM, Hochmair ES (1999) Influence of automatic gain control parameter settings on speech understanding of cochlear implant users employing the continuous interleaved sampling strategy. Ear and Hearing 20: 104-16.

Summerfield AQ, Marshall DH (1995) Cochlear implantation in the UK 1990-1994. Report by the MRC Institute of Hearing Research on the evaluation of the national cochlear implant programme. MRC Institute of Hearing Research, Nottingham, UK.

Summerfield AQ, Marshall DH (1999) Paediatric cochlear implantation and health-technology assessment. International Journal of Pediatric Otorhinolaryngology 47: 141-51.

Szilvassy J, Czigner J, Somogyi I, Jori, J, Kiss JG, Szilvassy Z (1998) Cochlear implantation in a patient with grand mal epilepsy. The Journal of Laryngology and Otology 112: 567-9.

Tait M, Lutman ME (1994) Comparison of early communicative behaviour in young children with cochlear implants and with hearing aids. Ear and Hearing 15: 352-61.

Teig E, Lindeman HH, Floltorp G, Tvete O, Hanche-Olsen S, Arntsen O (1992) Patient performance with two types of multiple electrode intracochlear implants. Scandinavian Audiology 21: 93-9.

Teissl C, Kremser C, Hochmair ES, Hochmair-Desoyer IJ (1998) Cochlear implants: in vitro investigation of electromagnetic interference at MR imaging – compatibility and safety aspects. Radiology 208: 700-8.

Terr LI, Sfogliano GA, Riley SL (1989) Effects of stimulation by cochlear implants on the cochlear nerve. The Laryngoscope 99: 1171-4.

Tucci DL, Lambert PR, Ruth RA (1990) Trends in rehabilitation after cochlear implantation. Archives of Otolaryngology Head and Neck Surgery 116: 571-4.

Tye-Murray N, Lowder M, Tyler RS (1990) Comparison of the F0F2 and F0F1F2 processing strategies for the Cochlear corporation cochlear implant. Ear and Hearing 11: 195-200.

Tye-Murray N, Tyler RS, Woodworth GG, Gantz BJ (1992) Performance over time with the Nucleus or Ineraid cochlear implant. Ear and Hearing 13: 200-9.

Tyler RS (1988) Open set word recognition with the 3M/Vienna single channel cochlear implant. Archives of Otolaryngology, Head and Neck Surgery 114: 1123-6.

Tyler RS (1993) Cochlear implants and deaf culture. The American Journal of Audiology March: 26-32.

Tyler RS, Summerfield AQ (1996) Cochlear implantation: relationships with research on auditory deprivation and acclimatization. Ear and Hearing 17: 38S-50S.

Tyler RS, Gantz BJ, Woodworth GG, Parkinson AJ, Lowder M, Schum LK (1996) Initial independent results with the Clarion cochlear implant. Ear and Hearing 17: 528-36.

Van Hoesel RJM, Clark GM (1999) Speech results with a bilateral multi-channel cochlear implant subject for spatially separated signal and noise. The Australian Journal of Audiology 21: 23-8.

Von Wallenberg EL, Battmer RD (1991) Comparative speech recognition results in eight subjects using two different coding strategies with the Nucleus 22 channel cochlear implant. British Journal of Audiology 25: 371-80.

Von Wallenberg EL, Laszig R, Gnadeberg D, Battmer R, Desloovere C, Kiefer J, Lehnhardt E, Von Ilberg C (1993) Initial findings with the modified Nucleus implant comprised of 20 active intracochlear and 2 extracochlear reference electrodes. In Hochmair-Desoyer IJ, Hochmair ES (eds) Advances in Cochlear Implants. Vienna: Manz, pp 186-92.

Von Wallenberg EL, Brinch JM (1995) Cochlear implant reliability. Annals of Otology, Rhinology and Laryngology 104 (suppl 166): 441-3.

Waltzman SB, Cohen NL, Shapiro WH (1991) Effects of chronic electrical stimulation on patients using a cochlear prosthesis. Otolaryngology, Head and Neck Surgery 105: 797-801.

Waltzman SB, Cohen NL, Gromolin RH, Shapiro WH, Ozdamar SR, Hoffman RA (1994) Long term results of early cochlear implantation in congenitally and prelingually deaf children. The American Journal of Otology 15 (suppl 2): 9-13.

Weber BP, Neuburger J, Koestler H, Goldring JE, Battmer R, Santogrossi T, Lenarz T (1999) Clinical results of the Clarion magnetless cochlear implant. Annals of Otology, Rhinology and Laryngology 108: 22-6.

Weston SC, Waltzman SB (1995) Performance as a function of time: a study of three cochlear implant devices. Annals of Otology, Rhinology and Laryngology 104 (suppl 165): 19-24.

Wilson BS, Finley CC, Lawson DT, Wolford RD, Eddington DK, Rabinowitz WM (1991) Better speech recognition with cochlear implants. Nature 352: 236-8.

Wilson BS (1993) Signal processing. In Tyler RS (ed.) Cochlear Implants Audiological Foundations. London: Whurr, pp 35-86.

Wilson BS, Lawson DT, Zerbi M, Finley CC, Wolford RD (1995) New processing strategies in cochlear implantation. The American Journal of Otology 16: 669-75.

Wilson BS (1997) The future of cochlear implants. British Journal of Audiology 31: 205–25.

Zeng F-G, Galvin III JJ (1999) Amplitude mapping and phoneme recognition in cochlear implant listeners. Ear and Hearing 20: 60–74.

Zeng F-G, Shannon RV (1993) Loudness growth in electrical stimulation. In Hochmair-Desoyer IJ, Hochmair ES (eds) Advances in Cochlear Implants. Vienna: Manz, pp. 339–41.

Zimmerman-Phillips MS, Murad C (1999) Programming features of the Clarion multi-strategy cochlear implant. Annals of Otology, Rhinology and Laryngology 108: 17–21.

Chapter 3
A paediatric cochlear implant programme: current and future challenges

SUE ARCHBOLD

This chapter describes one model of a paediatric cochlear implant programme, discussing the rationale on which it is based and its response to the changing demands of the children, their families and the local professionals who work with them. It gives protocols that have been developed for the assessment, implantation, rehabilitation and maintenance phases, reflecting on the changes in practice over time in response to changing demands. Over the 10 years following the programme's establishment, the long-term infrastructure required to support the future needs of these children has become increasingly evident, with the consequent staffing and costing implications; these will be discussed with a view to future planning.

Paediatric cochlear implantation: its development

Chapter 2 describes the history of the development of cochlear implantation more fully and there are many accounts of the development of cochlear implantation for the interested reader (Mecklenburg and Lehnhardt, 1991; Nevins and Chute, 1996; Clark in Clark, Cowan and Dowell, 1997; Niparko and Wilson in Niparko et al., 2000, Chapter 2). In a survey of European cochlear implant centres in 1996 (Archbold and Robinson, 1997) cochlear implantation was revealed as growing rapidly, with increasing interest in implanting children under the age of two. However, the study also revealed the discrepancies in practice between various European countries; for example paediatric cochlear implantation was much more common in Germany, France and the UK than in Sweden, Norway or Portugal.

Several influences on the development of paediatric implantation can be identified, some of which moved implantation forward, and some of which appeared to delay progress. Amongst these influences were:

- availability of child appropriate technology;
- parental pressure;
- deaf culture pressure;
- educational issues;
- evidence of outcomes from adults;
- restricted financial resources;
- individual endeavours.

(Archbold, 1997)

For example, it was not possible to move forward with implantation for young children until it was proven safe with adults and the technology was suitable in size and robustness for children. As the evidence grew from adults that cochlear implantation was able to provide useful hearing for those unable to benefit from conventional hearing aids, and some were even able to use the telephone, the pressure from parents of profoundly deaf children increased. The enthusiasm of individual scientists and surgeons, frustrated by the difficulties of fitting effective hearing aids to the deafest children, also influenced the development of cochlear implantation for children. However, with young children unable to make the decision for this elective procedure themselves, there were major concerns in the minds of many about proceeding.

For many years paediatric implantation, particularly in the case of congenitally deaf children, has been opposed by some of the groups involved with deaf children and adults. The controversy led to an unfortunate polarization of views and delayed the development of a rational approach to implantation in which parents could make an informed decision on behalf of their children (McCormick, 1991). At the time of writing, this controversy continues. Beard (1999) wrote that 'cochlear implantation may be an expensive white elephant, pushed forward by the drive for normalization through technical innovation in medicine.' She questions the tackling of what she sees as a socio-educational issue by surgery. Those involved in cochlear implantation have not always understood that paediatric implantation involves broader issues than implantation in a deafened adult. Inevitably an implant team working with children must consider how they are to address these issues but first they must attempt to understand them. This chapter will consider some of these issues: many are not new in the management of deaf children but are familiar to those with experience of hearing-aided children.

An understanding of deaf issues is often limited amongst professionals working with deaf children (Tyler, 1999) and the views of deaf people about cochlear implantation have often not been explored fully by implant teams. Deafness and disability can be seen according to medical, social or educational models (Knight, 1998); cochlear implantation is clearly seen as coming from a medical model. However, those who view themselves as members of the deaf community do not see deafness as a medical condition requiring treatment but as a linguistic and cultural identity (Power and Hyde, 1992; Knight in Gregory et al., 1998; Nevins and Chute, 1996; Niparko, 2000). Cochlear implantation may be seen as a threat to this identity and as an attempt to effect a 'cure' (Niparko, 2000; Tyler, 1993; Cayton, 1991; Lea, 1991). Much of the publicity which has accompanied implantation and the use of terms such as 'bionic ear' promote this myth (Laurenzi, 1993; Power and Hyde, 1992). Cochlear implantation in children is not merely an audiological or medical process but one which, as there is growing evidence to demonstrate, will affect a child's relationships with others, educational and communication options, and self image as a deaf person. It is vital that those professionals involved in paediatric implantation become familiar with issues associated with deafness, and ensure that parents of implant candidates also consider them in order that they can make an informed decision about implantation, understanding the implications of their decision for their children's future.

Despite the varying trends in practice and the lasting controversy in paediatric cochlear implantation, it is now widely accepted as a safe procedure (Summerfield and Marshall, 1995) and one in which the outcomes are increasingly well documented (Waltzman et al., 1994; Dowell in Clark, Cowan and Dowell, 1997; Uziel et al., 1996; Nikolopoulos, O'Donoghue and Archbold, 1999; O'Donoghue et al., 1999). These reports have their critics: Lane (1994) criticized them for lack of objectivity, and for self-selection, for example. Measuring outcomes objectively from the implementation of an evolving technology in a heterogeneous group such as deaf children inevitably has its difficulties, as described in Chapter 1, but this is a challenge that implant programmes must address.

With deafened adults, the aim of implantation is to restore a channel of audition to facilitate communication in one who has already established language skills. With children born deaf or deafened at an early age, we are aiming for more than this: we are aiming to provide audition, to facilitate the development of spoken language. For children without material auditory input, spoken language acquisition is likely to be grossly delayed (Mellon in Niparko et al., 2000) and even those deafened after the initial development of spoken language may lose the communication skills previously acquired. As discussed in Chapter 8, cochlear implants have provided profoundly deaf children with the opportunity for 'incidental learning' through the hearing they provide (Robbins in Niparko et al., 2000) and the accumulated evidence shows that cochlear implantation can provide significant number of profoundly deaf children with the opportunity to develop effective spoken language skills.

Kirk and Hill-Brown (1985) give a useful summary of published works on the adverse effects of profound hearing loss on the development of spoken language, explaining the influence of age at onset and degree of loss in predicting the severity of effect. The primary channel by which communication skills and thus spoken language are usually acquired is hearing; profound hearing loss can have a devastating effect on a child's linguistic development (Wood et al., 1986; Quigley and Kretschmer, 1984) and the resulting poor educational achievements are also well documented (Wood et al., 1986; Conrad, 1979). There are many complex influences on a deaf child's progress, but the degree of hearing loss was considered critical (Bamford and Saunders, 1985; Quigley and Kretschmer, 1984); however, recent work has shown that the age of intervention may also be significant (Yoshinaga-Itano et al., 1998).

Early amplification has been a desired goal for deaf children, but for some children conventional hearing aids will provide little benefit or auditory access to speech. Children under the age of three are the most rapidly expanding group to be implanted, including those below the age of two and in the first year of life. This is the group that will demand the greatest expertise on the part of the implant team and is likely to grow further with the advent of Universal Neonatal Hearing Screening and the earlier diagnosis of deafness. These children are unlikely to have developed age-appropriate communication skills, are likely to be difficult to test audiologically and, should implantation take place, are unlikely to show immediate post-operative benefit and be difficult to monitor. While age at onset, length of deafness and communication mode have all been considered predictors of positive outcomes from implantation, there remains a great deal of unexplained variance in outcome in children. This makes candidate selection and prediction of benefit accordingly more difficult than in the adult population. In the already complex picture of paediatric implantation, the emphasis on the implantation of young infants raises further issues. Tobey (1999) identified five questions with regard to the implantation of children under the age of two:

- the accurate identification of the hearing loss;
- the identification of other problems;
- the ability to tune in the device satisfactorily;
- the ability to monitor functioning effectively;
- the adjustment of parents to the hearing loss and the ability to make a fully informed decision at such an early stage.

Although difficult to assess, two of the most important factors in facilitating the effective use of a cochlear implant system, whatever the age of the child, may well be parental support and educational management. Family responsibilities will be discussed more fully later in the chapter and in the final chapter in this book. There is also a growing acknowledgement of the influence of family expectations on progress and, particularly with the implantation of very young children, of the role of parents in the rehabilitation process. Following early diagnosis of deafness, the issue of cochlear implantation may well not be one that parents feel ready to consider fully, or be able to make an informed decision.

For children with conventional hearing aids, educational management, regardless of communication strategy, is a vital factor in influencing educational achievements (Wood et al., 1986; Boothroyd in Owens and Kessler, 1989) and this is likely to be true for those with cochlear implants. The role of the child's educational management has long been emphasized by those with paediatric experience (Geers and Moog, 1991; Beiter, Staller and Dowell, 1991); the major long-term support for the child will be provided in the child's educational setting. Cochlear implantation has brought together the influences of medicine and education in a unique way which will be considered more fully later.

Experience has confirmed the challenges of child implantation, which need to be addressed by paediatric teams and which can be summarized as follows:

- the greater variability in outcome as opposed to the adult population;
- the correspondingly greater difficulty in pre-implant assessment and prediction of benefit;
- the need for appropriate outcome measures;
- the number of variables influencing outcomes: age of onset, aetiology, length of deafness, parental influence, educational management;
- the recognition of the various models of deafness and an understanding of deaf issues;
- the greater length of time taken to show benefit;
- the life-time commitment required for these children by the implant team;
- the role of parental responsibility in the decision-making process and long-term parental commitment necessary;
- the wide range of professionals required to work together as a team, often based in different geographical centres;
- the importance of educational liaison;
- the greater time-consuming nature of paediatric implantation;
- the long-term staffing and funding implications.

Any paediatric implant team should consider these issues and the way in which they will meet the particular needs of the child, family and local professionals involved with the child. In establishing a paediatric team, the management of the following issues must be addressed:

- multi-professional teamwork, including issues of roles, responsibilities, and decision making;
- differing professional structures and relationships;
- full involvement of parents, including facilitating informed decision making;

- involvement of local professionals, including provision of accessible information and appropriate training;
- involvement of deaf adults;
- provision of long-term infrastructure providing technical support;
- provision of long-term expertise – identifying what is necessary and where and how it should be provided.

Addressing these issues, including the necessary long-term funding, influences the staffing and management of the team formed; implant teams are usually managed within a medical context and such a team will demand more flexible management structures than are usually found there.

A paediatric cochlear implant team: structure and relationships

Summerfield and Marshall (1995) recommended that paediatric implantation should take place in clinics that are sufficiently large to maintain a centre of expertise in all required disciplines and that these centres should provide outcome data to inform parental and professional decisions. The teams established must be interdisciplinary rather than multidisciplinary (Nevins and Chute, 1996) and may challenge the usual medical frameworks, where the surgeon is conventionally the leader of the team. An implant team may need different leaders at different times: the differing professional views must be explored and valued in the team framework, but there may be increased emphasis on the opinion of one particular member at different times, according to changing circumstances. In order to avoid the situation in which the family may have conflicting views from different members of the team a key worker may be appointed for each child so that one person on the team is seen as the liaison person via whom the family relates to the team. Figure 3.1 illustrates the typical membership of a paediatric cochlear implant team.

However, the cochlear implant team that only considers the personnel at the implant centre is only considering part of the picture. While the expertise of the implant clinic is clearly vital, equally influential to the long-term successful use of the implant system may be the team at the child's home – the family and local supporting professionals. This chapter will now discuss the roles of the team supporting the child at home, followed by

	Radiologists	
Educational Psychologist		**Audiological Scientists**
Implanted Adults		**Surgeons and**
Nursing Staff	**THE COCHLEAR IMPLANT TEAM**	**ENT Staff**
Medical Physicists		**Administrators**
Speech and Language Therapists		**Teachers of the Deaf**
	Deaf Adults	

Figure 3.1. A typical paediatric cochlear implant team.

those of the clinic-based team, and then go on to consider ways of managing positive liaison and transfer of expertise.

The child and family

The most important members of any implant team are not the professionals but the child and his family. The child and his long-term needs must be the focus of any cochlear implant programme; as Staller, Beiter and Brimacombe in Cooper (1991) state, paediatric implantation 'creates a life-long relationship between the implant team and the patient'. In order that productive relationships can be established between the child and the implant clinic, a member of the clinic team, usually the implant clinic teacher of the deaf, must meet the child on his own ground – at school or nursery, and at home. Close observation of the child in his familiar setting will help assess the child's suitability for implantation, and baselines of functioning to be established (Nevins and Chute, 1996; Schopmeyer in Niparko et al., 2000).

Parents are usually the best guides as to their children's likely needs for preparation, which may depend on linguistic functioning, and in Chapter 11 parents describe their experiences of preparing children for operation. The use of videos, photographs and colouring books may be helpful, together with contact with other children wearing the device (Downs in Mecklenburg, 1986); practical advice is given in Chapter 8. Older children need to be given explanations for the operation and some reasonable expectations; it can be difficult to balance giving an explanation for the operation with the possibility of raising false expectations within the child. If good relations have been established with child and family from the outset then it should prove possible to prepare the child appropriately and to establish a basis for the 'life-long relationships' that may follow implantation. Clearly for many young infants the preparation possible for cochlear implantation is inevitably limited.

Deafness in one member of the family affects the others (Luterman, 1987; Gregory and Knight, 1998) and cochlear implantation too does not merely affect the recipient. The needs of other members of the family must be considered and balanced in meeting the needs of the child receiving the cochlear implant. All too often, the needs of siblings may be overlooked as the family prepares the deaf child for implantation. Cochlear implantation and the rehabilitation period can be stressful for the whole family (Downs in Mecklenburg, 1986; Archbold et al., 2002) and the support of other relatives or friends will be vital for parents during the operative period and ensuing tuning and rehabilitation. Travelling long distances to the implant centre, as frequently occurs, will require the support of family or friends so that the effects on the other members are minimized.

Studies by Quittner, Thompson Steck and Rouiller (1991) show high levels of stress in parents of deaf children before and after implantation, as some of the parents' comments in Chapter 11 illustrate. Levels of parental responsibility are high and the counselling towards realistic expectations must include the whole family. If early benefit is not seen following implantation (as is likely with young children) disappointment expressed by other members of the family is most unhelpful. Similarly, if expected benefits are not observed then the child must not feel responsible and parents must remain supportive (Evans in Owens and Kessler, 1989). Grandparents are often a useful source of support for parents of deaf children (Luterman, 1987) and if they have been involved during the preparation period by inclusion in visits and the loan of information materials, their support is likely to be realistic during the post-operative phase.

Parents, however, remain the strongest source of support for their child (Evans in Owens and Kessler, 1989). Contact with other parents has been found to promote greater understanding of the likely difficulties and a sharing of feelings that is not possible with implant professionals; this is the most frequently mentioned factor that parents found helpful prior to implantation. The implant clinic bears some responsibility for facilitating this contact; several teams have active parents' support groups and newsletters and in many countries, parents run their own support groups, which are good sources of independent information. In Europe the Euro CI Users' Group includes active participation by parents.

The local team supporting the child and family

The child's local teachers: mainstream and specialist

The long-term management of the child has long been recognized as falling largely on the teacher in the child's educational setting (Somers in Cooper, 1991; Geers and Moog, 1991; Goin and Parisier, 1991) and experience is bearing this out. With young children this may be a qualified teacher of the deaf visiting at home or in a nursery setting; it may be a non-specialist teacher working in a mainstream class receiving support from a visiting teacher of the deaf. Whatever the child's educational setting, teaching staff must be involved from the beginning in the assessment of the child for suitability and in the discussion of the child's long-term rehabilitation needs should implantation proceed. The child's local teacher of the deaf will see the child on a more regular basis than the implant clinic teacher and brings insights into the child's everyday functioning and a knowledge of the local educational options for that child, which is invaluable to the implant team (Robbins in Niparko et al., 2000). Establishing the co-operation of the child's educational staff for the ongoing rehabilitation of a child will involve discussing communication and educational management styles, as well as practical issues such as the suitability of the acoustic environment for developing listening skills (Nevins and Chute, 1996). However, this may need a sensitive approach by the implant team; there are major areas of tension for teachers of the deaf. Cochlear implantation may be seen to be intrusive on educational time and to raise issues of equity of support and provision for all the children in the teacher's care (Archbold and Robinson, 1997). Moreover, teachers may be seen to be responsible for many of the outcomes from cochlear implantation yet feel that they have not been fully included in the assessment process or feel that they have not supported the intervention.

Local speech and language therapist

In the UK the amount and type of speech and language therapy offered to hearing impaired children varies widely. Where available, close co-operation must be established from the outset between the implant team speech and language therapists and local therapist, and the roles are discussed in Chapter 11. Assessments before and after implantation must be made in collaboration with the local therapist as well as educator, and future rehabilitation and assessment planned jointly.

Local audiological scientist

The child's local audiological scientist may have been closely involved in the audiological management of the child prior to implantation; following implantation, there may be little that the audiological scientist can do beyond simple trouble-shooting of the system because of the complex programming equipment required for most devices. The provision of spares, replacements and repairs will usually be managed by the implant centre, as will the tuning of the device and monitoring of the system. An interested audiologist may find it difficult to have little professional responsibility, and the implant centre should involve the child's scientist, where possible, by organized visits and regular reports. Future developments in sharing expertise between the implant centre and local professionals, such as video conferencing networks, may facilitate greater participation locally, not only by the audiological scientist.

Prior to implantation, particularly with changing audiological criteria, the local audiologist may feel his or her own assessments are being questioned as the implant team carries out its own evaluations. However, it is vital that, with the legal responsibility carried by the implant team, the implant team should complete its own audiological assessment in order to inform the decision making process, particularly if difficult decisions need to be made about which ear to implant.

Local consultant in otorhinolaryngology

In the UK, the referral to the implant centre will generally be made by the child's local consultant or audiological physician, and the implant surgeon may well need to consult with the local specialists about medical and surgical assessments, particularly if the child has complex needs. Where the child lives at some distance from the implant centre, the local consultant should be asked to co-operate in the post-operative care and long-term medical support of the child. Parents find it reassuring to know that local medical support and co-operation have been established between the implanting surgeon and local otolaryngologist prior to implantation.

Local educational psychologist

Most hearing impaired children in the UK will have an educational psychologist responsible for ensuring that a statutory Statement of Special Educational Needs (SEN) is completed as appropriate, outlining their special educational needs and ensuring that these needs are met. This is equivalent to the IEP (Individualized Education Plan) in the US. During the assessment period, contact should be made with the local psychologist to ask for a contribution to the child's assessment. It is important that all areas of a child's development are explored as any other learning difficulties may influence rehabilitation and the likely benefits from the implant system. A cochlear implant is likely to influence future educational placement and management and an educational psychologist who shares the responsibility for the decisions made about educational choices for the child must have realistic expectations of implantation.

Local social worker for the deaf

Any social worker for the deaf appointed to the child and family must be involved in the assessment of a child for implantation. In practice, in the UK, comparatively few deaf children have an assigned social worker for the deaf, but where a social worker, generic or specialist, is supporting child and family he or she must share in the preparation period and also be made aware of the implications of implantation. A social worker for the deaf will often be in contact with the local deaf community and have insights into the deaf culture that are useful to the family considering implantation. This contact, if available, is an important one for the clinic team to develop, in order to strengthen understanding about implantation within the deaf community and overcome the problems of misinformation amongst the deaf people.

Deaf adults

In the UK, as in other countries, deaf adults are often involved in the education of deaf children, and in the home from an early age, working with parents from diagnosis, particularly in Scandinavia. Deaf adults need up-to-date information about cochlear implantation in an accessible format and should be included in the process, according to their particular responsibilities in their roles.

Other carers

Deaf children are the concern of many other carers during the course of their day. These may be both professional and non-professional and it is important that all are included in the pre-implant information-sharing process. This serves two purposes; it ensures that the child wears the system effectively at all times and receives appropriate management, and it ensures that all concerned with the child share realistic expectations.

The team at the implant clinic

The amount of work involved in paediatric implantation has been emphasized (Kileny, Kemink and Zimmerman-Phillips, 1991; Goin and Parisier, 1991) and is becoming increasingly evident. Staff at the clinic should have prior experience in the paediatric aspects of their work to enable close co-operation to be readily established with the team at the child's home, and to establish their own credibility.

Team co-ordinator/administrator

The difficulties of multi-disciplinary work are well known (Warnock in Cohen and Cohen, 1982; Haggard, 1993), with misunderstandings arising between team members from different professions, but it is vital that effective co-ordination is achieved so that the team is seen to be providing consistent support and advice and maintains professional credibility. With rapidly growing numbers of implanted children, often travelling long distances to the implant centres, and from a wide variety of educational programmes, the problems of co-ordination become accordingly more complex. The co-ordinator's role encompasses the co-ordination of the role of each team member at the implant centre as well as the interaction between the implant clinic team and those supporting the child locally. The typical tasks of a co-ordinator are:

- to respond to referrals, send out and request information;
- to manage appointments, assessments, evaluations and data-base;
- to co-ordinate audiological, medical and rehabilitation follow-up;
- to manage the budget, order equipment and control stock;
- to co-ordinate team decisions, sharing information amongst team members;
- to co-ordinate professional development within the team, through meetings and professional visits;
- to liaise with other teams to develop 'best practice'.

The co-ordinator of a paediatric cochlear implant team is required to liaise with a large range of people for each child, both at the implant centre and at the child's home. It is important that parents and local professionals talking to cochlear implant team members receive consistent information and that decisions are co-ordinated in order to ensure the integrity of the programme. The co-ordinator should ensure that time is made for team meetings and for sharing professional experiences to develop a fuller understanding of the differing roles of members. In this way implant team decisions can be made with appropriate recognition and respect for other professional viewpoints, and professional development can take place within the team.

The issues of managing staff in a multi-professional team, with attendant demands of equity of pay, conditions and responsibilities is a sensitive one, which each team must address within its own structure. This complex co-ordinating role can only be achieved with a large degree of secretarial and management support.

Implant clinic otolaryngologists/surgeons

With young children, the surgeon has an important counselling role in addition to carrying out medical assessment prior to the decision to implant (Gibbin, 1992; O'Donoghue, 1992). The importance of parents' understanding of the future implications of their decision has been stressed but parents must also make the decision to implant their child in full knowledge of the risks involved. Chapter 5 describes more fully the role of the surgeon throughout the management of the child. Although the shared responsibility of the team is stressed throughout this chapter, the surgeon carries overall clinical responsibility for the implanted child (Fraser in Cooper, 1991) and there are many issues to be considered in dealing with young children. The issue of informed consent is particularly relevant to paediatric implantation, where parents are deciding about an elective operation with life-long consequences for their child. Dawes and Kitcher (1999) revealed greater awareness on the part of consultants in the importance of their role in this process, rather than leaving the job to junior doctors. In paediatric implantation it is vital that enough time is given to parents to discuss the risks of the procedure with those who can answer the questions at first hand.

Paediatric teams find it helpful to have two surgeons and to ensure that other members of their medical staff develop the necessary skills to provide appropriate medical cover for children; this requires continuing professional development for all staff. As more children are implanted who may have other disabilities, the medical assessments become more complex and it may become necessary to liaise with other medical specialities, for example paediatricians, cardiologists or neurologists.

Nursing staff

The nursing staff in the hospital have a vital role to play in a paediatric implant programme; they will meet the parents and children during the assessment period, when parents may be experiencing doubts about putting their children through the tests and procedures and when the parents are concerned that their children may not be suitable for cochlear implantation. Parents may use the hospital staff to ask many of the worrying practical questions that concern them; the nursing staff must feel part of the implant programme, being aware of current thinking and involved in development within the programme. In some paediatric programmes members of the nursing staff attend team meetings to ensure full participation in the programme.

Implant clinic audiological scientists

The audiological scientists at the clinic take responsibility for full audiological assessment prior to implantation, including the evaluation of hearing aid use. Post-implantation, the responsibilities include the fitting and tuning of the external parts, refinements of tuning and long-term maintenance of the implant system. Further audiological investigations with and without the implant device, including sound field investigations and speech audiometry, are carried out. The scientist must discuss the external equipment and its controls and the programming process; this information must be disseminated to others in daily contact with the child. Scientists must be up-to-date with all the information about current devices and systems and be able to convey this clearly to parents and children.

For young children with few or no communication skills, who are unable to give verbal feedback during tuning sessions, it is important that the rehabilitation team and audiological scientist work closely together in order that changes in listening skills, or vocalization, for example, are reported to the scientist. The role of the audiological scientist is developed fully in Chapters 4 and 7.

Implant clinic medical physicist

The medical physicist works in conjunction with the audiological scientist, and in some programmes takes responsibility for electrophysiological investigation of children. Evoked response audiometry is an essential part of the overall audiological assessment prior to implantation in young children, and such investigations provide an objective measure of hearing in support of behavioural tests. There is also an important role for the physicist during implant surgery and after implantation regarding the development of the recording technique for the electrically evoked auditory brainstem response (EABR) and stapedial reflexes. Electrical stimulation of the cochlea by the implant can be used to elicit the EABR. This investigation can provide valuable objective information about the functioning of the implant, which can also be used to assist the later tuning-in procedure. These electrophysiological investigations are described more fully in Chapter 6.

Implant clinic technician

As large numbers of children are implanted, technical support becomes crucial. Devices break down and need repair, children need spare equipment and an efficient maintenance service must be developed. Children become dependent upon the auditory signal provided by the implant to monitor their environment as well as to access speech, and they may become very distressed if without their implant system for any length of time. This creates a great responsibility for the implant clinic to ensure reliability of technical support and its financial backing. Implant clinics must consider warranty issues, and the establishment of maintenance contracts with the supplying companies. Most breakdown problems will involve returning the processor to the company and this entails further expenditure by the team on a supply of spares. In some countries, this role is carried out by external companies or suppliers; if this is the case, care must be taken in its organization. It is absolutely vital that the correct parts are sent and these are regularly updated in order to ensure the system is working optimally. Moreover, requests for more frequent support may indicate potential problems with the device itself to which the implant programme must be alert.

Implant clinic teacher of the deaf

Teachers working at an implant programme must have wide previous experience of the different approaches and educational settings in which deaf children are placed in order to establish credibility in the classroom and acceptance by the child's local teacher of the deaf. Prior to implantation, the teacher will visit the local teacher to:

- establish liaison and a working relationship;
- ensure information is understood about cochlear implantation;
- assess the educational environment;
- assess the child's functioning in everyday settings (Nevins and Chute, 1996).

Should implantation proceed, the implant clinic teacher of the deaf may be required to fulfil various roles on visits to the child's school:

- monitoring device functioning in non-clinical settings;
- monitoring the development of listening and communication skills;
- trouble-shooting any minor problems with the device;
- ensuring all concerned are able to troubleshoot the device and that spares are available;
- discussing specific listening conditions and difficulties ensuring all are aware of the potential of the implant system;
- observing the child in class and individual situations;
- liaising between implant centre clinic, home and school;

- discussing individual progress and sharing in identification of any other learning difficulties which may become apparent after implantation.

These roles must be carried out sensitively; for children who have been without useful residual hearing, management styles may have been established that are counterproductive to the development of post-implant auditory competence. The objective is to ensure that the management of the child at home and at school facilitate the child's use of the auditory potential from the device.

Implant clinic speech and language therapist (SLT)

The work of the speech and language therapist (SLT) at the implant clinic is described in Chapter 10. As with the implant clinic teacher of the deaf, the clinic SLT visits and works with the child and the family at a local level. The SLT carries out pre-implant assessments of the child's functioning in communication skills and spoken language, with the help of parents and local professionals.

The roles outlined below are elaborated in Chapter 10:

- to describe and explain the implanted child's current communication skills;
- to demonstrate the child's readiness for speech training after implantation;
- to update the team SLT assessment procedure;
- to allow time for feedback on reports and for joint planning of immediate goals at all linguistic levels;
- to provide advice on appropriate materials and strategies to local professionals.

Implant clinic educational psychologist

Implant teams vary in their use of clinical as well as educational psychologists. In the early days of implantation, implant candidates were expected to be of at least average intellectual ability in order that they could cope with the extensive pre- and post-operative testing (Aplin, 1993). As Laurenzi (1993) points out, however, it would be considered unethical to deny a conventional hearing aid to a child of below average intellectual ability, and this criterion has assumed less importance. Children with significant developmental delay and complex disabilities are now being implanted and the educational psychologist will be helpful in identifying those that may preclude proceeding with implantation. Where there is a concern about a child's cognitive functioning in areas unrelated to deafness, and there is difficulty in assessing this, then the services of an educational psychologist, familiar with working with deaf children, must be obtained. With the growing emphasis on the implantation of very young children, this role is likely to become more important. It should be remembered that significant numbers of deaf children will have other learning difficulties, some of which are difficult to identify in infancy or prior to implantation.

Following implantation, the opinion of an experienced educational psychologist may be useful in cases where a child, with lengthy access to useful audition, is not developing spoken language as expected, to determine if there is a specific learning difficulty present influencing progress.

Implant clinic social worker for the deaf

The literature reports wide variability regarding the remit of a social worker in the field of cochlear implantation. In practice few deaf children in the UK will have access to their own social worker for the deaf, but it is important that the role is recognized by implant clinics, and some use the skills of a social worker.

Deaf adults

Deaf adults as part of an implant team can add significantly to the team's understanding of deaf issues and in working with parents and the children themselves as they grow up with or without an implant. In some centres, deaf adults act as a deaf advocate, and in other centres deaf adults with cochlear implants are used to talk to families about the reality of living with an implant.

Implant clinic team and the local team: working together

Figure 3.2 illustrates the family between the local team and the implant clinic team; how to manage the shared support in a seamless fashion is a major challenge. A comprehensive paediatric team including both the clinic-based team and the local professionals will only be effective if ways of working together are established. With growing numbers of children receiving cochlear implants an implant team which is solely clinic based will be unable to provide efficient management of the children.

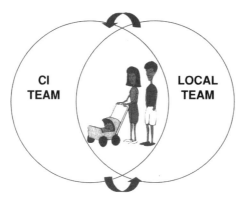

Figure 3.2. The child and family, situated between the local and clinic-based teams.

As local services have become more experienced in dealing with children with cochlear implants, the expertise which can be transferred to the local service and that which must remain at the implant centre has become clearer.

In the National Health Service in the UK, the 'hub and spoke' model of service delivery has been promoted (Audit Commission, 1997). This model of working is illustrated in Figure 3.3; the implant centre can be viewed as the 'centre of expertise' or the 'hub' and the local services at the end of the 'spokes' along which expertise and knowledge is transmitted. This, however, is rather a narrow and elitist view; dissension can arise as to which expertise remains at the centre and which can be transferred, and the process should not be viewed as one way. Undoubtedly the implant centre needs to retain the clinical experience about implantation and its direct management, but the local services may well know more about the child and his or her daily functioning, and have much to offer the implant team. A more even approach is illustrated in Figure 3.4, where the two teams are working together and the exchange of information and expertise is seen as a two-way process. The figure suggests written communication, telephone calls and visits are essential. In future, teleconferencing systems may be an efficient way of managing children and advising on their difficulties at a distance.

Wootton (1998) describes developments in telemedicine, enabling patients to access specialist expertise at a distance, and having great potential for decentralizing health care. This approach has much to commend it for the future of management of those with implants, perhaps enabling complex technical difficulties to be managed in non-specialist centres at a distance

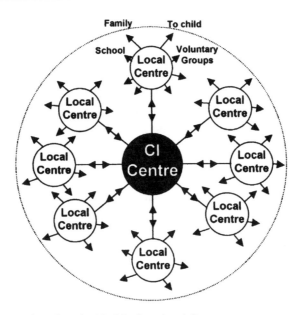

Figure 3.3. Hub and Spoke Model of service delivery.

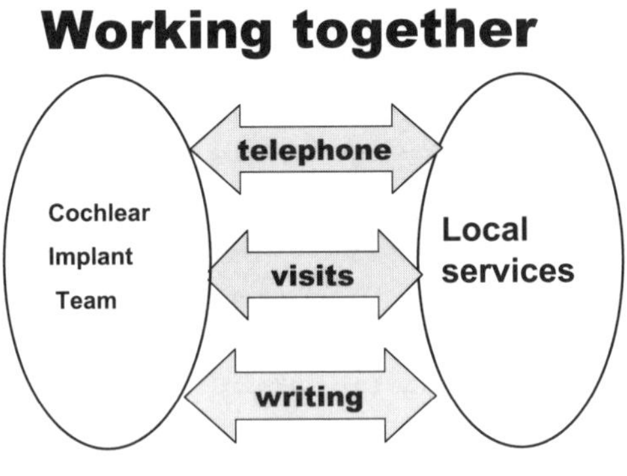

Working together

Figure 3.4. Working together – clinic-based team and local team, supporting child and family.

from the implant centre, having access to the expertise there through excellent communication systems.

Fundamental to developing efficient models of working together is a mutual regard for roles and responsibilities. Paediatric cochlear implantation has brought together the medical and educational management of deafness more directly than previously; a survey of European cochlear implant centres revealed that educational support of children after implantation was seen as the biggest problem centres faced after funding issues (Archbold and Robinson, 1997). Experienced implant centres have long recognized the importance of the interface between those working in the clinic and those working locally with the child, particularly the child's educators. The House Ear Institute (HEI) initiated the School Contact Programme in 1982, with the educators on the staff of the HEI acting in a liaison role between school and clinic (Selmi, 1985). This recognized, at an early stage in paediatric implantation, the crucial role of educators of the deaf and the value of their observations. Other implant teams in Australia, the US, the UK and Holland, have developed close links with schools for the deaf, and work with teachers in their classrooms on a regular basis. The relationship between implant centres and local educators varies considerably. It ranges from rehabilitation being carried out mainly in the clinic with regular attendance there by parents and child, with only telephone and written contacts with the child's local professionals, to the major responsibility for rehabilitation and ongoing support being provided by the child's family and teacher.

In some instances, schools or classes have been established for children with cochlear implants, with teachers in charge who have specific expertise in the management of cochlear implant systems. It is arguable whether this is necessary or advisable; rehabilitation appropriate for children with cochlear implants may well be appropriate for many hearing-aided children. Implanted children do not present new problems; they are children who have useful audition following implantation, as do many hearing-aided children (Tyler, 1993) and, as described in Chapter 8, many activities currently being used by teachers of the deaf with hearing-aided children will be suitable.

Somers in Cooper (1991) recommended that implant centres in the US should bring teachers of the deaf into programmes more actively than was currently being done and Osberger et al. (1991) describe the frustration experienced by many teachers of the deaf faced with unrealized expectations of devices and technical problems; these frustrations have not changed over the years and may well have increased. These issues must be addressed by the implant clinic during the preparation period so that the local teacher of the deaf who is likely to be dealing with the daily management of the system feels confident in handling problems and does not feel that the child has been 'dumped on them' (Beiter, Staller and Dowell, 1991). They may well feel that they are responsible for the daily management of the child, but were not involved in the decision to proceed with cochlear implantation (Archbold, 2000).

Teachers of the deaf are commonly responsible for the daily checking of hearing-aid systems. Although simple checks can be carried out (Chapter 7), they cannot 'listen' to the quality of the signal from the child's processor. In addition to giving input to the rehabilitation programme, the implant centre must provide information about the system's management and maintenance and expectations of its use. Moog and Geers (1991) give an excellent description of the in-service training that must be provided by the implant centre and, more recently, cochlear implant companies have taken on a major role in providing this training. The Network of Educators of Children with Cochlear Implants (NECCI) disseminates practical information for teachers of implanted children in the US and provides a forum for discussion. In the UK the British Association of Teachers of the Deaf and the National Deaf Children's Society encourage the sharing of expertise amongst teachers of the deaf. Nottingham Paediatric Cochlear Implant Programme and Birmingham University have developed distance learning courses at Master's degree level for those wishing to specialize in the management of children with cochlear implants.

These sources are useful but it is still necessary for there to be direct contact between implant centre and local professionals about the management of each specific situation: each child presents differently and each educational setting and communication style will vary. As the need to provide long-term care for implanted children has become apparent, a variety of models of service delivery have been developed in order to address these issues (Chute, Nevins and Parisier in Allum, 1996; Cowan in Clark, Cowan and Dowell, 1997). Cowan in Clark, Cowan and Dowell (1997) identifies three different ways of working:

- rehabilitation provided solely within the clinic;
- specialized educational settings incorporating or liaising directly with a cochlear implant clinic;
- professionals from the cochlear implant clinic liaising with local educators directly.

Robbins in Niparko et al. (2000) describes how information between centre and local educator can be transmitted in creative ways. An innovative model of service delivery is given by Muller, Allum and Allum in Allum (1996) in which the emphasis is to provide a complete cochlear implant support system. To achieve this, a unique collaboration between an implant centre and school has been established, with shared facilities and personnel. Bertram in Allum (1996) and Sillon et al. (1996) describe two examples of effective clinic-based rehabilitation services and Archbold in McCormick et al. (1994) and Nevins et al. (1991) describe the educational liaison model, in which educational consultants from the implant centre visit the child's own teachers. In the UK this concept of the educational outreach model is well established.

An educational outreach programme

One way in which direct contact can be developed and ongoing in-service training carried out, appropriate to the child's educational setting, is through an educational outreach programme carried out by the implant clinic teachers of the deaf and speech and language therapists. In the author's programme, this outreach programme was established at the outset, although many children live several hundred miles away. Initially, visits were made by clinic staff to home and school twice prior to surgery and then approximately monthly in the first year after implantation, bi-monthly in the second and third years, and annually thereafter. Over time, as liaison and experience of local staff have developed, these visits have become more flexible and are not as frequent. Having established working relationships, it is possible for visits to vary as needed. For example, they can be increased at appropriate times, when there is a transfer to a new school or teacher, or when there is a problem with a device and more support is required from the implant centre.

The aims of this educational outreach programme are:

- to provide direct contact between implant clinic and home and school, before and after implant;
- to gain insight into the child's home and educational setting;
- to ensure the support programme is appropriate for the child's educational setting; for example, whatever the mode of communication;
- to ensure that the implant system is managed appropriately at home and school, so that it functions optimally at all times;
- to provide direct support and feedback for parents and local professionals;

- to monitor the development of listening skills in 'everyday' settings;
- to ensure that there are shared realistic expectations.

Providing direct contact with home and school can be time consuming and costly in terms of travel for the implant clinic team. However, by focusing support in the child's home and school, it ensures that it is appropriate throughout the child's waking hours, rather than only during clinic visits. In the author's programme, less than 1% of the child's waking hours in the first year after implantation are spent in the clinic; 99% are spent at home and school. This is likely to be a similar figure in other centres; it is essential that the implant clinic team can directly influence the use of the system during the 99% of waking hours spent away from the clinic. Working in this way can prove an effective use of the implant clinic team's time, as well as being a means of limiting the disruption to the child's family and school life, experienced when a long stay or frequent visits to the clinic are required. With more programmes in the UK working in this way, the need for the co-ordination of these educational outreach programmes provided by clinics to schools is becoming very evident. Staff from more than one implant centre may be working in a particular educational setting, and in order to maintain the co-operation of hard-pressed educators, it is essential to ensure that visits, requests and advice are co-ordinated. Guidelines for teachers of the deaf working with children with cochlear implants were developed in the UK with the support of the British Cochlear Implant Group, the Department for Education and Employment, the British Association of Teachers of the Deaf and the National Deaf Children's Society in order to promote consistency of practice.

The implant clinic staff on outreach visits will be required to deal sensitively with a diversity of educational settings and communication philosophies. In the UK, communication styles will range from those that are strongly oral/aural through those in which there is use of oral/aural, written and manual components (Total Communication) to those in which British Sign Language, with its own syntax, is considered to be the first language of the deaf child. These differing communication settings may be found in a variety of educational management settings, summarized in Table 3.1, adding to the difficulties of an implant clinic team liaising with the local professionals.

In the first three placements in Table 3.1, the residential and day schools for the deaf and a unit, or resource base, without integration, there is likely to be one teacher of the deaf responsible for the child who will maintain the primary role in liaison with the implant centre. In the other settings, where some element of mainstreaming is taking place, the implant clinic teacher of the deaf will be required to liaise with several teachers and carers who will be responsible for the child during the course of his day. In recent years the inclusion of children with disabilities has become common – that is, the placement of these children within their local school rather than in a special school, with specialist expertise. Many of their teachers and carers may have little expertise in the management of deafness, hearing aids or cochlear implants and may have unrealistic expectations of a child with a cochlear implant, making direct support from the implant centre even more valuable.

Table 3.1. Range of educational management systems

Educational placement	Professional support
Residential school for the deaf	
Day school for the deaf	One teacher of the deaf
Unit for the hearing impaired	
Without integration	
With integration	
Mainstream with teacher of the deaf support/ withdrawal	
Mainstream with other support/withdrawal	Range of staff working with child
Mainstream without withdrawal	
Pre-school/nursery	

A paediatric cochlear implant programme: schedules

An example of the overall stages of a paediatric implant programme is given in Figure 3.5, showing progress from the initial referral through assessment, implantation, programming of the device and rehabilitation to life-long maintenance. The rest of this chapter will discuss the management of the programme with implications for future planning.

Timescale   **Process**

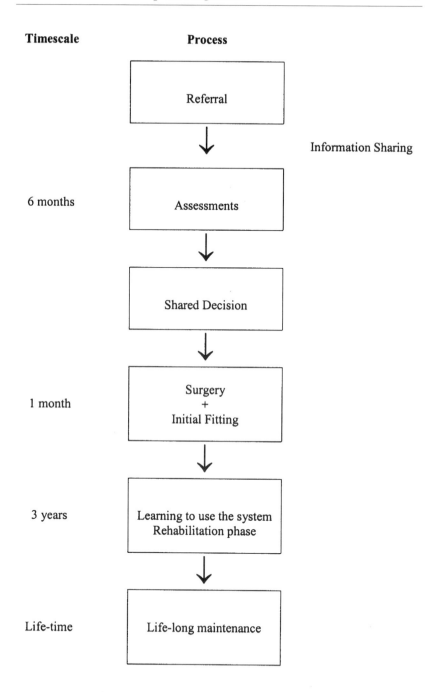

Figure 3.5. Schedule of a paediatric cochlear implant programme.

Assessment and preparation for implantation

The traditional guidelines for children given by Staller, Beiter and Brimacombe in Cooper (1991) were:

- bilateral profound deafness;
- age two to 17 years;
- no radiological contraindications;
- no medical contraindications.

Additionally, candidates at that time should:

- demonstrate little or no benefit from conventional amplification;
- receive educational support that includes a strong auditory/ oral component;
- be psychologically and motivationally suitable;
- have appropriate family and educational expectations and support.

There have been marked changes in candidature as experience has grown, particularly as discussed in Chapters 3 and 4 in the relaxation of audiological criteria. The changes in candidature include the implantation of:

- children with greater residual hearing;
- children with other disabilities;
- younger children, including infants;
- older children, particularly those with more residual hearing;
- more children of deaf parents.

Implantation of children with greater residual hearing, infants and those with significant other disabilities has added to the responsibilities of the implant team during the period of assessment, and the care which must be taken in making decisions about these children.

Figure 3.6 breaks down the assessment period, illustrating the process leading to a decision shared by all about the appropriateness of implantation for the child. At all stages, information should be shared with family and local professionals, and documented, so that the decision making process is clearly articulated to all.

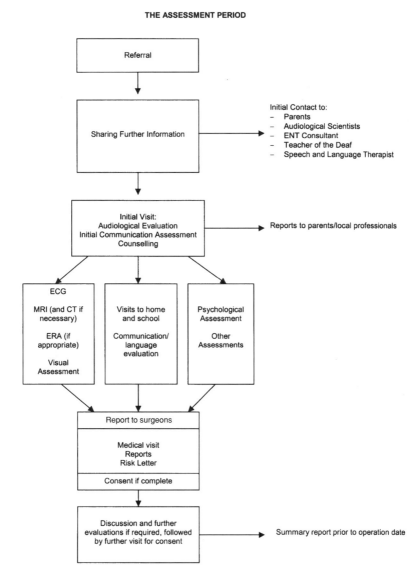

Figure 3.6. The assessment schedule of the Nottingham Paediatric Cochlear Implant Programme.

Prior to beginning formal assessment, the co-ordinator at the implant clinic sends information to the child, his parents and local professionals, outlining the process of implantation, briefly describing a cochlear implant, the likely needs for rehabilitation and reasonable expectations from the device (Archbold, 1992; Tye-Murray in Tyler, 1993). In addition, it will be important for the co-ordinator to obtain as much information as possible about the child, so that inappropriate cases are not brought forward for assessment and parental expectations are not raised unnecessarily. Parents may well wish to discuss issues with the implant co-ordinator prior to the first visit: Tye-Murray in Tyler (1993) summarizes the most commonly asked questions, which include the practical issues of time and financial commitments required, as well as the reliability of the device and the benefits that might be expected. Parents considering implantation for their child will be particularly anxious to find out about long-term effects of the implant system, long-term support and future educational management. Parents at this stage often wish to be put in contact with parents of implanted children to discuss issues with them. Independent information will be particularly valued, and the role of organizations such as the National Deaf Children's Society in the UK in producing such information in a variety of languages is invaluable. As more deaf parents are pursuing the option of cochlear implantation for their children, information needs to be available in video format with signs and subtitles.

The audiological evaluation is usually carried out during the initial visit to the clinic and is fully described in Chapter 4. This evaluation is the assessment at which cochlear implantation is most likely to be found to be inappropriate, and it gives parents time to discuss implantation with team members prior to any medical intervention. It also provides a situation in which rehabilitation staff can observe the child's interaction with parents, style of learning and communication, begin baseline assessments and identify areas of development which may need later scrutiny.

Following the discussion after the evaluation, arrangements are made for the next assessments as identified in Figure 3.6. Magnetic resonance imaging (MRI) is routinely used at the author's programme, with computed tomography (CT) carried out in addition if indicated. If there is good reason, however, for MRI or CT scanning to take place early (for example following meningitis to consider the onset of ossification), then this procedure may be brought forward.

As Schopmeyer in Niparko et al. (2000) describes, it is important to assess the vision of deaf children considered for implantation: significant numbers of deaf children are likely to have vision problems and it is important that this is assessed. Other assessments, such as psychological assessments, occupational therapy and further medical investigations will be carried out on an individual basis.

At the Nottingham programme, the assessments are deliberately spaced out at intervals so that parents have to return to the implant centre on several occasions; this gives parents time to reconsider their options, to formulate questions and receive answers, and to understand a little of the long-term commitment which will be expected of them. Parents have practical issues to consider in addition to those of an ethical nature: the time, travel and financial commitments required following implantation need careful thought. Problems that are likely to occur later, for example in the keeping of appointments, may be brought to light during this period, as parents experience some of the difficulties that may occur in travelling to the implant centre, in organizing leave from work, and arranging for the needs of other members of the family to be met.

It is important during this phase that the local professionals are involved so that, should implantation not be appropriate, an informed support system is available to consider the future options for the child and to support the family to make appropriate decisions. Local professionals are welcomed at assessment appointments to ensure a shared understanding of the issues discussed. It is also important that the family meets members of the deaf community and parents who have decided against implantation, so that all options are considered rationally. If implantation is not appropriate, this should not be considered 'failure', but rather there may be other more appropriate options for the child.

Tye-Murray in Tyler (1993) lists the topics covered during counselling sessions at this stage: audiological and medical candidacy criteria, cochlear implant hardware, cost and insurance reimbursement, realistic expectations, commitment, social considerations, communication mode and educational placement. A systematic means of considering these issues and guiding decisions about candidacy has been developed by the Children's Hearing Institute, Manhattan Eye, Ear and Throat Hospital in the form of the Children's Implant Profile (ChIP) (Hellman et al., 1991) and discussed further in Chapter 10. It itemizes 11 factors to be considered in assessing suitability for implantation:

- chronological age;
- duration of deafness;

- medical/radiological indications;
- multiple handicapping conditions;
- functional hearing;
- speech and language abilities;
- family support and structure;
- family expectations;
- educational environment;
- availability of support services;
- cognitive learning style.

This has been adapted by the Nottingham team and now includes 'cognitive ability' and 'learning style', giving 12 factors (see Chapter 10). Each factor is given a rating from a scale of 'no concern', 'mild-to-moderate concern' and 'great concern'. The ChIP is seen as a tool in the process of decision making, not as a 'pass or fail' test of suitability. As Schopmeyer in Niparko et al. (2000) comments, the audiological and medical assessments are those that are likely to be the deciding factors; other issues may influence discussions, but not prevent implantation proceeding. It is useful, however, to document all these issues, anticipate potential difficulties, and remedy those that it is possible to remedy. Some difficulties may not have a possible solution but there may be alternatives available that will ameliorate the worst effects.

Included during this period are visits by teachers and therapists from the implant centre to the child's home and local professionals; it is vital that these visits are carried out in order to assess the child functioning in non-clinical settings and to establish the context of ongoing support following implantation. Implantation requires a long-term commitment by both the clinic team and the local team, so the assessment phase must be given priority and all concerned should feel that they can contribute to the final decision and feel comfortable with it. The three main aims during this period are:

- to assess the child's appropriateness for implantation;
- to enable parents to make an informed decision regarding implantation;
- to establish the basis for future co-operative relationships should implantation proceed (Archbold, 1992).

Before the final consent to proceed is given by parents, it is important to ensure that the team and the surgeon who has medico-legal responsibility ensure that parents are fully informed. Experience is showing that this is becoming more important rather than less. As children with more residual hearing and those with more complex needs are receiving implants, and as there are greater choices available as to which device to implant, parents are faced with more difficult choices than previously. Dawes and Kitcher (1999) report that patients (and parents) often do not understand the terms used by the medical profession. Implant teams have a responsibility to ensure that information is clear and relevant and that time is made for full discussion with those who know the issues.

When the decision to implant has been taken by parents and implant team, further and more vigorous assessments of the child's functioning are made; baselines of language and communication skills are established using standardized tests where appropriate, video analysis and observation, questionnaire and interview material. This period builds on the previous relationships already developed with child, family and local professionals, and enables full preparation of the whole team to take place prior to implantation.

Surgery and initial fitting

Particularly for those parents of children with hearing loss acquired through meningitis, the hospital stay may be traumatic. Parents may experience reawakened memories of the feelings of bereavement and loss experienced at the time of the acquisition of deafness. In spite of an emphasis on the development of realistic expectations, parents may still hope for a full return of hearing. As one parent commented to the author, 'My head listened to you, but my heart didn't.' The responsibility for the decision to implant may weigh heavily at this time; parents bring a healthy child to hospital and choose for him or her to undergo surgery entailing some discomfort and risk. It might be difficult for them to share their feelings with professionals; Chapter 11 provides some insights into their thoughts at this time. The nursing staff have a crucial role, and they need to understand the nature of the whole process, and the comparatively brief, but vital, role of the surgery in the programme. This can be a useful period for developing a further understanding of family dynamics, which may later influence the support the family require. This support is particularly important if post-operative complications develop.

After discharge, the children in the Nottingham programme are visited at home by the implant clinic teacher of the deaf, and prepared, with their families, for the next stage – the initial tuning of the device. They are able to familiarize themselves with the equipment and its controls, decide how they will wear the processor, see photographs of other children, share books about it and prepare for listening experiences in a realistic way. Older children may be prepared more specifically for the activities that tuning in the device will require of them; highly structured preparation for the tasks ahead, however, is not necessary and the child may well not understand the concepts involved in tuning the device without the experience of sound stimulation.

The initial tuning session is often called 'switch on'. This is rather a misnomer, but is taken to mean the time at which the external parts of the device are fitted – microphone, transmitter and processor – and is described fully in Chapter 7. This takes place some four weeks after surgery, and with young children the initial tuning period is generally two days. As Osberger in Mecklenburg (1986) clarifies, there are three main aims at this time:

- to set the device
- to assess the responses of the child
- to enable parents and professionals to plan the programme for the development of listening skills.

The rehabilitation staff and audiological scientists liaise closely; it is mutually useful to share the child's responses in clinic and in the outside world. The final day of the initial tuning visit may involve the child's local teacher of the deaf, speech therapist and audiologist so that they can learn how to manage the system and promote its use at home and share the early responses and realistic expectations.

Rehabilitation and evaluation

With the benefits of implantation only being seen in the long term, the importance of the entire team and the preparation phase is now 'tested' as the team begins to function. The rehabilitation phase involves implant clinic scientists, teachers and speech and language therapists working with the family and local professionals to ensure optimum use of the device. Whether rehabilitation is the most appropriate term to use to cover this period is discussed in Chapter 8, together with appropriate activities. It may be more appropriate to call it a support programme. During this time, the implant clinic team must ensure that:

- parents and teachers are able to maintain the device appropriately;
- spares are available at all times and that everyone knows how to trouble-shoot the device;
- the child is in optimum conditions to use the new sense of audition, bearing in mind the educational setting and style of communication.

Although we have emphasized the importance of the implant clinic team's visits to home and school, the child and family will need to visit the implant centre at regular intervals. During these visits (usually eight days in the first year in the Nottingham programme) the child will see the surgeon, audiological scientist, speech and language therapist and teacher of the deaf at the clinic, and will have, at regular intervals:

- a medical check;
- further tuning of the device;
- monitoring of the system;
- evaluation of listening skills;
- evaluation of spoken language skills;
- discussions of progress so far and guidelines for further progress.

Experience has shown that, for many children, it is two or three years after implantation before predictions can be made with any certainty about outcomes. It is therefore important to keep up regular contact during this phase, when difficulties in developing the use of the system, or the presence of other learning difficulties may come to light. This phase with close contact should last for at least three years; others have recommended five years. Educators express the need for continued liaison as children change teachers or schools (Moog and Geers, 1991); as described earlier, this contact is provided at the author's programme by a combination of clinic visits, the educational outreach programme and by the provision of training materials and courses to share expertise.

Maintenance period: for life

Implantation may result in the altering of communication style, educational management, career options and how the child later perceives himself (Tyler, 1993) so the statement that implantation involves a commitment for life (Goin and Parisier, 1991) is not far from the truth. The maintenance phase must last for the life of the child with, at the very least, regular maintenance of the system, the availability of spares, repairs and a trouble-shooting service. With growing recognition of some of the technical problems encountered with internal and external equipment, the organization of this maintenance period is vital. Children reliant on their cochlear implant systems for access to the educational curriculum demand urgent technical support when necessary and this may be complex to arrange. Problems with devices may not be straightforward. The problem may lie with external equipment, the internal device, with the child's changing circumstances at home or school, or be a medical problem. The appropriate infrastructure must be in place to provide this inter-disciplinary service and the local support team must know how to access it. The development of 'hub and spoke' models of working where some of the expertise is transferred to the local service is likely to be helpful to facilitate this.

Following the three-year post-operative rehabilitation programme, the Nottingham team provides at least an annual clinic visit, together with a maintenance contract for all hardware problems, a contact service for local professionals, and medical cover. It has proved essential to staff clinics to provide for emergency sessions, where children can access scientific expertise if experiencing device problems. We have found it useful to provide the child with an identity bracelet from a medical security firm, which makes details of the child's implant and any medical conditions the child may have available anywhere in the world in the case of an emergency.

Programmes of a paediatric nature, such as the Nottingham one, need to consider the children's support as they become teenagers and then adults. Some programmes have established adolescent programmes to meet the needs of this group – as described in Chapter 8, this group has specific needs for support. The liaison established with educational services should continue as these children go to higher education with the changing demands there, and an interim programme of support is invaluable as the children become responsible for their own equipment and develop their own identities as deaf adults with cochlear implants. In the Nottingham programme, as this group is growing, the associated adult programme works with the paediatric programme during this transition period as the teenagers become independent adults. The maintenance needs of this group continue throughout adulthood.

Paediatric cochlear implant programme: long-term funding

Having established the life-long support needed by implanted children, and the increasing awareness of the complexities of maintaining implanted devices, it is essential that paediatric implant programmes look to their long-term funding and staffing to provide the necessary infrastructure. It is equally important that, in order to cost their programme accurately, all elements of the service are included and that purchasers of the programme, whether health authorities, insurance companies or individuals, know what they are buying and the length of the financial commitment. Many healthcare purchasers may be just realizing the long-term financial implications of cochlear implantation as those already implanted require continued maintenance, in addition to those requesting new funding for implantation.

Figure 3.7 shows one example of information material available for purchasers: this was sent, with brochure, to all healthcare purchasers in the UK by the Nottingham programme. It itemizes costs for 2001/2002 and the service provided. These costs provide the level of support described in this chapter, including rehabilitation and full maintenance of the device, and includes replacement processors. In order to produce accurate information of this kind, the financial and time implications of the programme need to be considered in some detail. A database has been developed at the author's programme, initially in collaboration with the Medical Research Council's Institute of Hearing Research, which enables staffing, time and equipment cost inputs to be monitored, as well as maintaining biographical data and outcome measures on children.

In addition to staff time, allowances must be made for equipment, spares and the cost of reimplantation if necessary. The development of new technology by implant companies raises

QUEEN'S MEDICAL CENTRE

Nottingham University Hospital NHS Trust

NOTTINGHAM PAEDIATRIC COCHLEAR IMPLANT PROGRAMME
Ropewalk House, 113 The Ropewalk, Nottingham NG1 6HA

FINANCIAL YEAR 2001/02 - PROGRAMME & COSTS

REFERRAL: PRE ASSESSMENT INFORMATION COLLECTION

Background information from parents plus audiological and educational history from
local professionals is essential information for the patient's file prior to 1st appointment

* Waiting time may be extended if response to request for information is slow

ASSESSMENT

Audiological/medical evaluation and counselling
MRI scan
Evoked Response Audiometry - ERA
Educational/speech and language assessments involving visits to home and school
Preparation of the child, family and local professionals by the implant team
Decision to Implant

Time taken to assess depends upon the individual needs of each child

YEAR 1: IMPLANT AND REHABILITATION

Surgical implantation
Switch on, setting up and tuning of the device
Medical checks
Rehabilitation and monitoring of the child's progress and functioning of the device
Monthly visits to home and school by members of the implant rehabilitation team

Normally involves eight full-day visits to Nottingham during the year

YEARS 2 & 3: ONGOING REHABILITATION

Tuning and monitoring of the device
Medical checks
Rehabilitation and monitoring of the child's progress and functioning of the device
Visits to home and school by members of the implant rehabilitation team every two months

Normally involves three full-day visits to Nottingham each year

FROM YEAR 4: ANNUAL REVIEW AND MAINTENANCE

Audiological and medical checks
Annual visit to home and school by members of the implant rehabilitation team
Emergency Service: Spares/supplies/reasonable maintenance costs
A replacement speech processor every 6 years as recommended by the manufacturer

Normally involves one full-day visit to Nottingham each year

		INVOICE TIMETABLE	COST £
YEAR 1	Assessment, Implant and Rehabilitation	Month of Implant	32,368.00
YEAR 2	Ongoing Rehabilitation/maintenance	1st anniversary	5023.00
YEAR 3	Ongoing Rehabilitation/maintenance	2nd anniversary	5023.00
Year 4 on	Annual review and maintenance ongoing	Each Anniversary	2678.00

Figure 3.7. An example of a description of paediatric cochlear implant programme contents and costs, for healthcare purchasers.

parental and child expectation; each new innovation demands implementation with hardware costs, software costs and staff time to be funded. Children make heavy use of technology and more sophisticated technology may not necessarily be more robust. As the programme has grown over time, the proportion of time and money spent maintaining those implanted, compared with the newly implanted, has changed drastically. Figure 3.8 shows, for the Nottingham programme, the changing proportions of children over 10 years. Similarly, Figure 3.9 shows the changing proportions of staff costs, costs of new devices and costs of maintaining devices (spares and replacements) over 10 years of the programme. It can be seen that, as cochlear implant programmes grow, plans must be made for the funding of long-term maintenance of devices.

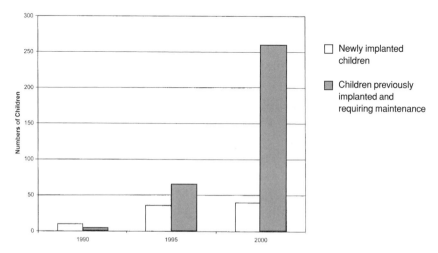

Figure 3.8. Changing proportions of the newly implanted to those maintained over 10 years.

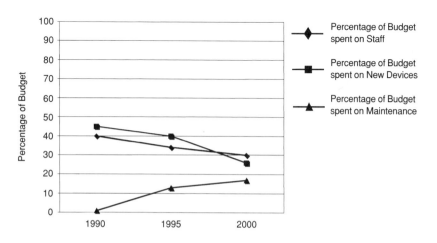

Figure 3.9. The changing proportions of costs as a percentage of budget over 10 years.

Many studies are looking at the economic evaluation of cochlear implantation. It is no longer enough to present safety and efficacy outcomes; economic evaluations are now demanded (Niparko et al., 2000). Initial studies seem to indicate that paediatric cochlear implantation represents reasonable value for money (O'Neill et al., 2000); Cowan in Clark, Cowan and Dowell (1997) commented that this was influenced by the amount of rehabilitation support given and whether the children attended mainstream schooling. There has been a great deal of interest shown in the educational support required by children following cochlear implantation with regard to studies of cost-effectiveness (O'Neill et al., 2000). However, the situation is complex; the Educational Resource Matrix developed by Koch et al. (1997) to map the changing resources used by the child with an implant over time is immensely useful. It plots both educational placement and the use of support services on the matrix, allowing complex situations to be fully illustrated. Although children with implants may move towards a mainstream setting, they may, in fact, initially, use more support services in order to move successfully. A large-scale study currently in progress in the UK, Support Options for Hearing Impaired Children, being carried out by the Medical Research Council's Institute of Hearing Research, may provide some answers to these questions in the long term.

The use of accessible outcome measures for healthcare purchasers

Whilst recognizing the need for rigorous outcome measures in children, conventional measures of speech perception and production do not enable a health service purchaser or financial advisor to comprehend what an implant may offer a deaf child. Implant programmes must provide evidence of the efficacy of implantation in an accessible form to purchasers in order to obtain long-term funding.

Measures such as Categories of Auditory Performance (Archbold, Lutman and Nikolopoulos, 1998) and Speech Intelligibility Rating (Allen, Nikolopoulos and O'Donoghue, 1998) were developed to provide such accessible information to purchasers. These measures, illustrated in Chapter 1, have proved useful, not only in the UK, but elsewhere, to demonstrate outcomes from different populations over extended time-scales.

Categories of Auditory Performance (CAP) is a scale used to rate outcomes in everyday life, and is easily understood by non-specialists. It contains eight categories with criteria for completion, and has been found to have high inter-user reliability (Archbold, Lutman and Nikolopoulos, 1998). The categories are:

- no awareness of environmental sounds;
- awareness of environmental sounds;
- response to speech sounds (for example, 'go');
- identification of environmental sounds;
- discrimination of some speech sounds without lipreading;
- understanding of common phrases without lipreading;
- understanding of conversation without lipreading;
- use of telephone with known speaker.

The speech intelligibility rating (SIR) is a similar rating scale, looking at speech intelligibility rather than perception; it too has been found to be reliable (Allen et al., 2001) and is discussed further in Chapter 10.

Purchasers are also interested in such measures of outcome as long-term usage rates: high levels of elective use over long timeframes indicate satisfaction with the intervention as discussed in Chapter 1. Implant programmes have a responsibility to provide details of:

- costings;
- candidature;
- safety outcomes;
- long-term usage rates;
- long-term accessible outcomes.

These are not only useful to purchasers, but also to parents to provide informed decision making.

Comment

Taking the child as the focus of the programme, Figure 3.10 illustrates the triangle of support that remains necessary to ensure the long-term effectiveness of the device, with the local team of professionals, implant clinic team and family working together with the child. Paediatric implantation involves a long-term commitment of finance, expertise and time. Its extent is only

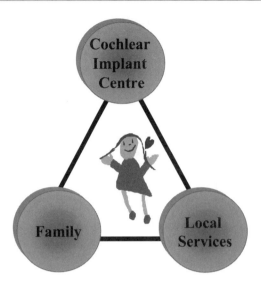

Figure 3.10. The triangle of support necessary for the child.

recognized with experience, and a paediatric programme must be based on sound management to ensure its future viability for all implanted children.

In the UK, in order to ensure that best practice prevails, Quality Standards have been published by the National Deaf Children's Society (NDCS, 1999) and the British Cochlear Implant Group and include the following recommendations:

• multi-disciplinary teams with relevant paediatric experience;
• specialist centres, implanting at least 10 children per annum;
• established educational networks;
• long-term commitment and funding;
• dedicated staff for the paediatric teams.

Cochlear implantation has been criticized for being a magnet for support services for deaf children and of creating rather than saving costs. However, it may be that the provision of specialist teams for paediatric implantation has had some beneficial effects on provision for all deaf children. It may be that, in raising awareness of the needs of these children and in opening up services for all deaf children to external scrutiny, cochlear implantation in young children has broken down some of the professional barriers that have existed for years. Some of the questions asked may have led to improved services for all deaf children rather than only those with cochlear implants. Many of the issues discussed in this book, such as the establishment of support structures, are relevant to all deaf children and raise concerns common to all.

What of future challenges? Each new development in technology or change in candidature places new demands on implant teams. Growing pressure for bilateral implants, for wholly implantable devices, and for the implementation of increasingly sophisticated technology requires expertise, staffing, time and money. Each new innovation raises expectations. The successful future of cochlear implantation for children requires stable, well-staffed, clinic-based implant teams, working with local teams and the implant companies to ensure a secure future for those already implanted, as well as those who will continue to be candidates.

References

Allen C, Nikolopoulos TP, Dyar D, O'Donoghue GM (2001) The reliability of a rating scale for measuring speech intelligibility following pediatric cochlear implantation. Otology and Neurology 22: 631–3.

Allen C, Nikolopoulos T, O'Donoghue GM (1998) Speech intelligibility in children after cochlear implantation. The American Journal of Otology 19: 742–6.

Aplin DY (1993) Psychological assessment of multi-channel cochlear implant patients. Journal of Laryngology and Otology 107: 298–304.

Archbold S (1992) The development of a paediatric cochlear implant programme: a case study. British Journal Association of Teachers of the Deaf 16(1): 17–26.

Archbold S (1994) Implementing a paediatric cochlear implant programme. In McCormick B, Archbold S, Sheppard S (eds) Cochlear Implants for Young Children. London: Whurr, pp. 25–59.

Archbold S (1997) Development of a paediatric cochlear implant programme. Paper presented at 17th Danavox Symposium, Kolding, Denmark, 9–12 September.

Archbold SM (2000) Cochlear implantation in children – influencing educational choices. Paper presented at 19th International Congress on Education of the Deaf, Sydney, 9–13 July.

Archbold SM, Lutman ME, Gregory S, O'Neill C (2002) Parents and their deaf child: their perceptions three years after cochlear implantation. Deafness and Education International.

Archbold S, Lutman M, Nikolopoulos T (1998) Categories of auditory performance: inter-user reliability. British Journal of Audiology 32: 7–11.

Archbold S, Robinson K (1997) A European perspective on paediatric cochlear implantation, rehabilitation services and their educational implications. American Journal of Otology 18(6): s75–s78.

Audit Commission (1997) NHS Higher Purchase (Commissioning Specialised Services in the NHS) Department of Health.

Bamford J, Saunders E (1985) Hearing Impairment, Auditory Perception and Language Disability. London: Arnold.

Beard M (1999) Signs of the times. New Scientist (24 April) p. 52.

Beiter AL, Staller SJ, Dowell RC (1991) Evaluation and device programming in children. Ear and Hearing 12(4): 25S–33S.

Bertram B (1996) An integrated rehabilitation concept for cochlear implant children. In Allum DJ (ed.) Cochlear Implant Rehabilitation in Children and Adults. London: Whurr Publishers Ltd.

Boothroyd A (1989) Hearing aids, cochlear implants and profoundly deaf children. In Owens E, Kessler DK (eds) Cochlear Implants in Young Deaf Children. Boston, MA: Little, Brown & Co, pp. 81–100.

Cayton H (1991) Problems and issues in developing a cochlear implant programme for children. Journal of Medical Engineering and Technology 15(2): 49–52.

Chute PM, Nevins ME, Parisier SC (1996) Managing educational issues throughout the process of implantation. In Allum DJ (ed.) Cochlear Implant Rehabilitation in Children and Adults. London: Whurr, pp. 119–30.

Clark GM (1997) Historical perspectives. In Clark G, Cowan RSC, Dowell RC (eds) Cochlear Implantation for Infants and Children. San Diego, CA: Singular.

Conrad R (1979) The Deaf School Child. London: Harper & Row.

Cowan RSC (1997) Socio-economic and educational management issues. In Clark G, Cowan RSC, Dowell RC (eds) Cochlear Implantation for Infants and Children. San Diego, CA: Singular.

Dawes PJD, Kitcher E (1999) Informed consent: British otolaryngologists surveyed. Clinical Otolaryngology 24: 198–207.

Dowell RC (1997) Preoperative audiological, speech and language evaluation. In Clark G, Cowan RSC, Dowell RC (eds) Cochlear Implantation for Infants and Children. San Diego, CA: Singular, pp. 83–110.

Downs MP (1986) Psychological issues surrounding children receiving cochlear implants. In Mecklenburg DJ (ed.) Cochlear Implants in Children; Seminars in Hearing. New York: Thieme Medical Publishers.

Evans JW (1989) Thoughts on the psychological implications of cochlear implantation in children. In Owens E, Kessler DK (eds) (1989) Cochlear Implants in Young Deaf Children. Boston, MA: Little, Brown & Co, pp. 307–14.

Fraser G (1991) The cochlear implant team. In Cooper H (ed.) Cochlear Implants; A Practical Guide. London: Whurr Publishers Ltd, pp. 84–91.

Geers AE, Moog JS (1991) Evaluating the benefits of cochlear implants in an educational setting. American Journal of Otology 12: 116–25.

Gibbin KP (1992) Paediatric cochlear implantation. Archives of Disease in Childhood 65(6): 669–71.

Goin DW, Parisier SC (1991) Implementing a cochlear implant team in private practice or academic setting. American Journal of Otology 12: 213–17.

Gregory S, Knight P (1998) Social development and family life. In Gregory S, Knight P, McCracken W, Powers S, Watson L (eds) Issues in Deaf Education. London: Fulton, pp. 3–11.

Haggard M (1993) Research in the Development of Effective Services for Hearing Impaired People. Fifth HM Queen Elizabeth the Queen Mother Fellowship, The Nuffield Provincial Hospital Trust, London.

Hellman SA, Chute PM, Kretschmer RE, Nevins ME, Parisier SC, Thurston LC (1991) The development of a children's implant profile. American Annals of the Deaf 136(2): 77–81.

Kileny PR, Kemink JL, Zimmerman-Phillips S (1991) Cochlear implants in children. American Journal of Otology 12(2): 144–6.

Kirk KI, Hill-Brown C (1985) Speech and language results in children with a cochlear implant. Ear and Hearing 6(3): 36S–47S.

Knight P (1998) Deafness and disability. In Gregory S, Knight P, McCracken W, Powers S, Watson L (eds) Issues in Deaf Education. London: Fulton, pp. 215-24.

Koch ME, Wyatt JR, Francis HW, Niparko JK (1997) A model of educational resource use by children with cochlear implants. Otolaryngology Head and Neck Surgery 117: 1-6.

Lane H (1994) The cochlear implant controversy. World Federation of the Deaf News. No. 2-3.

Laurenzi C (1993) The bionic ear and the mythology of paediatric implants. British Journal of Audiology 27: 1-5.

Lea AR (1991) Cochlear Implants: Australian Institute of Health. Health Care Technology Services 6. Canberra: AGPS.

Luterman D (1987) Deafness in the Family. Boston, MA: Little, Brown & Co.

McCormick B (1991) Paediatric cochlear implantation in the UK - a delayed journey on a well marked route. British Journal of Audiology 25: 145-9.

Mecklenburg D, Lehnhardt E (1991) The development of cochlear implants in Europe, Asia and Australia. In Cooper H (ed) Cochlear Implants: A Practical Guide. London: Whurr pp. 34-57.

Mellon NK (2000) Language acquisition. In Niparko JK, Iler Kirk K, Mellon NK, Robbins AM, Tucci DL, Wilson B (eds) Cochlear Implants: Principles and Practice. Philadelphia, PA: Lippincott Williams & Wilkins, pp. 291-314.

Moog JS, Geers AE (1991) Educational management of children with cochlear implants. American Annals of the Deaf 136(2): 69-70.

Muller R, Allum DJ, Allum JHJ (1996) A service network for rehabilitation of cochlear implant users. In Allum DJ (ed.) Cochlear Implant Rehabilitation in Children and Adults. London: Whurr Publishers Ltd.

National Deaf Children's Society and British Cochlear Implant Group (1999) Quality Standards in Cochlear Implants for Children. London: National Deaf Children's Society.

Nevins M, Chute P (1996) Children with Cochlear Implants. San Diego, CA: Singular.

Nevins ME, Kretschmer RE, Chute PM, Hellman SA, Parisier SC (1991) The role of an educational consultant in a paediatric cochlear implant programme. Volta 93: 197-204.

Nikolopoulos TP, O'Donoghue GM, Archbold S (1999) Age at implantation; its importance in paediatric cochlear implantation. Laryngoscope 109: 595-9.

Niparko JK (2000) Culture and cochlear implants. In Niparko JK, Iler Kirk K, Mellon NK, Robbins AM, Tucci DL, Wilson B (eds) Cochlear Implants: Principles and Practice. Philadelphia, PA: Lippincott Williams & Wilkins, pp. 371-8.

Niparko JK, Iler Kirk K, Mellon NK, Robbins AM, Tucci DL, Wilson B (eds) (2000) Cochlear Implants: Principles and Practice. Philadelphia, PA: Lippincott Williams & Wilkins.

Niparko JK, Wilson BS (2000) History of cochlear implants. In Niparko JK, Iler Kirk K, Mellon NK, Robbins AM, Tucci DL, Wilson B (eds) Cochlear Implants: Principles and Practice. Philadelphia, PA: Lippincott Williams & Wilkins, pp. 103-8.

O'Donoghue GM (1992) Cochlear Implants in Children. Journal of the Royal Society of Medicine 85: 655-7.

O'Donoghue GM, Nikolopoulos TP, Archbold SM, Tait M (1999) Cochlear implants in young children: the relationship between speech perception and intelligibility. Ear and Hearing 20(5): 419-25.

O'Neill C, O'Donoghue GM, Archbold SM, Normand C (2000) A cost-utility analysis of pediatric cochlear implantion. The Laryngoscope 110: 156-60.

Osberger MJ (1986) Auditory skill development in children with cochlear implants. In Mecklenburg DJ (ed.) Cochlear Implants in Children: Seminars in Hearing 7, 4. New York: Thieme Medical Publishers.

Osberger MJ, Dettman SJ, Daniel K, Moog JS, Siebert R, Stone P, Jorgenson S (1991) Rehabilitation and education issues with implanted children; perspectives from a panel of clinicians and educators. American Journal of Otology 12: 205-12.

Power DJ, Hyde MB (1992) The cochlear implant and the deaf community. Medical Journal of Australia 157: 421-22.

Quigley SP, Kretschmer RE (1984) Language and Deafness. London: Croom Helm.

Quittner AL, Thompson Steck J, Rouiller RL (1991) Cochlear implants in children: a study of parental stress and adjustment. American Journal of Otology 12.

Robbins AM (2000) Rehabilitation after cochlear implantation. In Niparko JK, Iler Kirk K, Mellon NK, Robbins AM, Tucci DL, Wilson B (eds) Cochlear Implants: Principles and Practice. Philadelphia, PA: Lippincott Williams & Wilkins, pp. 323-62.

Schopmeyer B (2000) Professional roles in multi-disciplinary assessment of candidacy. In JK Niparko, K Iler Kirk, NK Mellon, AM Robbins, DL Tucci, BS Wilson (eds) Cochlear Implants: Principles and Practice. Philadelphia, PA: Lippincott Williams & Wilkins.

Selmi A (1985) Monitoring and evaluating the educational effect of the cochlear implant. Ear & Hearing 6(3): 52S-59S.

Sillon M, Vieu A, Piron JP, Rougier R, Broche M, Artieres-Rouillard F, Mondain M, Uziel A (1996) The management of cochlear implant children. In Allum DJ (ed.) Cochlear Implant Rehabilitation in Children and Adults. London: Whurr, pp. 83-101.

Somers MN (1991) Effects of cochlear implants in children: implications for rehabilitation. In Cooper H (ed.) Cochlear Implants: A Practical Guide. London: Whurr, pp. 322-45.

Staller SJ, Beiter AL, Brimacombe JA (1991) Children and multichannel cochlear implants. In Cooper H (ed.) Cochlear Implants: A Practical Guide. London: Whurr, pp. 283-321.

Summerfield AQ, Marshall D (1995) Cochlear Implantation in the UK: 1990-1994. London: HMSO.

Tobey EA (1999) Paper presented at Under Twos meeting, Nottingham, 29 October.

Tye-Murray N (1993) Aural rehabilitation and patient management. In Tyler RS (ed.) Cochlear Implants: Audiological Foundations. San Diego, CA: Singular Publishing Group Inc, pp. 87-144.

Tyler RS (1993) Speech perception by children. In Tyler RS (ed.) Cochlear Implants: Audiological Foundations. San Diego, CA: Singular Publishing Group Inc, pp. 191-256.

Tyler RS (1999) Cochlear implants and the deaf culture. American Journal of Audiology March, pp. 26-32.

Uziel AS, Reuillard-Artieres F, Sillon M, Vieu A, Mondain M, Prion JP, Tobey EA (1996) Speech-perception performance in prelingually deafened French children using the Nucleus multichannel implant. American Journal of Otology 17: 559-68.

Waltzman SB, Cohen NC, Gomolin RH, Shapiro WH, Ozdamar SR, Hoffman RA (1994) Long-term results of early cochlear implantation in congenitally and prelingually deafened children. American Journal of Otology 15: (Suppl. 2) pp. 9-13.

Warnock M (1982) Children with special needs in ordinary schools: integration revisited. In Cohen A, Cohen L (eds) (1986) Special Educational Needs in the Ordinary School. London: Harper & Row.

Wood DJ, Wood HA, Griffiths AJ, Howarth CI (1986) Teaching and Talking with Deaf Children. London & New York: John Wiley.

Wootton R (1998) Telemedicine in the National Health Service. Journal of the Royal Society of Medicine Vol. 91: 614–21.

Yoshinaga-Itano C, Sedey A, Coulter D, Mehl A. (1998) Language of early- and later-identified children with hearing loss. Paediatrics 102: 1161–71.

Chapter 4

Assessing audiological suitability of cochlear implants for children below the age of five years

BARRY MCCORMICK

Introduction

Over the 10 years from 1990 to 2000 cochlear implant systems advanced to such a degree that many implanted children out-perform children with considerable amounts of residual hearing who use conventional hearing aids. As a consequence of this the audiological criteria for cochlear implant consideration have progressively relaxed and children with significant amounts of residual hearing are now being considered for the technique. This situation could not have been envisaged a decade ago when the technique could only be undertaken with children who had no usable hearing and the primary aim was to give them a rudimentary sensation of hearing. Interest now centres on what hearing aids cannot do that cochlear implants can do, and do very well. This represents a total change of emphasis and the situation arises because of the remarkable progress of many children with cochlear implants.

A notable trend to have emerged in recent years is the implantation of babies and very young children. This trend can be expected to increase very significantly over the next decade with the widespread introduction of neonatal hearing screening. Implantation of very young children requires special candidacy consideration and although this has been given some attention in the literature (for example Osberger, 1997) there is a need for more detailed coverage. This chapter will address this issue.

Progressive improvements in cochlear implant design have resulted in better outcomes for users. These technological advances have, however, also been shadowed in the hearing aid market. Following a decade of little significant advancement in hearing aid design the situation is now changing with the widespread introduction of 'digital' instruments. Digitally programmable hearing aids enable better and more flexible matches to be made to compensate for differing audiometric configurations, and fully digital processing systems provide additional benefits with better loudness mapping capabilities. These advances should improve the performance of those with moderate or severe hearing losses more than those with profound losses but the new technology may also provide benefits to the profoundly deaf. Digital feedback management systems may enable some profoundly deaf children to make better use of acoustic hearing aids and due cognizance must be paid to such advances when considering likely implant candidature.

These advances pose special challenges to the paediatric audiologist because it is now necessary to obtain very early and accurate measurements of hearing function in babies if the full advantages of the new technologies are to be gained in the early formative months of life. The problem of who to refer for cochlear implant assessment and who to accept on audiological grounds has to be tackled at much earlier ages now than a decade ago. Cochlear implant selection guidelines with specific application for very young children, who cannot perform speech testing, are difficult to find in the professional literature and yet such children will be the main cochlear implant candidates in the future.

Selection criteria have been changing so rapidly over the past decade that it has been difficult to publish timely guidelines – by the time the articles appear in print their contents are out of date because of the pace of change. The situation has, however, become more stable recently and it must now remain stable because of the need to evaluate the performance of children with the new digital hearing aid technology and to compare their progress with that of children using cochlear implants. For several years we have had to collect and analyse data for children who have received this new technology and who approach the present audiological borderline criteria for cochlear implantation. Until this has been completed there should be only very cautious relaxation of the cochlear implant selection criteria for children

For the reader's convenience this chapter is divided into two parts. Section one gives a clear description of the criteria now being adopted within the Nottingham programme and includes brief coverage of the audiological test techniques needed to assess cochlear implant suitability. The second section provides the rationale for the present stance backed by the findings from a series of studies that have been undertaken in the Nottingham programme over the past decade. These studies influenced the shifting trends in audiological selection criteria over this period, and they provide a useful historical overview, which is then brought up to date with a review of other recommendations from the field. Readers without a scientific background might gain all they need from the first section and they might wish to be spared the scientific details in section two.

Section 1

The findings from an audiological assessment might determine whether a baby/child continues to use hearing aids or progresses to cochlear implantation during the most important years for establishing spoken language skills. A wrong decision at this stage will influence the individual's progress for the rest of their lives and considerable responsibility does, therefore, rest on the shoulders of the paediatric audiologist.

The following audiological selection criteria have been derived over the past decade during which time the progress of hearing aid users and cochlear implant users within the Nottingham audiology and implant services has been subject to constant scrutiny. The criteria will determine whether a child is to be referred for full evaluation by the rest of the cochlear implant team and the audiological assessment effectively acts as a gateway to the programme.

Pure tone audiometric selection criteria for typical sloping hearing losses

- Full cochlear implant evaluation will be considered if the better ear audiometric thresholds at 2 kHz and 4 kHz are 105 dB HL or more.

Pure tone audiometric selection criteria for flat or slightly rising hearing losses

- Full cochlear implant evaluation will be considered if the averaged thresholds for 500 Hz, 1 kHz and 2 kHz are 90 dB or more and the threshold at 4 kHz is 95 dB or more.

Aided threshold criteria

If there are doubts about the reliability of the pure tone thresholds with very young or very difficult-to-test children it is useful to assess the child's aided thresholds when wearing high powered analogue hearing aids. If the aided thresholds at 2 kHz and 4 kHz are greater than 50 dB(A) then a programme of full cochlear implant evaluation should be considered.

Speech tests

If the child has developed some spoken language and is mature enough to undertake speech discrimination testing then the results of such testing may also be taken into account. With very young babies/infants speech testing might not be possible.

The Nottingham programme has access to a very refined speech discrimination test developed by the Medical Research Council's Institute of Hearing Research and this is, unfortunately, only available in a few sites in the UK. This test enables an additional selection criterion to be used if the child is able to perform speech discrimination testing. A child will be referred for full assessment by other members of the team if:

- unable to obtain the optimum 71% speech discrimination score below a listening level of 65 dB(A) in the Institute of Hearing Research/McCormick Automated Toy Discrimination Test.

For those who do not have access to this test procedure, cochlear implantation should be considered if:

- a score of less than 30% is obtained for open-set speech discrimination tests in the listening only condition.

Special cases

- Asymmetrical hearing losses. For children with asymmetrical hearing losses there could be a slight concession to the normal rules if one ear shows virtually no benefit from hearing aids. In these cases the poorer ear only should be considered for implantation.
- Progressive hearing losses. Children with progressive hearing losses can sometimes perform much better in speech discrimination tasks than might be expected for their current

hearing levels because they benefit from strategies they developed when they had better hearing. Although they can obtain respectable scores in such tests they often cannot perform the tasks comfortably and this needs to be taken into account. Implant users can often obtain the same scores but with ease. Thus a sensible concession to the above criteria might be applied in such cases if there is a definite pattern of progressive deterioration of hearing.

These criteria serve as general guidelines and it must be acknowledged that there will be exceptions to the general rules. There must, however, be good justification, backed by multidisciplinary opinion, if the normal guidelines are not being applied.

A particularly useful feature of the Nottingham approach is that the audiological guidelines are flexible enough to be used with babies in their first year of life. The minimum audiological information required is that of high-frequency unaided thresholds preferably backed by aided thresholds. Such measures can normally be obtained, even in the very young, with application of visual reinforcement audiometry. If there are doubts about the reliability of the findings the measurements can also be obtained using electrophysiological methods described in Chapter 6. In both cases it will be essential to ensure that the child does not have any superimposed temporary conductive hearing loss at the time when the measurements are undertaken. Otitis media with effusion is very common in the very young. It will be wise to have a locally arranged otological check prior to making what might be a long and potentially wasted journey to the implant centre. If evidence of middle-ear effusion is noted then arrangements should be made to treat the condition and to reschedule the audiological assessment for a later date when the treatment has the desired effect.

Audiological assessment

Audiological test techniques are described in detail in a sister publication entitled *Paediatric Audiology 0-5 years* (McCormick 1993 – third edition in press for 2003) and only a very brief description of the techniques will be given here. The approach adopted within the Nottingham programme is that the paediatric audiological assessment should precede and not follow the medical, radiological and electrophysiological testing (with the exception of checks and treatment for conductive hearing loss). Although cochlear implantation can now be considered very early in the child's life it is still important to arrange a trial with appropriate hearing aids and to document the progress or lack of progress with the instruments in consultation with the parents and the rehabilitation team.

An exception to the test sequence might be made in cases of babies/children deafened by meningitis for whom the risk of new fibrous growth (ossification) within the cochlea might prevent the later insertion of an electrode array. In these cases early radiology might be indicated with fast tracking through the programme if structural changes are occurring. If ossification is not present a period of watchful waiting with hearing aid use can be justified. Partial recovery of hearing following total meningitic deafness has been documented by McCormick et al. (1993) and, although such recovery is thought to be very rare, the possibility should be considered. Beiter, Staller and Dowell (1991) suggested that a hearing aid trial extending to a minimum of six months is desirable for all children regardless of the cause of deafness and although neonatal hearing screening offers an opportunity to implant babies of a few weeks of age the actual wisdom of a rushed approach, in any case other than meningitis (with ossification formation), must be questioned. Apart from the need for a sensible hearing aid trial there are issues of parental acceptance of, and adjustment to, their baby's deafness. Parents may need time to form a balanced and informed appreciation of the variety of remedial options available for their child of which cochlear implantation is just one.

The investigations

A 90-minute session is recommended for the first appointment to allow sufficient time to obtain a comprehensive audiological profile.

Hearing aid condition and technical performance

The state and physical condition of the hearing aid might indicate the extent of its use. Suspicions of lack of use might be raised if the aids show no signs of wear and tear despite having been issued some time previously without replacement. It is vital to know that hearing aids have been given a fair trial and most parents accept this requirement. Sometimes, however, the parents might have foreshortened the trial because no obvious benefit has been observed, particularly if there has been a battle of acceptance on the part of the child.

The condition of the earmould and tubing should be inspected to see if the tubing is loose or has hardened or become discoloured with age and to check that the mould is not blocked with wax or debris. It might be necessary to retube the mould or to clean it in an ultrasonic cleaner. The performance of the hearing aids should be checked against the manufacturer's specifications using a well calibrated test station.

Assessing hearing thresholds

The techniques for measuring hearing thresholds will vary according to the age and maturity of the baby/child. The basic techniques will include distraction testing and/or visual reinforcement audiometry for infants below two years of age with the introduction also of performance testing (play audiometry) for those above the age of two years.

The distraction test

Most audiology clinics in the UK have adopted visual reinforcement audiometry (VRA) as their primary assessment technique with the very young. It is worth remembering, however, that additional useful information can sometimes be obtained from the distraction test if a child is too young for, or is disinterested in, the VRA procedure. The distraction test illustrated in Figure 4.1 can be used with babies from five months of age and sometimes below this age if the baby's head and spine are suitably supported. One tester attracts and then controls the baby's attention at the front whilst a second tester remains out of vision to present sound or other stimuli at the appropriate time rewarding any turns to locate the stimuli with, for example, a smile or a tickle on the arm. The baby's responses in the form of head turns or other subtle reactions are observed by the distractor at the front. A particular merit of the distraction test is that the baby's responsiveness to sounds, touch and vision can be assessed in a quick sequence and this affords an opportunity to determine the general state of responsiveness. For example, if the baby turns quickly to visual stimulation, to touch or to vibrotactile stimuli, but not to sound then the tester can be certain that the attention state is optimum and the baby is ready to respond if given sufficient stimulation. If the baby fails to respond to sound, touch or vision, great care will be needed in interpreting the lack of responsiveness to sound. Another merit of the distraction test situation is that the stimuli (sound or vibrotactile) can be presented very close to each ear thus enabling each ear to be tested separately without the need for the baby to wear any disturbing equipment. Because of the close proximity to the ear the stimuli can be very intense with levels in excess of 110 dB being easily attainable. Such levels would not be achievable with a typical VRA sound field speaker system. With the routine availability of VRA equipment it is very tempting to dispense with the distraction test but it can still contribute useful information when applied skilfully in a diagnostic setting.

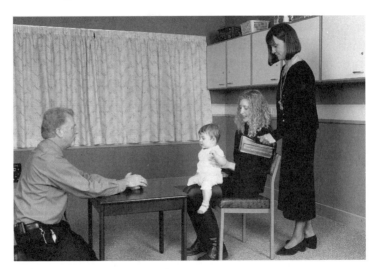

Figure 4.1. The arrangement for a distraction test.

Visual reinforcement audiometry

Visual reinforcement audiometry is a powerful technique for application with babies from as young as six to eight months and its application can be extended to children of three or four years or more. It works on the principle of reinforcing responses to sounds (such as head turns) with interesting visual displays such as the lighting up of a puppet in a cabinet (Figure 4.2a). Careful application of the technique in a well-calibrated sound field set up can enable 20–30 responses to be obtained in a single test session and with the programming of occasional breaks it should be possible to determine aided and unaided hearing thresholds for a few frequencies in each ear during a single appointment. The use of insert phones (Figure 4.2b), if tolerated by the baby, will enable independent unaided hearing thresholds to be obtained for each ear and bone conduction thresholds can be assessed with the use of a normal bone conduction transducer. Profoundly deaf babies might show some responses to vibrotactile signals from bone conduction transducers at the low 250 Hz and 500 Hz frequencies and observation of responsiveness to vibration provides useful information about the baby's general state of attention and also about the nature of the response that might be expected to sound, if indeed the baby can hear. The significance of any lack of

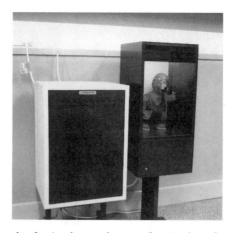

Figure 4.2a. Example of a visual reward system for visual reinforcement audiometry.

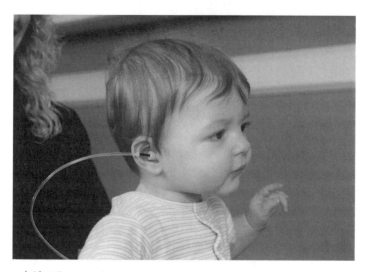

Figure 4.2b. The use of insert phones for visual reinforcement audiometry.

reaction to sound can be judged by inserting vibrotactile signals at intervals during the testing to ensure that the baby is still in a responsive state.

The performance test and pure tone audiometry

For children above the age of two years it might be possible to undertake conditioning for play audiometry (Figure 4.3). The child is conditioned to wait for a sound stimulus and then to respond with some play activity such as placing a man in a boat or a ball on a stick when the sound is presented in the absence of any visual or other clue. A skilled tester can keep a child's interest for a considerable time by introducing new and novel play activities and by including appropriate task reinforcements and encouragements. It should be possible to record a number of aided and unaided hearing thresholds in a single session, using well calibrated sound field stimuli for aided threshold measurements and headphones or insert phones for unaided thresholds. Vibrotactile (low frequency) bone conduction stimuli can be useful for helping to establish conditioning for the play task knowing that the child should definitely 'feel' a 250 Hz stimulus at around 25–40 dB(A) and a 500 Hz stimulus at around 55–70 dB(A) (Boothroyd and Cawkwell, 1970). Once having established a reliable pattern of conditioning the significance of any lack of response to sound will become apparent and hearing thresholds can be recorded using the standard Hughson and Westlake ascending threshold chasing techniques (described by

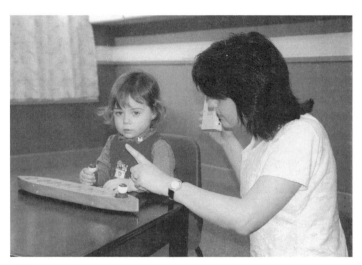

Figure 4.3. Conditioning for a performance test (play audiometry).

Carhart and Jerger, 1959). If at any time the child becomes unresponsive it will be useful to introduce further vibrotactile stimuli to ensure that attention is still on the task.

Speech discrimination testing

It might not be possible to undertake this type of testing with very young candidates for cochlear implantation. Nevertheless attempts should be made to assess auditory and audio-visual speech discrimination performance to establish a baseline measure from which to judge future progress. If formal speech audiometry cannot be performed it will be necessary to use measures from the video analysis techniques described in Chapter 9 together with other ratings outlined in Chapters 8 and 10 to establish baseline measures of communication ability prior to implantation.

The McCormick Toy Discrimination Test (McCormick, 1977) is an example of a test designed for application with the very young. The test has been designed for application in children with a mental age of two years and above but in a simplified form it can be used with children as young as 18 months. It consists of a series of seven paired toy items that have been chosen to have similar sounding names within the pairs. The vocabulary content is known, either through the spoken word or through sign, to a child of two years of age for the full set and 18 months for the sub-set cup/duck spoon/shoe. The paired items known to the child are displayed and the child is prompted to point to each item on request. The listening level required to obtain an 80% score (four correct responses out of five requests) is recorded in dB(A) for the live mode of presentation thus giving a reference measure against which future performance can be assessed. The test can be undertaken in the listening only mode or with the aid of signing or lipreading to sample alternative communication modes.

An advanced version of the test known as the Institute of Hearing Research/McCormick Automated Toy Discrimination Test (Ousey et al., 1989; Palmer, Sheppard and Marshall, 1991), illustrated in Figure 4.4, permits the recording of a very precise and repeatable measure of speech discrimination and, because of the way it is designed, it is free from the floor and ceiling scoring effects that often limit the usefulness of other tests. This automated version of the test procedure considerably enhanced precision in terms of standardized presentation and scoring. In this

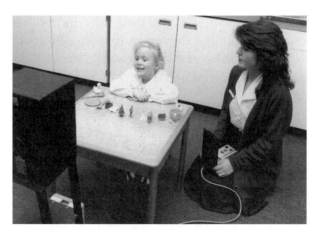

Figure 4.4. The Medical Research Council Institute of Hearing Research/McCormick Automated Toy Discrimination Test.

recorded test the words are digitized at 20 Hz and low pass filtered at 8.5 kHz. They are played through a loudspeaker in random order (selecting only the words known to the child). The threshold in dB(A) at which the child obtains a 71% discrimination score is then calculated using a two-down, one-up adaptive procedure based on six reversals (Levitt, 1971). The Automated Toy Test has a dual advantage in that it is free from language constraints that can influence scores on sentence material in very young children, and it provides a good measure of the functional use of hearing. Any child who has the linguistic capacity for the test but cannot perform the test with hearing aid use in the listening only mode below a conversational listening level of 65 dB(A) is considered to have a significant hearing disability of sufficient magnitude to warrant cochlear implantation consideration. Justification for this criteria will be given in part two of this chapter.

Tympanometry

Tympanometry must be undertaken routinely during each session to ensure that there is no evidence of middle-ear dysfunction. This should have been detected during the local otological check the week or so before the appointment but it will still be wise to ensure that everything is clear on the day of the audiological investigation.

Otoacoustic emissions

Otoacoustic emission recording can help to delineate the possibility of the presence of retrocochlear lesions (auditory neuropathy).

The absence of otoacoustic emission activity will offer some degree of reassurance that the lesion is within the cochlea. This test can be performed very rapidly with the latest recording systems and it should be undertaken routinely either during the initial audiological session or at a later stage if necessary.

Assessing the audiological profile

Following the administration of the above test battery it should be possible to form an opinion about the appropriateness of further cochlear implant evaluations for the child. It will be necessary to allow time to counsel the family and to explain the significance of the findings in relation to the child's needs. No family should leave the clinic feeling abandoned or rejected by the implant programme because the child does not fit within the implant criteria. The positive side of continued hearing aid use should be stressed and of a signing approach if that is the parents' first choice. It is inevitable that some parents will have focused their attention on an implant but they must be advised that it is not in the child's best interest to consider this route if the child has too much residual hearing or does not meet the criteria for other good reasons. Some families express relief that the implant route is not appropriate and they feel consoled by the fact that they have at least explored the possibility on behalf of their child.

In cases where the child clearly does not fit the audiological selection criteria it might not be necessary for other investigations to be undertaken by the rest of the cochlear implant team. There will, however, be many borderline cases for whom full investigations will be needed by the surgeons, teachers of the deaf, psychologists and speech and language therapists before sensible decisions can be made about the wisdom of implantation.

Section 2

In this section detailed justification for the Nottingham approach will be presented and an historical excursion through the investigations that were undertaken to justify the prevailing criteria will be included. This will be followed by a review of the literature on audiological candidacy issues leading to a summary of the existing stance and pointers for possible future approaches.

Teachers of the deaf and specialist speech and language therapists are accustomed to the fact that most profoundly deaf hearing aid users have great difficulty accessing high frequency information. Because they cannot hear the high frequency consonants they are not able to produce these consonants accurately: there are no surprises here. What does surprise the experienced professional who is used to working with the deaf and who meets cochlear implant users for the first time is the intelligibility of their speech and the ease with which they can identify and produce high frequency consonants. They can, for example, easily hear the difference between the /s/ and /sh/ sounds. This striking feature of the behaviour of cochlear implant users provides clear pointers to the fact that cochlear implant selection criteria should take account of the individual's capacity to access high frequency information through hearing aids and their potential to improve this ability with the aid of cochlear implants.

The potential offered by cochlear implants to enhance access to high frequency sounds is the primary consideration in the Nottingham audiological criteria and it represents a significant drift away from the most widely quoted criterion which averages only low and middle frequency hearing thresholds. Justification for this departure will be given in the studies that follow. Figure 4.5 shows mean and standard deviation values of the frequency content in the speech of four typical cochlear implant users (top tracings) and four platinum/gold (star) hearing aid users (lower traces) (attending the Nottingham service) when saying the word 'horse' (Durst, 1999 unpublished study). It can be seen that the cochlear implant users produce frequencies above 3 kHz that are not present to anything like the same degree in the speech of exceptionally good hearing aid users with severe/profound hearing losses. It is known that there is a link between speech production and speech perception skills (Tye-Murray, Spencer and Gilbert-Bedia, 1995; O'Donoghue et al., 1999) and if children are simply too deaf to hear particular speech frequencies it is not surprising that these frequencies are absent in their speech. The potential of cochlear implants to impart high frequency speech information does, therefore, become of paramount importance.

The justification for the establishment of the Nottingham high frequency audiological selection criteria for cochlear implantation in the mid-1990s was based on comparisons of the performance of hearing aid users and cochlear implant users.

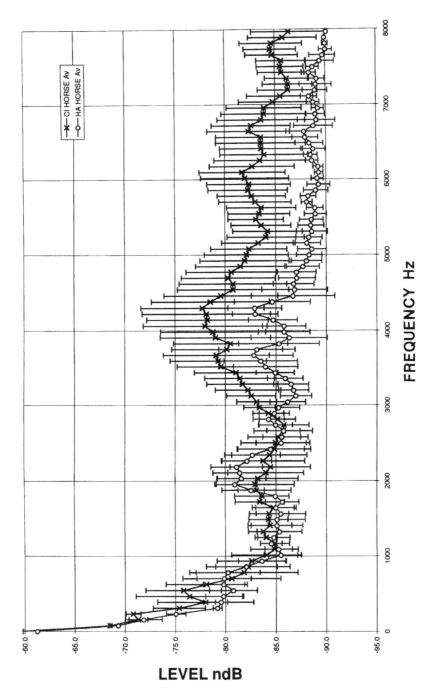

Figure 4.5. Frequency spectra for the word 'horse' spoken by profoundly deaf child hearing aid users (circles) and cochlear implant users (crosses) showing the higher and more natural presence of high frequencies above 3kHz in the speech of the cochlear implant users.

The recording of aided sound field threshold responses with hearing aids and with cochlear implants was, at the time, a novel approach but it was considered to be very desirable for two main reasons. Firstly, high frequency aided thresholds were actually accessible to measurement in the absence of any recordable unaided pure tone thresholds at high frequencies (early implant candidates were too deaf to show high frequency audiometric thresholds). Secondly, aided responses provided a measurement of functional performance with a device and enabled performances with hearing aids and cochlear implants to be compared.

Study 1- predicting speech discrimination from audiometric summary measures

In the first study (hitherto unpublished) the objective was to investigate the validity of using aided sound field warble tone thresholds to predict deaf children's speech discrimination performance. If a relationship could be established then the very accessible aided thresholds, which could be measured in babies, could be used to establish an audiological selection criterion at a time when speech discrimination measures could not be obtained for obvious reasons. This study was undertaken during 1997/8 by Robinson, McCormick, Cope and Twomey working in the Nottingham Paediatric Cochlear Implant Programme and in the Nottingham Children's Hearing Assessment Centre. The study was undertaken on retrospective data obtained from 74 hearing-aided children during the course of their routine reviews in clinic. Pure tone audiometry and aided sound field warble tone threshold recordings were undertaken in each session and speech discrimination performance was measured using the IHR/McCormick Automated Toy Discrimination Test referred to earlier in this chapter. The conditions under which the tests were presented were carefully controlled and are described below.

The subjects

The 74 children in this study were the entire population of children fitted with hearing aids over a 15-year period, the only exclusions being those with learning difficulties additional to those associated with deafness. They had been fitted with high-quality analogue hearing aids by the investigators or their colleagues and had been regularly reviewed over an extended period (range 2–15 years). Twenty-nine were moderately deaf

(41–70 dB HL), 19 were severely deaf (71–95 dB HL) and 26 were profoundly deaf (>95 dB HL). Their average ages at the time of the test was 10.4 years (SD 3.1) they had used their aids for an average of 6.8 years (SD 3.1) and the mean age of fitting was 2.2 years (SD 1.7). The group showed the typical trend of earlier detection of deafness for the deafer children with median age of detection being eight months for the profoundly deaf, 12 months for the severely deaf and 40 months for the moderately deaf.

Results

The first analysis determined the effect size (ES) based on the ability of the audiometric summary measure to discriminate between being able and unable to perform the IHR/McCormick Automated Toy Discrimination Test. The performance criterion on this test was taken to be 65 dB(A), being roughly the level of conversational speech. The inability to perform the test was scored at 66 dB(A) although it is worth noting that the test was measured to a maximum level of 78 dB(A). The effect size was calculated using Lipsey (1990), based on the difference in means between those able to perform the Automated Toy Test and those unable to perform the Automated Toy Test. To derive the effect size the difference score was then expressed as a function of the standard deviation for all of the hearing-aided children. This measures the power of an audiometric measure to discriminate between those hearing-aided children who obtained functional benefit from a hearing aid (better than or equal to 65 dB(A) on the Automated Toy Test) and those who do not obtain functional benefit (unable to perform the Automated Toy Test).

The analysis of effect size, or discriminatory power for audiometric variables, showed that the effect sizes of thresholds are highest for aided thresholds at 4 kHz (1.8 SD) followed by 2 kHz (1.7 SD), as may be seen in Table 4.1. In addition, of the summary audiometric measures, discriminatory power is highest (1.8 SD) for the high frequency aided thresholds (averaging 2 kHz and 4 kHz) hereafter known as the HAT.

Correlations

A second analysis involved the calculation of the Spearman ranked correlation coefficient between the summary audiometric measure and that of the Automated Toy Test. A non-parametric correlation was chosen to enable inclusion of those children who were unable to perform the Automated Toy Test. The

Table 4.1. Effect sizes for individual audiometric frequencies and for summary audiometric measures

Measure	Aided	Unaided
0.5 kHz threshold	0.98 SD	1.11 SD
1 kHz threshold	1.12 SD	1.29 SD
2 kHz threshold	1.70 SD	1.45 SD
4 kHz threshold	1.79 SD	1.51 SD
Four frequency average (0.5,1,2,4 kHz)	1.50 SD	1.49 SD
High Frequency Aided Threshold (2,4 kHz) (HAT)	1.80 SD	1.58 SD

results are given in Table 4.2 and they show that the best-ranked correlation between a summary audiometric measure and speech discrimination for children with severe/profound hearing losses was 0.85 achieved by the HAT.

Table 4.2. Spearman ranked correlations between speech discrimination and the summary audiometric measures for moderate and severe/profound hearing aid users.

	Moderate	Severe/profound
Better Hearing Ear Three Frequency Average (0.5, 1, 2 kHz)	0.58 (p=0.005)	0.58 (p<0.001)
Better Hearing Ear Four Frequency Average (0.5, 1, 2, 4 kHz)	0.54 (p=0.005)	0.82 (p<0.001)
Better Hearing Ear High Frequency Average (2, 4 kHz)	0.27 (p=0.189) not significant	0.79 (p<0.001)
Aided Three Frequency Average (0.5, 1, 2 kHz)	0.70 (p=0.001)	0.71 (p<0.001)
Aided Four Frequency Average (0.5, 1, 2, 4 kHz)	0.82 (p<0.001)	0.80 (p<0.001)
High Frequency Aided Threshold (HAT) (2, 4 kHz)	0.48 (p=0.016)	0.85 (p<0.001)

Study 2 – the relationship between the IHR/McCormick Automated Toy Discrimination Test speech discrimination measure and other measures of speech perception

A second hitherto unpublished study was undertaken in 1997/8 by Robinson, McCormick, Cope and Twomey and involved the undertaking of retrospective analysis of data obtained from 53 children with cochlear implants during the course of their routine reviews in clinic. All children in the implant programme who had used their devices for more than three years were included except those with additional learning difficulties and those for whom spoken English or British Sign Language were not used at home. The mean age of the children was 10.2 years (2.7 SD) and they had been implanted at 4.2 years of age (2.4 SD). They had used their devices for 5.5 years (2.4 SD).

In addition to the IHR/McCormick Automated Toy Discrimination Test, two additional tests were administered by the implant programme's teachers of the deaf. These were the Iowa Closed-set Speech Perception Sentence Test for Hearing-Impaired Children (Tyler and Holstad, 1987) and the Connected Discourse Tracking Open-set Test (De Filippo and Scott, 1978). The latter two tests were administered using live voice at a conversational level in a quiet room in the listening only mode. Neither of these tests had the rigorous control of the Automated Toy Test but they do sample aspects of everyday auditory communication skill in a form accessible to (re)habilitation services (see for example Tye-Murray and Tyler, 1988).

The Iowa test was administered with 4×4 picture matrices and the child had to point to the four pictures, from the total set of 16, which described the sentence that was presented. In the Connected Discourse Tracking task, simple stories were read to the child phrase by phrase and the child had to repeat them verbatim. The exercise was timed and the number of words repeated correctly per minute was calculated. The test is open set.

Results

Correlation analysis was performed on the data. Spearman ranked correlations were calculated to enable inclusion of those children who scored worse than 65 dB(A) on the Automated Toy Test. The results revealed that the Automated Toy Test correlated well with the two tests of speech perception. The ranked correlation with the closed-set Iowa Matrix Test was 0.59, and it was 0.71 with performance on the Connected Discourse Tracking task. Both correlations were significant ($p < 0.50$).

Discussion

The most important findings from these studies were:

- that the averaged high frequency aided threshold for 2 kHz and 4 kHz was an acceptable (and for severely/profoundly deaf children the best) discriminating variable in predicting the ability to perform speech discrimination;
- the speech discrimination score obtained from the IHR/McCormick Automated Toy Discrimination Test correlated well with open-set sentence performance (Connected Discourse Tracking) and with closed-set speech perception performance (Iowa Matrix Test). The good correlations between these tests indicate that the Automated Toy Test samples an aspect of speech perception that relates to everyday communication ability.

Combining these two findings it can be deduced that a simple and very accessible measurement of hearing sensitivity (aided high frequency thresholds) can indicate potential for speech discrimination and for open-set perception. This is very important information to consider when assessing babies or the very young for whom speech discrimination testing cannot be performed. This opened the way for establishing an audiological guideline for cochlear implant candidacy based on a measure of hearing sensitivity. This was the focus of the next study and it addressed the issue of what constituted satisfactory hearing aid performance and what level of performance should warrant cochlear implant consideration.

Before describing that study it is of interest to discuss a subsidiary finding that emerged from the data presented so far that showed there was a marked difference between the moderate and profound hearing aid users in the pattern of correlations between the summary audiometric measures and the speech discrimination scores. This difference concerns the importance of the high frequencies (2 and 4 kHz). For severe/profound hearing-aid users the high frequency aided and unaided thresholds were either better correlated with speech discrimination score or as good as the aided and unaided three and four frequency averages (Table 4.2). In contrast, for moderately deaf hearing aid users the aided and unaided three and four frequency averages had better correlations with the speech discrimination scores than either the aided or unaided high frequency averaged thresholds for 2 kHz and 4 kHz. Results from previous research relating speech discrimination with audiometric measures in children with mild losses (Palmer et al., 1991; Summerfield et al., 1994) is consistent with the pattern shown for moderate hearing aid users in this study. Why, then, do the high frequencies at 2 kHz and 4 kHz have such a marked importance for speech discrimination for severe/profound hearing aid users? One explanation might be that with increased hearing loss the importance of the frequency weightings for speech discrimination changes. Further work relating degree of hearing loss with audiometric configuration, speech discrimination and speech perception is required before an adequate explanation is possible.

Study 3 – establishing an audiometric selection criterion for paediatric cochlear implantation with data from hearing aid users

This third study was undertaken by McCormick, Cope and Robinson (1998a, 1998b).The findings have had far reaching consequences for paediatric cochlear implant programmes in the UK and in other European countries.

Having established that the high frequency aided threshold (HAT) was a good predictor of speech discrimination performance and the IHR/McCormick Toy Discrimination Test result had a strong association with wider measures of speech perception, the pathway was open to the establishment, from these simple measures, of an indicator of efficiency of hearing aid use that could be used to form an audiological selection criterion for cochlear implantation.

The aim of this third study was to establish an audiometric selection criterion for cochlear implantation that was generally suitable for all children but with equal application to those in the first year of life. This was an important clinical and research consideration because of the inaccessibility of routine clinical speech perception tests to the increasingly younger children who were being referred as candidates for cochlear implantation. Moreover there are severe limitations in the spoken language development in severe/profoundly deaf children which makes speech perception testing more difficult. In contrast sound field warble tone thresholds are relatively simple and swift to undertake and can be accurate and repeatable in some children as young as six months of age. Aided thresholds provide a measure of the child's functional use of hearing aids and the degree of access to the speech spectrum.

In this study the High Frequency Aided Threshold averaged over 2 kHz and 4 kHz (HAT) was used to predict speech discrimination scores in the IHR/McCormick Automated Toy Discrimination Test enabling the definition of a boundary area that marked the limits of acoustic amplification for analogue aids beyond which electrical stimulation of the hearing system could be considered. At the time the data were collected digital processing hearing aids were not available routinely in the UK and bilateral fitting of good quality high power analogue instruments was the norm for children. Retrospective data were analysed from a population of children from an audiology service that was considered to be a model for practice in the UK (McCormick et al., 1984; McCormick, 1988). Children in the study were managed in the service and received high quality hearing aid support from the day of initial fitting. They received regular audiological reviews in the same centre over the years to ensure that optimum benefit was maintained. It is worth noting that such a study could not now be undertaken on a prospective basis because cochlear implants would be provided as an alternative to hearing aids for many of the profoundly deaf children.

Subjects

The hearing-aided group comprised the 74 children referred to in Study 1 above . Their performance was compared with that of the 53 cochlear implanted children referred to in Study 2 above. The age of the children in the two groups at the time of the data collection was comparable with a mean age of 10.4 years for the hearing-aided children (SD 3.1) and 10.2 years for the cochlear implanted children (SD 2.7). The children with cochlear implants had less experience of using their devices (5.5 years; SD 2.4) than the children with hearing aids (6.8 years; SD 3.1). The children with hearing aids were fitted at 2.2 years (SD 1.7 years) and the implanted children were implanted later (4.2 years; SD 2.4). The cochlear implanted children had initially been fitted with hearing aids and they were referred for cochlear implantation because of lack of progress. This study was undertaken at a time when the majority of cochlear implant candidates had virtually no residual hearing (as will be seen from the data) and the objective was to determine how far the boundaries could be moved forward to accommodate children with usable residual hearing in the implant programme.

One difference between the groups that must be mentioned was that the dominant cause of deafness for the cochlear implant group was meningitis whereas the children with hearing aids were mostly congenitally deaf. This reflected the trends in cochlear implantation at the time and the situation has changed dramatically since then with the majority of cochlear implant candidates now being congenitally deaf. (Subsequent analysis revealed that cause of deafness did not influence the eventual outcome for the particular children in this study possibly because the meningitis occurred mostly at the pre-lingual stage.)

An interesting feature of this study was that the same staff had fitted and evaluated the hearing aids and also fitted and tuned the cochlear implant speech processors over the years thus ensuring continuity in quality of care. Hearing aid fitting was checked with the aid of the Seewald Desired Sensation Level technique where possible (Seewald et al., 1996) and the hearing aid performance was checked using a Fonix 6500-C Hearing Aid Test System.

Children with cochlear implants used the Nucleus 22 channel intra-cochlear implant system with the SPEAK speech processing strategy.

All testing was undertaken in identical sound-attenuated clinics and the positioning of loudspeakers and calibrating microphones was identical in each test room. The loudspeaker was placed so that its central axis was aligned with the microphone one meter away. Calibration was achieved by positioning a microphone where the child's head was located during the test.

Audiometric testing used the manual method recommended by the British Society of Audiology/British Association of Otolaryngologists (1981). This is a modified Hughson-Westlake procedure using 5 dB steps. Aided sound field threshold measurements were undertaken using the IHR/McCormick Automated Toy Test warble tone facility, which covered a range from 0 dB to 78 dB in steps down to 1 dB. The frequency modulation depth was 10% and the modulation rate was 10 Hz.

Speech discrimination scores were collected using the IHR/McCormick Automated Toy Discrimination Test as described in the previous studies.

Results – establishing the clinical criterion for paediatric cochlear implantation

Figure 4.6 shows a plot of hearing sensitivity (aided HAT) against speech discrimination ability (IHR/McCormick Toy Test result) for the moderate, severe and profound hearing aid users.

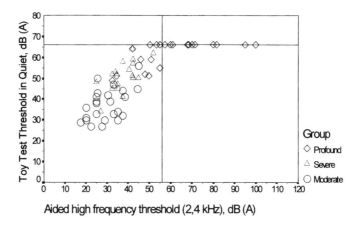

Figure 4.6. Discrimogram plots for moderately, severely and profoundly deaf hearing aid users showing aided high frequency averaged thresholds for 2 kHz and 4kHz against the listening levels required to obtain the optimum 71% discrimination score in the MRC Institute of Hearing Research/McCormick Automated Toy Discrimination Test.

This graphical representation is particularly interesting because it informs us not only about the child's access to sound but also how the child actually uses the hearing for speech discrimination purposes. This graph is much more informative than an aided or unaided audiogram and the term Discrimogram is an appropriate description of the chart. Children who perform well approach the origin of each scale – that is, the best performers have a low hearing threshold and they obtain the 71% speech discrimination score at a quiet level. In contrast the higher the values the greater the difficulty with performance. Not surprisingly, most of the children with moderate degrees of hearing loss perform better than those with severe losses although there is an overlap of performance. Similarly those with severe hearing losses tend to outperform those with profound losses but, again, there is an overlap. The fact that children with the same degree of hearing loss have different speech discrimination abilities is clearly displayed. It is of interest to note that up to the 65 dB line for the Toy Test threshold it would be possible to draw a line of linear regression showing a strong correlation between the two measures. The HAT could easily predict the Toy Test score within 10 dB or so. This is not the intention of the exercise, however, and it is more important for this study to view each point on the discrimogram as a unique identifier of a child's performance on two separate, albeit related, measures.

The horizontal reference line is set at 66 dB(A). Children who cannot discriminate speech at the conversational level of 65 dB(A) are considered to have a serious disadvantage and for convenience all values above 65 dB(A) have been plotted as 66 dB(A) even though levels up to the maximum of 78 dB(A) were used. To achieve the selection criterion for cochlear implantation the HAT that correctly classifies all hearing-aided children who are able to perform the Automated Toy Test was determined. A vertical reference line has been drawn at 56 dB(A), which shows that hearing-aided children with a HAT of 55 dB(A) or better are generally able to perform the Auto-mated Toy Test at conversational listening levels of voice.

Sensitivity analysis

For this analysis 'condition presence' is considered to be the inability to perform speech discrimination at the conversational listening level of 65 dB(A). An audiometric criterion set at a HAT worse than 55 dB(A) will ensure that there are no children selected who are able to perform the Automated Toy Test with hearing aids (specificity of 100%). Hence if the criterion for paediatric cochlear implantation is set at a HAT of worse than 55 dB(A) then none of the hearing-impaired children who were able to perform the Automated Toy Test would have been implanted.

Turning to detecting those children who were unable to perform speech discrimination (sensitivity) a HAT of worse that 55 dB(A) would detect 83% of children who were unable to perform the Automated Toy Discrimination Test criterion with hearing aids. The balance of 17% (3/18) of children who were unable to perform the Automated Toy Test with a HAT of 55 dB(A) or less are shown on the horizontal line to the left of the vertical HAT criterion line in Figure 4.6. Table 4.3 shows the detailed analysis of specificity and sensitivity.

Further inspection of the data revealed that the equivalent threshold for the better hearing ear unaided three frequency average (0.5, 1, 2 kHz) was 105 dB HL and it was 45 dB(A) for the aided thresholds averaged for these same frequencies.

A less stringent criterion is the point at which children who were unable to perform the Automated Toy Test are potentially selected for cochlear implantation. In this case the vertical line in Figure 4.6 would be set at a HAT of worse than 50 dB(A). In this situation the specificity is 95% and there is a 5% (3/56)

Table 4.3. Specificity and sensitivity for criterion set at worse than 55 dB(A)

Test Result	Condition status	
	Unable to perform	Able to perform
Positive	15 True positive (TP)	0 False positive (FP)
Negative	3 False negative (FN)	56 True negative (TN)
Specificity = TN/ (FP + TN) = 56/56 = 100%	Sensitivity = TP/ (TP + FN) = 15/18 = 83%	

chance that a child with a HAT worse than 50 dB(A) would be able to perform the Automated Toy Test. The sensitivity remains at 100% (all those unable to perform the Automated Toy Test would have been implanted). Table 4.4 shows the detailed calculations of sensitivity and specificity for the 50 dB(A) HAT criterion.

Further inspection of the data revealed that the equivalent thresholds for the better ear unaided three frequency average (0.5, 1, 2 kHz) was 97 dB HL.

Table 4.4. Specificity and sensitivity for criterion set at worse than 50 dB(A)

Test Result	Condition status	
	Unable to perform	Able to perform
Positive	18 True positive (TP)	3 False positive (FP)
Negative	0 False negative (FN)	53 True negative (TN)
Specificity = TN/ (FP + TN) = 53/56 = 95%	Sensitivity = TP/ (TP + FN) = 18/18 = 100%	

Performance of children with cochlear implants

The performance of the 53 children with cochlear implants was compared with that for the hearing-aided children to provide confirmation of the clinical criterion for paediatric cochlear implantation. It will be recalled that these were all of the children in the implant programme at that time who had at least three years experience with their devices and who were exposed to spoken English or British Sign Language as their first language. Children with learning difficulties in addition to those associated with their deafness were excluded from the study.

Figure 4.7 shows the performance of the cochlear implant children prior to implantation (filled triangles) and following experience with their implants (open triangles). Note that some of the pre-implant data points overlap and 45 children showed a high frequency average of 120 dB(A) or more (plotted at 120 for convenience). Prior to implantation none of the children could obtain a score in the Automated Toy Test not because of vocabulary constraints, because the items were mostly known through sign and/or lipreading, but because they were too deaf to discriminate the words in the listening-only mode. As already indicated, their aided thresholds (HATs) prior to implantation were off the scale (worse than 120 dB(A)) for most of the children. Following implantation their aided thresholds (HATs) were all less than 50 dB(A), thus showing a considerable improvement and 79% (42/53) of the children were able to perform the Automated Toy Discrimination Test. It was interesting to note that, of the 11 children who were unable to perform the Automated Toy Discrimination Test, eight had greater than five years of virtually total deafness prior to implantation. In addition, one was later diagnosed with a central learning disability and a further two had problems with their implants, one of which required reimplantation. Table 4.5 describes each child and potential causes for the inability to perform the Automated Toy Test. Further analysis showed that the duration of deafness

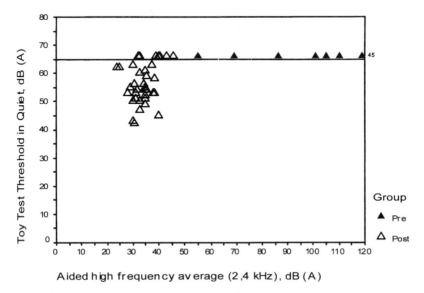

Figure 4.7. Discrimogram plots showing performance with hearing aids before implant (filled triangles) and the same children's performance with cochlear implants (unfilled triangles).

Table 4.5. Cochlear implant children unable to perform Automated Toy Test

1. Five electrodes deactivated in middle of array, sign dependent, > 5 years duration of deafness
2. Vestibular problems, neurological symptoms, speech/language impairment
3. Sign dominant school
4. > 5 years duration of deafness, epilepsy, vestibular problems, lipreading dependent, non-ideal home situation
5. 5 years duration of deafness, sign dependent, family difficulties, change in educational setting
6. > 5 years duration of deafness, possible dyslexia, attention poor, Usher's Syndrome
7. >5 years duration of deafness, lipreading dependent
8. > 5 years duration of deafness, global delay, Asperger's Syndrome
9. Implant failure (three channels functioning at the time of test)
10. > 5 years duration of deafness, sign dominant school, speech and language impairment
11. > 5 years duration of deafness, learning difficulties, possible central deficit

was predictive of ability to perform speech discrimination. The mean duration of deafness was 6.2 years (SD 2.3) for the 11 children who were unable to perform speech discrimination and 3.7 years (SD 2.2) for the 42 children who were able to perform the task (t50 = 3.36, p = 0.001).

Figure 4.8 shows the performance of the cochlear implanted children superimposed on that of the hearing aid users. There are a lot of overlapping data points on this chart and the very fact that

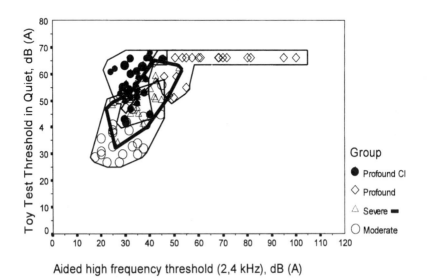

Figure 4.8. Discrimogram plots for cochlear implant users (filled circles) and moderately, severely and profoundly deaf hearing aid users.

they do overlap in this way is very interesting. It is, however, difficult to interpret the illustration by viewing the points in the overlapping regions, and so for convenience the boundaries of
performance for the four groups are drawn to aid interpretation. It
is immediately apparent that the cochlear implant users were
performing much better than the majority of the profoundly deaf
hearing aid users and there was also a large overlap in the performance of the cochlear implanted children and that of the hearing
aid users with severe and moderate hearing losses.

Odds ratios for clinical application

Given the conservative criterion of a HAT worse than 55 dB(A),
the odds of the cochlear implant candidates being able to
perform the Automated Toy Test if they continued with hearing
aids is zero. On the other hand the odds of the child being able
to perform the Automated Toy Test following implantation are
better than 5 in 7 or 79% (42/53).

Given the more relaxed criterion of a HAT worse than
50 dB(A) the odds of a hearing-aided child being able to perform
the Automated Toy Discrimination Test after a mean of 6.8 years
continued experience with hearing aids is 1 in 7 (3/18, 17%). The
odds that the child would be able to perform the Automated Toy
Test with a cochlear implant are better than 5 in 7 (42/53, 79%).

Discussion

The finding from this study showed that cochlear implant selection candidacy could be based on a simple measure of aided
high frequency hearing at 2 kHz and 4 kHz. Implant consideration could safely be given to any child whose aided thresholds at
these two frequencies were 55 dB(A) or more. Adoption of this
criterion would ensure that no hearing-impaired child who was
able to discriminate speech at conversational listening levels
would be selected. Adoption of a less stringent criterion of aided
thresholds at these two frequencies being 50 dB(A) or more
could also be applied but there would be an increased risk (from
zero to a 1 in 7 chance) that an implanted child might do no
better with the implant than with continued hearing aid use. To
some people this risk might be acceptable.

Progressive revision of the audiological criterion

The aided threshold criterion established above served the
Nottingham programme very well for a number of years. It did,

however, differ significantly from the more commonly adopted National Institute of Health/United States Food and Drug Administration (FDA) criterion (NIH, 1995) in two respects. Firstly, it used aided thresholds. Secondly, it concentrated on high frequency hearing. The NIH criterion required the unaided hearing thresholds averaged across 500 Hz, 1 kHz and 2 kHz to be greater than 90 dB HL. The HAT criterion was less stringent for steeply sloping losses but more stringent for flatter losses. None of the hearing-aided children in the above study with steeply sloping losses and HATs greater than 55 dB(A) could perform the speech discrimination task thus supporting the notion that 2 kHz and 4 kHz have great significance for speech tasks. Some of these children would not meet the NIH pure tone criterion because of their reasonable low frequency thresholds. On the other hand the HAT criterion may have been too strict for profound losses with a flat configuration which would easily fit the NIH criterion.

With the passage of time cochlear implant speech processing strategies improved and it became clear that there was a need for further relaxation to be made to the audiological selection criterion. Further observations of the relative progress of implanted children and children with hearing aids supported this need. Of particular importance when evaluating the significance of the above studies was the fact that the implanted children included in the studies came from an early cohort of candidates and they had virtually no residual hearing. Adoption of the 55 dB(A) HAT criterion did, however, permit the implantation of many children with very significant amounts of residual hearing in the low and middle frequency regions over the succeeding years. After several years experience with their implants these children showed advantages over hearing aid users who approached but did not quite meet the borderline criterion for implantation. Unlike their hearing-aided peers the cochlear implant users could often use normal telephones (Tait et al., 2001) and they developed clearer speech with better pronunciation of high frequency consonants. Lack of ability to use a telephone and lack of clear speech production could be taken into account and could tip the balance in favour of cochlear implantation when assessing older borderline candidates.

A third noticeable feature of the behaviour of hearing aid users who approached, but did not quite meet, the borderline criterion was the degree of effort and concentration needed to obtain a score in the Automated Toy Discrimination Test as determined by their hesitancy and delayed reaction when undertaking the test. The response of cochlear implantees after a few years experience with the use of their devices was normally quick and positive in marked contrast to the experienced profoundly deaf hearing aid users (who approached the borderline) who managed to obtain a score below 65 dB(A) but only with difficulty. In this respect the implant users' behaviour was more like that of severely deaf hearing aid users and this is borne out also by the pattern of the actual scores in Figure 4.8. The distribution of scores for the experienced cochlear implant users more closely resembles that of the severely deaf hearing aid users than that of the best scoring profoundly deaf hearing aid users; this applies for high frequency aided thresholds down to 45/50 dB(A). It became clear that this third subtle aspect of a child's behaviour could be taken into account to further relax the selection criteria. Account must, however, be taken of possible future improvements in digital hearing aid technology that might prove to be beneficial to borderline candidates. Any further relaxation must, therefore, be introduced with considerable caution.

With the increasing availability of newer generations of digital processing hearing aids with non-linear processing characteristics and with active sound management features it is difficult to interpret the significance of aided thresholds and less reliance can be placed on such measurements in the future. Unaided thresholds are much easier to interpret because they are independent of hearing aid use or type. Previously the children had been too deaf to show any measurable high frequency thresholds on the audiogram and aided thresholds were the only ones that were accessible to analysis. With progressive relaxations in the criteria it became feasible to base the criteria on unaided thresholds. Extracting the data from the children included in the above studies who were using state of the art analogue hearing aids (mostly the Phonak PPCL4+ instrument on volume setting 3/3.5) the 50/55 dB(A) aided warble tone thresholds for the 2 kHz and 4 kHz frequencies obtained under these conditions corresponded to audiometric unaided thresholds of 105/110 dB HL. This became the new criterion, leaving open the possibility of recording aided thresholds with analogue hearing aid fitting to cross check the eligibility for very young or difficult-to-test children. As has already been indicated there may be scope for further relaxation of the criteria in the future but possibly not much more than 10dB or so.

Review of trends and suggestions from other programmes

It is interesting to note that the NIH/FDA criterion has relaxed over recent years from originally specifying pure tone averages (0.5, 1, 2 kHz) of 100 dB to the present 90 dB and originally only accepting an absence of open-set speech recognition to now accepting understanding of up to 60% on recorded open-set sentence testing. Lenarz (1998) points out that the borderline between hearing aids and cochlear implants will shift further towards severe hearing loss as was predicted by Boothroyd and Eran (1994). Reports are beginning to appear in the literature of results for implanted children with severe hearing losses. The studies undertaken so far include data on very small numbers of children and they must be interpreted with considerable caution.

One of the best controlled studies to have been undertaken on the statistical justification for selection criteria for adults was reported by Rubinstein et al. (1999) and, although the findings may not be directly applicable to children with pre-lingual deafness, it is of interest to note that the general findings support the notion that there is scope for introducing a general relaxation of the audiological selection criteria. Their study aimed to determine the effects of pre-operative speech reception on post-operative speech recognition with a cochlear implant and a well conducted statistical modelling approach was used. Their main findings were that duration of deafness and pre-operative sentence recognition were both significant predictors of word recognition with a cochlear implant and these two factors alone accounted for 80% of the variance in word recognition. It is universally accepted that shorter durations of deafness correlate with better outcomes in cochlear implant users (Gantz et al., 1993) and this applies to both adults and children. Their second finding was that patients with good levels of pre-operative sentence recognition ability performed extremely well in the more demanding tests of word recognition following cochlear implantation. A test of sentence recognition was used before surgery to avoid floor effects and a test of word recognition was used after surgery to avoid ceiling effects. The study provided compelling evidence for relaxing selection criteria to include patients with up to 40–60% pre-implant sentence recognition. To determine the duration of deafness, the point at which the subjects were no longer able to use a telephone was used as a reference marker for the onset of a serious disability. A particular strength of this study was the authors' derivation of a predictive index to facilitate the expansion of the selection criteria to include patients with greater amounts of residual hearing. Although their predictive tables cannot be used with children who are unable to perform sentence recognition tests, it is important to know that well-controlled studies of this nature are providing justification for the implantation of patients with increasing amounts of usable residual hearing.

The criteria for cochlear implantation have shifted over the years partly because the introduction of new speech processing strategies resulted in better reception and speech production skills. Numerous studies have compared the speech production performance of children with cochlear implants, conventional hearing aids and tactile aids (including Tobey et al., 1994; Ertmer et al., 1997; Geers, 1997; Schgal et al., 1997) but limited follow-up data are presented for users with five or more years of experience with implants. Tobey et al. (1994) did demonstrate progressive improvement beyond the three years of cochlear implant use and found that performance of implanted children was similar to that of hearing aid users with losses greater than 100 dB HL up to three years post-implant but it matched the performance of the hearing aid users with 90–100 dB HL hearing losses after three years of device use. A similar trend in speech perception performance was recorded by Meyer et al. (1998). In this study speech perception scores of implanted children were similar to those of hearing aid users with losses of 101 dB after two years of implant use and equivalent to the scores of hearing aid users with average losses of less than 90 dB after four years of implant use. Data from the Nottingham programme presented in this and other chapters of the present book demonstrate continuing progress up to five years after implantation and it is unlikely that the performance has peaked even at this stage. The findings that are now emerging from longitudinal studies are reinforcing the need to re-examine the cochlear implant selection criteria.

An interesting study reported by Zwolan et al. (1997) compared post-operative performance of 12 children who demonstrated some open-set speech recognition before cochlear implantation (the borderline candidacy group) with that of 12 matched controls who had no pre-implant speech recognition (the traditional candidacy group). One year after implantation children in the borderline group had significantly higher scores on six speech perception measures. The conclusion was drawn that children with some residual hearing should be considered for cochlear implantation if their speech perception performance is less than that obtained by the average cochlear implant recipient. This is in total agreement with the data presented earlier in the present chapter and with the findings of Kiefer et al. (1998), Yaremko and Gibson (1995) and Cowan et al. (1997). Cowan et al. (1997) reported that 90% of their children with hearing thresholds of 70 dB up to 2 kHz had no pre-operative open-set understanding but after implantation they achieved scores of 20–50% in open-set word understanding. In another study Dolan-Ash et al. (2000) reported the results of 13 borderline candidates ranging in age from five to 14 years with mean pure-tone average (0.5, 1, 2 kHz) thresholds of 96 dB HL and mean aided thresholds of 41 dB HL. All 13 cases showed significant benefit from implantation and the investigators recommended the expansion of candidacy criteria to include children with more residual hearing.

Despite the recommendation from the National Institutes of Health Consensus Development Conference (1995) that children with profound losses greater than 90 dB HL should be considered for cochlear implantation, Geers (1997) questioned the wisdom of including children with losses in the 90–100 dB range and stated that 'We do not recommend an implant for children whose pure-tone average thresholds are less than 100 dB in the better ear regardless of their speech perception scores.' She went on to say that those who were beginning to implant children with hearing thresholds better than 90 dB should carefully evaluate this practice. Despite these cautions numerous workers have now implanted children with severe losses below 90 dB HL including children with unaided hearing thresholds in the 70 dB region (Cowan et al., 1997). Boothroyd's data (1997) from a thorough and well designed study showed that the distribution of scores in the Imitative Test of the Perception of Speech Pattern Contrasts Test (IMSPAC) for implanted children is similar to that of hearing aid users with losses in the 90–99 dB range and only the more successful implant users performed like hearing aid users with 70–89 dB hearing losses. It is apparent that relaxation of the criterion down to 70 dB does, therefore, demand extremely cautious consideration.

Eisenberg et al. (2000) compared open-set speech recognition performance of 'platinum' hearing aid users with that of cochlear implant users and concluded that children with three frequency pure tone averages (0.5, 1 and 2 kHz) between 60 and 82 dB HL produced higher mean scores on all measures than the cochlear implant group after two years experience with their devices. A group with pure tone averages between 82–98 dB yielded lower mean scores than the implanted children with oral backgrounds. They concluded that their findings lend some support to implanting 'select' patients who exhibit more residual hearing than do children who would typically be considered. Unfortunately, the study was performed on only nine hearing aid users and the generalization of their finding must be considered with caution. Even within such a small group one child with a pure tone average of 85 dB HL fitted with digital hearing aids showed performance comparable with the better (60–82 dB) group thus surpassing the performance of the cochlear implanted group.

A multicentre study by Gantz et al. (2000) was only able to include data on six implanted children who had some pre-implant residual hearing ranging from 98 to 120 dB and who had two years experience of cochlear implant use. This group exhibited speech perception scores similar to those of a group of hearing aid users with pure tone averages for 0.5, 1, and 2 kHz of 71 dB HL. The investigators concluded that it would be reasonable to study a larger cohort of children with pre-operative word scores up to 40% in the binaural aided condition. Furthermore, they specified that the children should be at least five years of age so that speech perception test materials are appropriate for their level of language development and implantation should be limited to the poorer ear.

Snik et al. (1997) introduced an interesting concept that they termed 'equivalent hearing loss'. This involved matching the speech perception scores of an individual with reference data based on the auditory speech perception of a group of hearing aid users. Their reference group consisted of 47 severely and profoundly deaf children with averaged hearing losses (0.5, 1, 2 kHz) in the range 70–135 dB and with an age span from four to eight years. When they assessed the performance of three post-meningitic deaf children they found that prior to cochlear implantation, and while using hearing aids, their equivalent hearing loss was above 120 dB HL. Three years after cochlear implantation these same children were performing as well as children in the reference group with a hearing loss of 70–80 dB HL. One-way analysis of variance showed that there was a significant relationship between all the test scores in their battery and the pure tone average thresholds (p<0.02). Their test battery included nine subtests sampling speech discrimination, speech identification and open-set speech recognition. The findings from this study, with data on a relatively large number of hearing aid users, are paralleled by those from the Nottingham studies reported earlier in this chapter.

The notion that speech intelligibility should be taken into consideration when considering borderline implant candidacy was introduced earlier in this chapter and this has also been given some support by Svirsky et al. (2000). These investigators observed that the differences in speech intelligibility as a function of implant use clearly exceed the changes over time predicted for profoundly deaf hearing aid users on the basis of maturation and training, even for hearing aid users with residual hearing in the 90-100 dB range.

Conclusion

It is clear that there is still considerable debate about the expansion of inclusion criteria for cochlear implantation. This debate will no doubt persist but having reviewed the literature it will be apparent to the reader that the Nottingham criterion presented in Section one of this chapter have been derived from large cohorts of child hearing aid users and cochlear implant users. The criteria presented have been derived from thorough investigations over many years and they can safely be applied to babies/children well before the age of five years. For older borderline children the decision as to whether to proceed with cochlear implantation may hinge on the sensitive issues of potential for speech intelligibility improvement and ability to use a telephone.

Very cautious thought should be given to any further relaxation of the criterion in the absence of long-term (at least five years) outcome data on children who have been well fitted with bilateral digital processing hearing aids.

References

Beiter AL, Staller SJ, Dowell RC (1991) Evaluation and device programming in children. Ear and Hearing 12(suppl.4): 25s–33s.

Boothroyd A (1997) Auditory capacity of hearing-impaired children using hearing aids and cochlear implants. Scandinavian Audiology 26(suppl. 46): 17–25.

Boothroyd A, Cawkwell S (1970) Vibrotactile thresholds in pure tone audiometry. Acta Oto-Laryngologica 69: 381–7.

Boothroyd A, Eran O (1994) Auditory speech capacity of child implant users expressed as equivalent hearing loss. Volta Review 96: 151–68.

British Society of Audiology/British Association of Otolaryngologists (1981) Recommended procedure for pure tone audiometry using a manually operated instrument. British Journal of Audiology 15: 213–16.

Carhart R, Jerger JF (1959) Preferred method for clinical determination of pure tone thresholds. Journal of Speech and Hearing Disorders 24: 330–45.

Cowan RSC, Deldot J, Barker EJ (1997) Speech perception results for children with implants with different levels of pre-operative residual hearing. American Journal of Otology 18: S125–S126.

De Filippo CL, Scott BL (1978) A method for training and evaluating the reception of ongoing speech. Journal of the Acoustical Society of America 63: 1186–92.

Dolan-Ash S, Hodges AV, Butts SL, Balkany TJ (2000) Borderline pediatric cochlear implant candidates: pre-operative and post-operative results. Annals of Otology, Rhinology and Laryngology 109(suppl. 185): 36–8.

Eisenberg LS, Martinez AAS, Sennaroglu G, Osberger MJ (2000) Establishing new criteria in selecting children for a cochlear implant: performance of 'platinum' hearing aid users. Annals of Otology, Rhinology and Laryngology 109(suppl. 185): 30–3.

Ertmer D, Kirk KI, Schgal ST, Riley AI, Osberger MJ (1997) A comparison of vowel production by children with multichannel cochlear implants of tactile aids: perceptual evidence. Ear and Hearing 18: 307–15.

Gantz BJ, Rubinstein JT, Tyler RS, Teagle HFB, Cohen NL, Waltzman SB, Miyamoto RT, Kirk KI (2000) Long-term results of cochlear implants in children with residual hearing. Annals of Otology, Rhinology and Laryngology 109(suppl. 185): 33–6.

Geers A (1997) Speech and language evaluation in aided and implanted children. Scandinavian Audiology 26 (suppl 46): 72–5.

Kiefer J, Von Ilberg C, Reimer B, Knecht R, Diller G, Sturzebecher E, Pfennigdorff T, Spelsberg A (1998) Results of cochlear implantation in patients with severe to profound hearing loss-implications for patient selection. Audiology 37: 382–95.

Lenarz T (1998) Cochlear implants: selection criteria and shifting borders. Acta Otorhinolaryngol Belg 52(3): 183–99.

Levitt H (1971) Transformed up-down methods in psychophysics. Journal of the Acoustical Society of America 49: 467–77.

Lipsey MW (1990) Design Sensitivity. Statistical Power for Experimental Research. London: Sage.

McCormick B (1977) The Toy Discrimination Test: an aid for screening the hearing of children above the mental age of two years. Public Health (London) 91: 67–73.

McCormick B (1988) The development of a model paediatric audiology service. In McCormick B, Medicine and Management. Nuffield Provincial Hospital Trust, London, Chapter 8.

McCormick B (ed.) (1993) Paediatric Audiology 0-5 Years. London: Whurr. (Third edition in press for 2002).

McCormick B, Cope Y, Robinson K (1998a) An audiometric criterion for paediatric cochlear implantation. Paper presented at the Seventh Symposium on Cochlear Implants in Children, University of Iowa.

McCormick B, Cope Y, Robinson K (1998b) An audiometric selection criterion for paediatric cochlear implantation. Paper presented at Fourth European Symposium on paediatric Cochlear Implantation, s'Hertogenbosch, The Netherlands.

McCormick B, Wood SA, Cope Y, Spavins FM (1984) Analysis of records from an open-access audiology service. British Journal of Audiology 18: 127-32.

McCormick B, Gibbin KP, Lutman ME, O'Donoghue GM (1993) Late partial recovery from meningitic deafness after cochlear implantation: a case study. American Journal of Otology 14(6): 1-3.

Meyer EA, Svirsky MA, Kirk KI, Miyamoto RT (1998) Improvements in speech perception by children with profound prelingual hearing loss: effects of device, communication mode and chronological age. Journal of Speech, Language and Hearing Research 41: 846-58.

NIH Consensus Statement (1995) Cochlear implants in adults and children. National Institute of Health Consensus Development Conference Statement 13(2): 1-30.

O'Donoghue GM, Nikolopoulos TP, Archbold A, Tait M (1999) Cochlear implants in young children: the relationship between speech perception and speech intelligibility. Ear and Hearing 20(5): 419-25.

Osberger MJ (1997) Cochlear implantation in children under the age of two years: candidacy considerations. Otolaryngol Head Neck Surg 117: 145-9.

Ousey J, Sheppard S, Twomey T, Palmer AR (1989) The IHR/McCormick Automated Toy Discrimination Test: description and initial evaluation. British Journal of Audiology 23: 245-9.

Palmer AR, Sheppard S, Marshall DM (1991) Prediction of hearing thresholds in children using an automated toy discrimination test. British Journal of Audiology 25: 351-6.

Rubinstein JT, Parkinson WS, Tyler RS, Gantz BJ (1999) Residual speech recognition and cochlear implant performance: effects of implantation criteria. The American Journal of Otology 20: 1-7.

Schgal ST, Kirk KI, Svirsky M, Ertmer DJ, Osberger MJ (1998) Imitative consonant feature productions by children with multichannel sensory aids. Ear and Hearing 19: 72-84.

Seewald RC, Cornelisse LE, Ramji KV, Sinclair ST, Moodie KS, Jamieson DGA (1996) Software Implementation of the Desired Sensation Level (DSL i/o) Method for Fitting Linear Gain and Wide-Dynamic-Range Compression Hearing Instruments. Hearing Health Care Research Unit. The University of Western Ontario.

Snik AFM, Vermeulen AM, Brokx JPL, Beijk C, Van Den Broek P (1997) Speech perception performance of children with a cochlear implant compared to that of children with conventional hearing aids. Acta Otolaryngol (Stockh) 117: 750-4.

Summerfield Q, Palmer AR, Foster JR, Marshall DH, Twomey T (1994) Clinical evaluation and test-retest reliability of the IHR/McCormick Automated Toy Discrimination Test. British Journal of Audiology 28: 165-79.

Svirsky MA, Sloan RB, Caldwell M, Miyamoto RT (2000) Speech intelligibility of prelingually deaf children with multichannel cochlear implants. Annals of Otology, Rhinology and Laryngology 109(suppl 185): 123-5.

Tait M, Nikolopoulos TP, Archbold S, O'Donoghue GM (2001) Use of the telephone in prelingually deaf children with a multichannel cochlear implant. Otology and Neurology 22: 47–52.

Tobey E, Geers A, Brenner C (1994) Speech production results: speech feature acquisition. Volta Review 96: 109–30.

Tye-Murray N, Tyler R (1988) A critique of continuous discourse tracking as a test procedure. Journal of Speech and Hearing Disorders 53: 226–31.

Tye-Murray N, Spencer L, Gilbert-Bedia EE (1995) Relationships between speech production and speech perception skills in young cochlear implant users. Journal Acoustical Society of America 98(5): 2454–60.

Tyler R, Holstad B (1987) A Closed-set Speech Perception Test for Hearing-impaired Children. Iowa City: University of Iowa.

Yaremko RL, Gibson WPR (1995) Cochlear implants in deaf children who previously utilised hearing aids successfully or suffered deteriorating loss. Annals of Otology Rhinology and Laryngology 104(suppl. 166): 217–19.

Zwolan TA, Zimmerman-Phillips S, Ashborough CJ, Hieber SJ, Kileny PR, Telian SA (1997) Cochlear implantation of children with minimal open-set speech recognition. Ear and Hearing 18: 240–51.

Chapter 5
Medical and surgical aspects of paediatric cochlear implantation

KEVIN P GIBBIN, GERARD M O'DONOGHUE,
THOMAS P NIKOLOPOULOS

The ultimate clinical and medico-legal responsibility for the welfare of the child undergoing cochlear implantation rests with the surgeon. The final decision to implant is that of the surgeon, although he or she will always be guided by the many other professionals associated with the assessment and future management of candidate children. The surgeon therefore needs to be assured of the quality of advice received from the many colleagues within the cochlear implant team.

The surgeon is also responsible for counselling of parents and carers, as well as the surgical and post-operative care of the child. It is essential, therefore, that the surgeon is intimately involved with the various phases of assessment during the build up towards offering a child an implant. This is particularly important in view of the move towards implantation of very young children. Only limited numbers of children under the age of one have so far been implanted but it is increasingly likely that the age at which cochlear implantation will be carried out will decline, particularly with the introduction of universal newborn hearing screening.

On the assumption that the audiological criteria have been satisfied, there are relatively few medical, radiological or otological reasons why a child should not undergo cochlear implantation. Age in itself should not be the sole factor other than for considerations of neural plasticity – congenitally and pre-lingually deaf children implanted over the age of three or four years tend to do less well than those implanted at a younger age (Lesinski et al., 1997; Waltzman et al., 1997; O'Donoghue et al., 2000). There is no absolute lower age limit for offering an implant to a child and

135

children as young as five months have now been implanted. This issue will be covered more extensively later in this chapter, and other aspects are addressed in other chapters.

Within the Nottingham Programme, audiological assessments are normally carried out as part of the preliminary assessment of a child, see Chapters 3 and 4. At this stage some children will be deemed unsuitable for implantation, either because their hearing is better than that considered appropriate for implantation or because of the lack of an adequate trial of appropriate hearing aids. Once the child has undergone audiological assessment and has been found appropriate for further investigation, radiological imaging will be carried out and the ENT surgeon will subsequently see the child. In a limited number of cases where there are other significant medical problems, the surgeon will see the child at a much earlier stage, with a view to involving his or her paediatric medical and anaesthetic colleagues in the management and decision-making process. It is also important to eliminate, as early as possible, any conductive component to the hearing loss in order to evaluate properly the true sensorineural hearing loss. Children with otitis media with effusion should be treated as appropriate with the insertion of grommets and possibly also adenoidectomy, before final audiological assessment is carried out.

The various factors that the surgeon will take into account in assessing any child for implantation may be summarized as follows:

- the degree and nature of the hearing loss;
- the aetiology of deafness;
- the duration of deafness;
- age at presentation;
- otological assessment (including the management of otitis media with effusion);
- radiological imaging;
- general medical evaluation, including assessment and management of other underlying general medical problems;
- general development assessment, including psychological evaluation where appropriate.

Otological assessment

In carrying out the otological evaluation of the child, a history or clinical signs and symptoms of otitis media with effusion and/or recurrent acute otitis media should be identified and recorded. Clinical examination will be followed by appropriate audiological testing including tympanometry and subsequent surgical management as appropriate. More rarely, there will be a history and findings of chronic suppurative otitis media and active middle-ear disease will require management. Cholesteatoma and other attico-antral disease may need ear exploration and tympanic perforation(s) may require surgical closure.

Radiological assessment

Radiology plays a major part in the assessment of a child for cochlear implantation. It is required in order to assess the cochlear patency and the general morphology of the inner ear, the presence or otherwise of an acoustic nerve, and the integrity of the central auditory pathways.

Historically, cochlear implant candidates were assessed radiologically using polytomography (Becker et al., 1984). However, because of the greater contrast resolution and increased sensitivity in depicting middle- and inner-ear abnormalities offered by high resolution computerized tomography (CT) scan, this became the investigative method of choice (Yune et al., 1991; Souliere et al., 1994). In addition, ultra-high resolution CT, using 1 mm sections, was frequently employed to give increased definition and detail to the areas studied (Phelps et al., 1990; Bath et al., 1993). However, CT scan has low sensitivity in detecting the growth of new bone in the cochlear lumen (cochlear ossification – Figure 5.1) in post-meningitic deafness when the radiological findings are compared with the surgical findings (Nikolopoulos et al., 1997 – Table 5.1).

Table 5.1. Diagnostic values for CT scan when the radiological findings are compared with the surgical findings with regard to cochlear obliteration in 44 post-meningitic children

Accuracy	75.0%
Sensitivity	62.5%
Specificity	82.1%
Positive predictive value	66.6%
Negative predictive value	79.3%

Moreover, a CT scan cannot detect the growth of soft-tissue in the cochlear lumen and has serious limitations in assessing the auditory nerve and the retrocochlear pathways. Therefore,

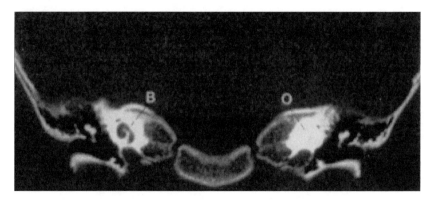

Figure 5.1. Left: partially obliterated cochlea (B). Right: totally obliterated cochlea (O) (high resolution CT scan).

in the Nottingham Programme, the CT scan has been replaced with modern magnetic resonance imaging (MRI) techniques (Constructive Interference in Steady State-CISS) developed initially by Casselman and his colleagues (1993), which allow a pseudo three-dimensional evaluation of the fluid compartments of the inner ear (the presence or otherwise of a normal cochlear lumen) – Figures 5.2 and 5.3.

These techniques also provide the possibility of assessing the development of the cochlea and detecting other congenital anomalies such as large vestibular aqueduct syndrome (Fahy et al., 2001) and other dysplasias (Figures 5.4 and 5.5). Moreover, they provide images of the internal auditory meatus in order to demonstrate the normal bundle of four nerves within the canal (facial nerve, cochlear nerve, superior and inferior vestibular

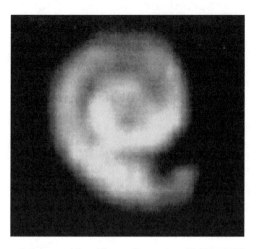

Figure 5.2. Normal right cochlea. Three dimensional MRI (CISS).

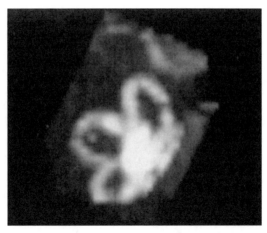

Figure 5.3. Normal vestibule and semicircular canals on three dimensional MRI (CISS).

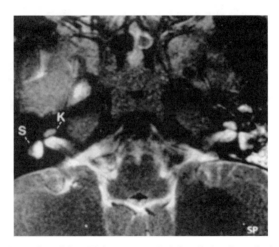

Figure 5.4. Normal cochlea (K) but congenital dysplasia of vestibule / semicircular canals (S) in MRI.

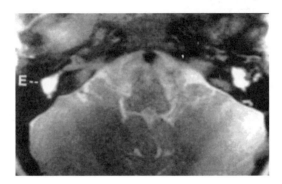

Figure 5.5. Congenital dysplasia of the inner ear (E) (primitive otocyst?) on MRI.

nerves) – Figures 5.6 and 5.7. This is extremely important in congenitally deaf children where a congenital aplasia or dysplasia of the cochlear nerve is suspected (Figure 5.8). In such cases, CT scan can only demonstrate asymmetry or stenosis of the bony internal auditory canal (Figure 5.9).

If when using MRI-CISS techniques it is not possible to identify four nerves in the internal auditory canal, it may be necessary to carry out electrophysiological testing via promontory stimulation in order to determine the presence of eighth nerve transmission. However, only positive results suggest that there is a functioning cochlear nerve whereas negative responses do not have any diagnostic value (Nikolopoulos et al., 2000).

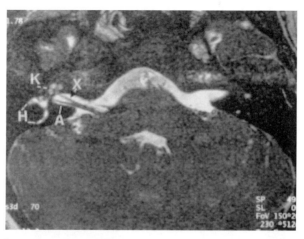

Figure 5.6. Cochlear nerve (X) and common vestibular nerve (A) cochlea (K) and semicircular canals (H) in MRI.

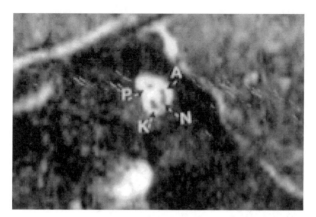

Figure 5.7. MRI (CISS). Right internal auditory canal in vertical plane: cochlear nerve (K), facial nerve (P) sup. vestibular nerve (A) and inf. vestibular nerve (N).

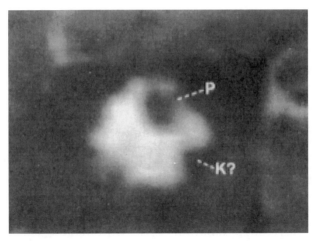

Figure 5.8. Vertical plane of internal auditory canal. Facial nerve (P) with probable aplasia of vestibular nerves and aplasia or dysplasia of cochlear nerve (K?) in MRI (CISS).

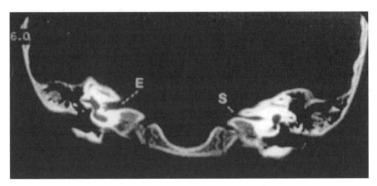

Figure 5.9. Asymmetrical stenotic internal auditory canals. Right (E) wider than the left (S) in CT scan.

If cochlear anomalies or obliteration are detected on MRI scanning, it may also be appropriate to carry out CT scanning in order to have a full radiological picture of the soft tissue and bony architecture of the ear; CT scanning may provide additional information with regard to the bony anatomy of the ear.

Finally, MRI techniques are able to detect the presence of abnormalities in the central pathways that may be crucial to the child's development not only with regard to language and communication skills but also to general motor and psychological development.

In cases of post-meningitic deafness, it is very important to assess the onset and degree of obliteration/ossification of the cochlea using MRI-CISS with or without a CT scan. If such changes are present, cochlear implantation should be considered as a matter of urgency. It is not known how soon after meningitis cochlear obliteration may develop. However, it may behave much like fracture callus after a bony fracture, with ossification starting to develop within a few weeks of the bacteriological insult. Reports have indeed demonstrated that almost complete obliteration of the cochlea may develop within few months following meningitis (Dodds et al., 1997). Therefore, children referred with a history of deafness following meningitis should be admitted through a 'fast-track' system with the radiology being carried out as a first step in the assessment. If these children do not show evidence of cochlear obliteration, regular follow-up scanning should be carried to enable early detection of the onset of such changes. In addition, MRI scanning of children with a history of meningitis may show abnormalities in the central nervous system as a result of the infective process.

For all these issues, close liaison with a neuro-radiologist is of paramount importance in the pre-operative assessment of a child for cochlear implantation.

General medical assessment

Apart from the hearing loss, the majority of the children undergoing cochlear implantation will be otherwise fit and healthy. It should, however, be borne in mind that these children will typically undergo at least two general anaesthetics and sometimes more; a general anaesthetic is required for the performance of MRI scanning in order to keep the child perfectly still. The cochlear implant operation itself requires a lengthy general anaesthetic, which can extend up to three hours. It is essential therefore to be sure that the child is otherwise well, with no other medical problems.

There are few absolute general medical contraindications to cochlear implantation: children with major cardiac and major respiratory disease have been successfully implanted within the Nottingham Paediatric Cochlear Implant Programme. It is in examples such as these that close liaison is required with the general medical paediatricians and of course with the paediatric anaesthetist. Such liaison is inherent in all paediatric surgical practice and the surgical team will liaise closely in the management of children. The surgical team includes the surgeon, the paediatric physician, paediatric anaesthetist, the ward staff, operating theatre and recovery staff.

Clearly, a small number of children may need their operation deferred if there is intercurrent disease at the time of the planned surgery and this intercurrent disease may be general medical, upper and lower respiratory infection, or may be otological – otitis media particularly. In these instances surgery will be deferred, appropriate treatment will be instituted and the child will be brought back for surgery once the intercurrent condition has been resolved.

General development/additional disabilities

The general development of the deaf child – neurological, motor, psychological, behavioural and social – may have serious implications for the development of communication skills and spoken language following implantation. Moreover, it is important that the child should be able to co-operate with the tuning, the rehabilitation process, and the various assessments involved before and after implantation. However, one of the most important extensions that has been made in the last years with regard to paediatric cochlear implant candidacy is the inclusion of deaf children with additional handicaps and disorders (Lenarz, 1998). The benefit that these children obtain from cochlear implantation has been confirmed although the rate of growth of perceptual skills is slower than that of the other deaf implanted children (Waltzman, Scalchunes and Cohen, 2000). The number of such candidates is expected to be quite considerable as it is well documented that additional disabilities are common in deaf children. In 1979, Martin assessed 3,000 pupils in schools for the deaf, in European Community countries, and found that 29% had other disabilities and 10% were mentally impaired (Martin, 1979). Another more recent study in UK found that almost 40% of hearing-impaired children had educationally relevant disabilities (Fortnum et al., 1996). Of course each child with additional disorders should be carefully evaluated from all the specialties involved (including paediatricians, neurologists, psychologists, and so forth) and the decision whether to proceed with implantation should be taken on an individual basis after extensive counselling of parents and carers in order to have realistic expectations. In general, such children should not be denied cochlear implantation even though the perceived benefits may be less evident or delayed. The acquisition of a limited vocabulary and the development of basic spoken language in a child with additional handicaps may contribute to a significant improvement in the child and family's quality of life, although the scoring in routine assessment tests may be poor.

It is perhaps not necessary for all paediatric candidates for cochlear implantation to be formally examined by a paediatric psychologist and neurologist, relying instead on the collective skills of the other members of the cochlear implant team. The otologists of the team usually have a wide experience in paediatric medical practice and similarly with the educators, speech and language therapists and others involved in the assessment (Gibbin, 1992). If any member of the team identifies a cause for concern, referral for formal pyschological evaluation should be arranged. In the case of the older, school-age child, an educational psychologist's report is sought.

A psychological and neurological assessment may be particularly important after meningitis. It should be remembered that meningitis may cause other brain injury, covert as well as overt, such damage sometimes being demonstrable radiologically although the findings in MRI scan may not be directly related to the clinical symptoms and signs (Pikis et al., 1996; Muller-Jensen, Harvarik and Valk, 1997). One example from the Nottingham Programme is of a child deafened by meningitis who developed good sound perception following cochlear implantation but who failed to develop spoken language skills even many years following implantation. Assessment by a clinical psychologist suggested that the child had developed a specific language disorder as a sequel of meningitis, which had only become revealed following cochlear implantation. Although suspicions were present, this condition could not be confirmed prior to implantation.

Aetiology of deafness

The cause of deafness very rarely makes a child unsuitable for cochlear implantation. One of the few such cases is the child with bilateral absence of the cochlear nerve. However, aetiology of deafness may be extremely important in all the phases of cochlear implantation; children with meningitis should be regularly monitored for cochlear ossification and thoroughly evaluated for additional neurological problems as a sequel from meningitis; those deafened after head injury with temporal bone fractures may have facial nerve problems; children with congenital or progressive hearing loss may have other dysplasias or disorders not necessarily as part of a particular syndrome. Those in whom a specific syndrome has been diagnosed may need different management in terms of anaesthesia, surgery and rehabilitation; those with acquired deafness due to chronic otitis media or previous operations may need modification of the cochlear implant surgery or even surgery in two stages. However difficult, time consuming or expensive is the identification of the cause of deafness, it may be very rewarding in terms of counselling, setting realistic expectations and planning surgery, and appropriate (re)habilitation. The most common factors that have been associated with severe and profound deafness in children are illustrated in Table 5.2 (Billings and Kenna, 1999; Rosen, 1999).

In a lot of cases the diagnosis is evident and has already been made before the referral to the cochlear implant programme, or the 'unknown' cause is supported by thorough evaluation coordinated by the local ENT consultant. In several instances, however, important clues from the history have not attracted proper attention and appropriate tests have not been carried out. In such cases the ENT surgeon of the cochlear implant programme has to thoroughly evaluate the child and ask for tests and referrals to other specialties.

Table 5.2. Factors or disorders associated with severe and profound deafness in children

Congenital malformations/syndromes/craniofacial dysplasias
Family history/genetics
Birth factors: prematurity, hypoxemia, elevated bilirubin levels, etc.
Maternal factors: substance abuse, placental abruption, toxemia, etc.
Infections: toxoplasmosis, rubella, cytomegalovirus, herpes, mumps, other
Extracorporeal membrane oxygenation
Chronic otitis media/surgical operations
Head injury/temporal bone fractures
Neurologic abnormalities: cerebral palsy, seizures, etc.
Meningitis/encephalitis
Ototoxic agents

Genetic assessment and its clinical/medical implications

Sometimes the difference between congenital and inherited deafness is confusing. Congenital simply means 'present at birth'; therefore deafness from maternal rubella is congenital but certainly not inherited. Conversely, a significant cause of hereditary deafness is that of autosomal non-syndromic delayed-onset. Individuals who are affected by this disorder are born with normal hearing and then begin to lose hearing between the second and third decade of life (Tomaski and Grundfast, 1999). Therefore genetic assessment should not be considered only in congenitally deaf children but in all children with an 'unknown' cause of deafness.

Approximately 80% of hereditary deafness is inherited as an autosomal recessive trait, 18% autosomal dominant, and 2% X-linked recessive (Grundfast, 1993). Approximately 200 genes have been estimated to be involved in hereditary deafness and significant progress is being made in locating these genes; more than 65 have been already identified and some of these are very common such as connexin 26 (Tranebjaerg, 2000).

Hereditary deafness can be syndromic (with associated anomalies in various organ systems such as the craniofacial, skeletal, ocular, neurological, renal, cardiovascular, or integumentary systems; anomalies that are part of a recognizable syndrome) and non-syndromic (isolated deafness without associated findings). Two thirds of cases of hereditary deafness are non-syndromic and one third of cases are syndromic (Tomaski and Grundfast, 1999; Mhatre and Lalwani, 1996; Grundfast, 1993).

Identification of hereditary deafness may be very important for parental counselling, family planning and setting realistic expectations. In syndromic deafness, identification of the particular syndrome and the organ systems involved may be very useful in order to manage properly the associated disorders; for example in the Nottingham Programme all deaf children routinely have ophthalmological assessment in order to identify Usher's syndrome and other visual disorders, and electro-cardiographic/cardiologic evaluation before their first general anaesthesia to exclude Jervell-Lange-Neilson syndrome or other cardiac anomalies. Moreover, various syndromes may have an effect on surgery itself; for example Klippel-Feil deformity could make a surgical approach to the cochlea difficult (Graham, Phelps and Michaels, 2000) and Pendred syndrome with large vestibular aqueduct could cause a perilymph leak during surgery although usually not very serious (Fahy et al., 2001). Finally, other associated neurologic and other medical conditions may have an effect in post-operative management and (re)habilitation as they could delay language development.

Counselling

Counselling of parents and carers of children who are candidates for cochlear implantation is an essential component of pre-operative work. This is an ongoing process and is not confined to one single episode during the assessment process. It is essential that all members of the team provide clear and consistent ongoing advice at all stages, although there is a clear onus of responsibility on the surgeon to ensure that the advice and counselling has been appropriate for the individual family, and that the family is fully aware of the long-term commitment required and the risks as outlined in the appendix. The surgeon and other members of the team need to be able to discuss practical, moral and ethical issues. Practical issues centre around the various assessments that the child will undergo during the process, including the medical, radiological and other investigations. Ethical and moral issues may be wide ranging and particular sensitivity is required in the case of profoundly deaf children of deaf parents. The other group of children for whom special sensitivity is required is that group of children whose hearing loss has been caused following meningitis. Parents of this particular group of children will already have had stressful dealings with hospitals and many will have experienced life-threatening illness as a result of the meningitis.

Parents need to be aware that cochlear implantation is not just the performance of an operation, but is very much a long-term commitment requiring integration of the skills of many professionals and the involvement of very many people, not only those within the immediate family. Counselling needs to ensure that parental expectation is realistic and parents should be given the opportunity of meeting other families whose children have already received a cochlear implant. Full and detailed literature should be made available to the families to give them the opportunity to reflect fully and comprehensively on the various issues.

Surgery

Consent for surgery

It is the clear and unambiguous responsibility of the surgeon to ensure that parents, and in the case of older children, the children themselves, are given a clear and detailed account of the risks of surgery and the possible complications, as well as the benefits that such surgery may bestow. Parents should be aware that neither the surgical outcome, nor any possible long-term benefits can be guaranteed. However, the record of the individual surgeon should help inform the parents of the likely result of the surgical procedure. The principles of Clinical Governance, the process by which doctors can demonstrate that best practice is being followed, should help reassure the parents and ensure that the trust they place in the surgeon is well founded. Finally, the surgeon must be aware of any legal requirements that influence the treatment and management of the child and family.

Pre-operative preparation

Once the decision to offer a cochlear implant has been taken, the date for surgery is set and arrangements are made for the child to be admitted. Children are usually admitted the day prior to surgery or on the day of surgery, at which stage the final assessment by the anaesthetist will be carried out and any final questions that the child or family may have can be answered. It is important to ensure that the child has no evidence of other intercurrent infection either in the ears or respiratory tract. In the small number of cases where this occurs, the surgery may need to be deferred. It is the practice of the Nottingham team to ensure that, if surgery is cancelled at a late stage, other parents are contacted in an endeavour to ensure that the operating 'slot' is not lost or wasted. It is important that any child for major surgery, such as cochlear implantation, is prepared in advance of the admission both physically and psychologically. The latter may be effected in a variety of ways, including provision of booklets and even dummy implants for the child's teddy to use.

The decision as to which side should be implanted will have been taken at a late stage in the evaluation process. A number of factors may determine which ear is to be implanted, such as residual hearing, hearing aid use and preference. Factors include radiological anomalies, contraindicating implantation of one or other ear, and otological abnormalities such as chronic infection and audiological factors. It is a general rule in otological surgery, when there is a choice of which ear to operate on, to select the worse hearing ear. However this rule does not always apply in cochlear implantation and there is still a considerable debate in the literature with regard to which ear should be implanted: the better or the poorer hearing ear. This is discussed in detail in Chapter 4.

The operation

Most children will receive pre-anaesthetic medication between one and two hours prior to the actual operation. One or other parent will usually accompany the child to the anaesthetic room and will be allowed to stay until the child is anaesthetized. A variety of surgical incisions and flaps may be used for cochlear implantation, including the extended endaural incision (the Hannover incision), the extended post-auricular incision, the straight oblique post-aural incision, the C-shaped incision, and the inverted U incision (Figures 5.10–5.14).

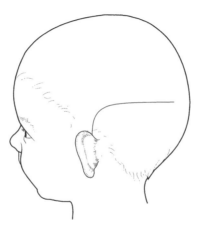

Figure 5.10. Diagram showing the extended endaural incision.

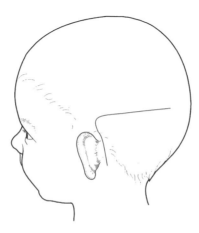

Figure 5.11. Diagram showing the extended post-auricular incision.

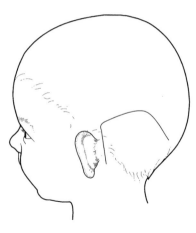

Figure 5.12. Diagram showing the inferior based inverted U flap.

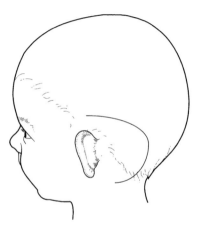

Figure 5.13. Diagram showing the anteriorly based C-shaped flap.

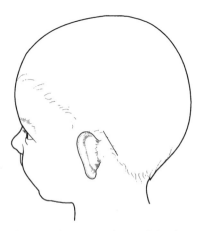

Figure 5.14. Diagram showing the Nottingham minimal access incision.

The head shave should now be obsolete and indeed the straight oblique post-aural incision requires no hair shaving. It is routine practice within the Nottingham Programme to attach facial nerve monitoring electrodes in order to be able to carry out monitoring during the whole operative period. Figures 5.15, 5.16, and 5.17 illustrate the operating theatre and the surgical team required.

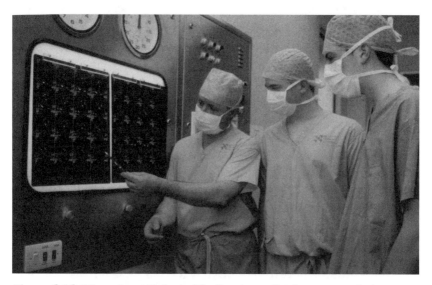

Figure 5.15. Discussing radiological findings immediately pre-operatively.

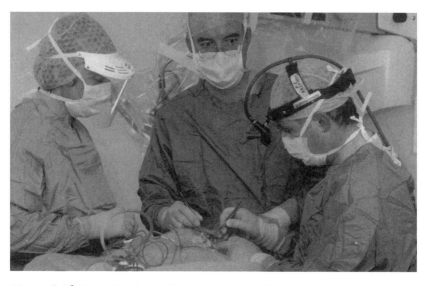

Figure 5.16. Preparing the site for the receiver package.

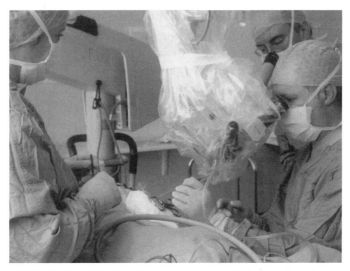

Figure 5.17. Much of the implant surgery is carried out using the operating microscope.

The operation and device testing typically take up to three hours, including time spent carrying out any perioperative electrophysiological testing. A simple mastoidectomy is performed. Then a well is created behind the mastoid to accommodate the receiver-stimulator portion of the internal device. The role of this well is to minimize protrusion, to reduce vulnerability to external trauma, and to restrict device movement, which can shear connecting leads. Through a careful posterior tympanotomy the facial recess is opened to visualize the incudostapedial joint, the promontory, and if possible the round window. The scala tympani may be opened in one of two ways: directly through the round window membrane or indirectly through the promontory. The latter approach involves a cochleostomy through the promontory, antero-inferior to the round window. After the cochleostomy is opened, the electrode array is advanced under direct visualization. If resistance to insertion is encountered, the array should be retracted slightly, rotated medially, and carefully advanced. Because buckling of the implant can produce damage to the cochlea aggressive insertion attempts should be avoided. Full insertion of the array within the basal turn of the cochlea represents an insertion depth of 25 to 30 mm, depending on array length (Figures 5.18 and 5.19).

For this depth, those electrodes placed deepest (apically) in the cochlea approach spiral ganglion cells subserving frequencies from 0.5 kHz to 1 kHz. The electrodes that are closer to the

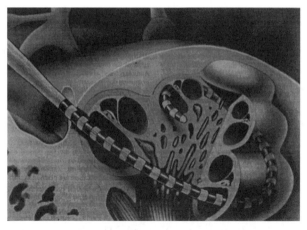

Figure 5.18. The electrodes of Nucleus implant system in place (scala tympani).

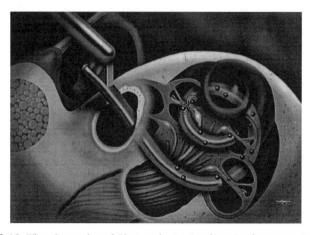

Figure 5.19. The electrodes of Clarion device in place (scala tympani).

(basal) insertion site lie adjacent to neurones subserving the highest frequency ranges of human hearing and convey higher formant information.

It is routine practice to close the wound with absorbent sutures placed under the skin obviating the need for suture removal. A firm crepe head bandage is usually placed on the head and left overnight following the operation, being removed the following morning.

Complications and other surgical considerations in children

In experienced hands, serious surgical complications are few (Johnson, Gibbin and O'Donoghue, 1997). A concern that parents have prior to implantation is the risk of facial nerve injury. No permanent facial nerve palsy has occurred within the Nottingham Programme with more than 300 children currently implanted. A great concern of any surgeon carrying out implant surgery is the risk of wound infection and flap necrosis. All operations carry the risk of possible wound infection but this becomes of great concern when implanting a foreign body, whether this be a cochlear implant, hip replacement prosthesis or pacemaker. If major infection supervenes in any of these cases, then, despite the use of modern powerful antibiotics, it may become necessary to remove the device in order to allow the infection to resolve. Such an instance has occurred within the Nottingham Programme twice in over 300 operations. Therefore the risk is less than 0.6% and this includes both immediate and long-term post-operative follow-up. Careful planning of the operation, an experienced surgical team, aseptic operative conditions, and close post-operative follow-up are essential to keep the rate of complications low. Other minor early post-operative complications like wound oedema, flap swelling, and haematoma are more common (reaching 4% of the 300 cases operated within the Nottingham Programme) but usually settle with no or conservative treatment.

Meningitis following cochlear implantation is rare despite the theoretical risk that a cochlear implant could act as a conduit for the spread of infection from the middle ear to the labyrinth. Middle-ear malformations like common cavity and Mondini dysplasia may increase this risk. However, very few cases of meningitis following cochlear implantation have been described (Daspit, 1991; Page and Eby, 1997); one possible case has been encountered in the Nottingham series.

The high prevalence of acute otitis media and otitis media with effusion in young children raises concerns about subsequent complications following cochlear implantation. The evidence is that the incidence of otitis media with effusion is lower in implanted children than non-implanted children and, interestingly, it seems to be the non-implanted ear that is more commonly affected (Cohen and Hoffman, 1993). The same was found with regard to acute otitis media as its incidence and severity decreased following implantation (Luntz et al., 1996). It has been suggested that the cortical mastoidectomy and removal of large areas of mucosa in the mastoid during cochlear implantation reduces the risk of post-operative mastoiditis and inflammation (Lenarz, 1997). Nonetheless, post-operative infections, especially in the vulnerable period during the healing process after implantation, should be immediately treated with antibiotics and carefully followed up. In addition, if persistent otitis media with effusion or recurrent acute otitis media is present during the pre-surgical evaluation of the child, grommet insertion and adenoidectomy at an early stage should be considered before proceeding with cochlear implantation because the rate of operative complication seems to increase if effusion is present at the peri-implantation time (Papsin et al., 1996).

Concern has been raised regarding the size of the skull and its growth in very young children both in respect of possible surgical difficulties and subsequent distraction of electrodes from within the cochlea as the child grows up. It is well known that the inner and middle ears are adult size at birth and the facial recess is also fully developed in neonates (Dahm et al., 1993). Therefore, surgery in children does not differ substantially from that in adults. However, the surgeon has to accommodate the relatively larger size of the receiver-stimulator portion of the internal device to a thinner scalp and calrarium; exposure of dura is sometimes needed. In addition, the significant post-natal growth of the mastoid and the external auditory canal should be taken into account so as the array fixation will allow up to 25 mm leadwire lengthening (O'Donoghue et al., 1986; Dahm et al., 1993). Otherwise, the operation is the same in children and adults. However, two common problems in childhood – post-meningitic ossification and congenital anomalies – need further consideration.

The surgical technique used for implantation of the ossified cochlea is a variation of the conventional technique. After the usual transmastoid-facial recess approach and confirmation of an ossified basal turn, the proximal cochlear turn is drilled with a microdrill to a depth of 6 to 8 mm. Further drilling has the risk of perforating the carotid artery. However, in certain cases with partial obliteration, after removal of a proximal segment of bony obstruction in the scala tympani, an open scalar lumen is discovered and full insertion of the electrode array can be accomplished. If this is not the case, there are further options:

- insertion of a limited number of electrodes into the lumen that was created through drilling;
- insertion of the electrode array into the scala vestibule through a cochleostomy anterior to the oval window;

- insertion of a double array cochlear implant; one array in the basal turn through the first cochleostomy (round window) and one array in the middle turn through a second cochleostomy (anterior to the oval window);
- insertion of the electrode array (single or double) through a middle fossa approach (Colletti, 1999), and other more extensive surgical techniques like the one proposed by Gantz et al. (1988) that creates a circum-modiolar trough for the electrode array.

Children with congenital deafness represent an increasingly large percentage of candidates for cochlear implantation and have become the majority of implanted children in our programme. Some children with deafness of congenital onset will exhibit a cochlear malformation. Common congenital malformations are the Mondini deformity in which the cochlea has a normal basal turn and a distal sac and the common cavity in which the cochlea and vestibule form a common cavity.

In some congenital malformations there is only a thin bony partition between the modiolus and the widened internal auditory canal (Jackler et al., 1987). The latter anomaly accounts for the cerebrospinal fluid leak that can occur when performing a cochleostomy for electrode insertion and the surgeon should be prepared for this problem during the operation. Other anomalies involving the round window niche and facial nerve have been observed in association with cochlear malformations (House and Luxford, 1993; Tucci et al., 1995). Despite associated anomalies, implantation of a significant number of electrodes (and often full insertion) within a malformed cochlea is feasible and can provide open-set speech perception in the majority of subjects (Niparko et al., 1998).

Moreover, special devices for certain malformations (for example, common cavity) have been developed in order to increase surgical safety and better functional results.

Total device failure may occur, but this is uncommon and has been encountered in less than 4% in the Nottingham series. In all cases, the faulty device was surgically replaced without any loss of functional performance. Partial failures (for example, of individual electrodes) or intermittent failure/malfunction are more common and require careful and regular tuning by experienced paediatric audiological scientists in order to sustain the maximum benefit from the device.

Post-operative care

Immediately following surgery, the child is brought to the recovery bay for initial post-operative care; nurses in the recovery suite need to be reminded that the child is deaf. The presence of the parents at an early stage during this period can be invaluable. This is the usual time for the surgeon to explain to the parents the relevant details of the operation. If the electrophysiological tests have been satisfactorily undertaken, confirmation of the functional integrity of the system can be conveyed to the parents.

The pressure dressing, which is aimed at preventing haematoma (a collection of blood clot) forming under the skin flap, is usually left in place overnight, being removed the following morning. In most implant centres it is standard practice to provide antibiotic cover during the operative period and this is usually given by intravenous cannula. This can be removed, typically the morning after implantation, once the child is eating and drinking satisfactorily. Implant surgery is not painful, requiring a simple analgesic such as paracetamol. Most children leave hospital within 24 hours of the surgery.

While the child remains on the ward, it is imperative that all members of staff should be aware of the particular communication difficulties of profoundly deaf children and also aware of the stress that any such surgery poses on the parents and family. It is important that the ward staff are educated about implant surgery to ensure that no misinformed comment is made to parents. The comments of a well-intentioned, but poorly informed professional, such as a junior nurse or junior doctor can have devastating consequences for the emotionally charged parent during this period.

On the morning following surgery, a check radiograph is taken (reverse Stenvers x-ray). This radiograph confirms satisfactory placement of the electrode array and provides a useful pictorial baseline of the position of the implant for possible future reference. An experienced radiographer who is prepared to communicate appropriately with the deaf child is a great help.

Communication

It is essential that all involved in the care of a child should know what is happening during the operative period and hospital stay. Clear and detailed discharge summaries should be sent to the family doctor and all local professionals, and in the case of children referred to the implant centre from elsewhere, to the local ENT surgeon. The standard practice of the Nottingham team is to arrange for a post-operative check locally approximately a week following surgery and a further medical check is scheduled at the implant centre approximately one month after the operation, at which point the external components are fitted and the tuning process begins.

The implant warranty must be completed and returned to the manufacturer. It is important that patient confidentiality be respected when completing this documentation.

The surgeon also has the responsibility to remind parents about the possible medical hazards associated with implantation. In particular they should be reminded of the child's inability to have MRI scanning, although it has been suggested that some devices are MRI compatible using weak MRI imagers and appropriate safety procedures (Teissi et al., 1998). It is also very important to make the parents and carers aware about the harmful effects of monopolar diathermy at any site on the body. It is the practice of the Nottingham team to offer all children a Medic Alert bracelet or necklace, which provides a telephone number accessible 24 hours a day to provide key information to any physician who may be about to undertake emergency treatment of a child with an implant.

Conclusions

The decision to implant is an exercise in collective decision making by experienced professionals in close discussion with parents, carers and, when possible, the child. The surgeon carries ultimate clinical responsibility for the care of the child and must be intimately involved in the whole decision-making process. The surgeon's role and responsibilities are clearly defined, ethically, morally and legally. Problems arising from cochlear implantation in young children are few, provided experienced surgeons undertake such surgery. Close involvement of parents and carers in the whole process is paramount. On the rare occasions that a complication occurs, it is particularly important to be completely open and honest with the family. An implant requires a lifetime commitment and should only be undertaken by those who have a genuine long-term professional commitment to these patients.

Appendix: risks/complications to be considered by parents

- *Infection of the wound:* this may resolve with medical treatment; the device may need to be removed.
- *Facial weakness:* a small risk of this attends any ear surgery. Most cases of weakness following implantation are transient.
- *Balance symptoms:* usually transient.
- *Taste disturbance:* an uncommon complication for a few weeks following surgery.
- *Device failure:* total implant failure may occur, but this is uncommon (less than 4% in Nottingham). It is usually possible to replace the implanted device without any loss of performance. Partial failures (for example, of individual electrodes) or intermittent failure/malfunction are more common.
- *Risk of meningitis with middle-ear infection:* this is a very uncommon occurence following implantations; vaccination is advised.
- *Electrochemical damage to the ear from long-term electrical stimulation.* The effects appear to be minimal based on current knowledge if the stimulation is appropriate.
- *Head growth:* fears that the electrode array would be pulled out of the cochlea due to head growth have not been founded in practice.
- *Limitation on certain activities:* activities that could damage or displace the device (such as rugby, boxing, squash) are best avoided. Swimming is possible if the external parts are removed.
- *Electrostatic damage:* this is possible and leaflets with appropriate information and precautions should be given to parents/carers/children.

Note: Normally only one ear will be implanted. This leaves the other ear available to benefit from future developments – bilateral implants may be a future option.

References

Bath AP, O'Donoghue GM, Holland IM, Gibbin KP (1993) Paediatric cochlear implantation: how reliable is computed tomography in assessing cochlear patency? Clin Otolaryngol 18: 475-9.

Becker TS, Eisenberg LS, Luxford WM, House WF (1984) Labyrinthine ossification secondary to childhood bacterial meningitis: implications for cochlear implant surgery. Am J Neuro Radiol 5: 739-71.

Billings KR, Kenna MA (1999) Causes of pediatric sensorineural hearing loss. Yesterday and today. Arch Otolaryngol Head Neck Surg 125: 517-21.

Casselman JW, Kuhweide R, Deimling M, Ampe W, Dehaene I, Meeus L (1993) Three-dimensional Fourier tranformation MR technique – constructive interference in steady state. Am J Neuroradiol 14(1): 47-57.

Cohen NL, Hoffman RA (1993) Surgical complications of multichannel cochlear implants in North America. Adv Oto-Rhino-Laryngol 43: 70-4.

Colletti V (1999) Improved auditory performance of cochlear implant patients using the middle fossa approach. Audiology 38(4): 225-34.

Dahm MC, Shepherd RK, Clark GM (1993) The postnatal growth of the temporal bone and its implications for cochlear implantation in children. Acta Otolaryngol suppl. 505: 1-39.

Daspit CP (1991) Meningitis as a result of a cochlear implant: case report. Otolaryngol Head Neck Surg 105(1): 115-16.

Dodds A, Tyszkiewicz E, Ramsden R (1997) Cochlear implantation after bacterial meningitis: the danger of delay. Arch Dis Child 76: 139-40.

Fahy CP, Carney AS, Nikolopoulos TP, Ludman CN, Gibbin KP (2001) Cochlear implantation in children with large vestibular aqueduct and a review of the syndrome. Intern J Pediatr Otorhinolaryngol 59: 207-15.

Fortnum H, Davis A, Butler A, Stevens J (1996) Health sevice implications of changes in aetiology and referral patterns of hearing impaired children in Trent 1985-1993. Report to Trent Health. Nottingham and Sheffield: MRC Institute of Hearing Research and Trent Health.

Gantz BJ, McCabe BF, Tyler RS (1988) Use of multichannel cochlear implants in obstructed and obliterated cochleas. Otolaryngol Head Neck Surg 98: 72-81.

Gibbin KP (1992) Paediatric cochlear implantation. Arch Dis Child 67(6): 669-71.

Graham JM, Phelps PD, Michaels L (2000) Congenital malformations of the ear and cochlear implantation in children: review and temporal bone report of common cavity. J Laryngol Otol Suppl 25: 1-14.

Grundfast KM (1993) Hereditary hearing impairment in children. Adv Otolaryngol Head Neck Surg 7: 29-43.

House J, Luxford W (1993) Facial nerve injury in cochlear implantation. Otolaryngol Head Neck Surg 109: 1078.

Jackler RK, Luxford WM, Schindler RA, Mckerrow WS (1987) Cochlear patency problems in cochlear implantation. Laryngoscope 97: 801-5.

Johnson IJ, Gibbin KP, O'Donoghue GM (1997) Surgical aspects of cochlear implantation in young children: a review of 115 cases. Am J Otol 18(6 Suppl): S69-70.

Lenarz T (1997) Cochlear implantation in children under the age of two years. In Honjo I, Takahashi H (eds) Cochlear Implant and Related Sciences Update. Adv Otorhinolaryngol. Basel. Karger 52: 204-10.

Lenarz T (1998) Cochlear implants: selection criteria and shifting borders. Acta Otorhinolaryngol Belg 52(3):183-99.

Lesinski A., Battmer R-D, Bertram B., Lenarz T (1997) Appropriate age for cochlear implantation in children – Experience since 1986 with 359 implanted children. In Honjo I, Takahashi H (eds) Cochlear Implant and Related Sciences Update. Adv Otorhinolaryngol 52: 214-17.

Luntz M, Hodges AV, Balkany T, Dolan-Ash S, Schloffman J (1996) Otitis media in children with cochlear implants. Laryngoscope 106(11): 1403-5.

Martin JAM (1979) Childhood Deafness in the European Community. Brussels/Luxembourg: Commission of the European Communities.

Mhatre AN, Lalwani AK (1996) Molecular genetics of deafness. Otolaryngol Clin North Am 29: 421-35.

Muller-Jensen A, Harvarik R, Valk J (1997) Bilateral white matter lesions following severe meningococcal meningoencephalitis. Neuroradiology 39(1): 23-4.

Nikolopoulos TP, O'Donoghue GM, Robinson KL, Holland IM, Gibbin KP (1997) Preoperative radiological evaluation in cochlear implantation. Am J Otol 18(6): supplement: s73-s74.

Nikolopoulos TP, Mason SM, O'Donoghue GM, Gibbin KP (2000) The prognostic value of Promontory EABR. Ear and Hearing 21(3): 236-41.

Niparko J (1998) Cochlear Implants, Auditory Brainstem Implants, and Surgically-Implantable Hearing Aids. In Cummings et al. (Eds.) Otolaryngology/Head & Neck Surgery, London.

O'Donoghue GM, Jackler RK, Jenkins WM, ScIndler RA (1986) Cochlear implantation in children. The problem of head growth. Otolaryngol Head Neck Surg 94(1): 78-81.

O'Donoghue GM, Nikolopoulos TP, Archbold S (2000) Determinants of speech perception in children following cochlear implantation.The Lancet 356(9228): 466-8.

Page EL, Eby TL (1997) Meningitis after cochlear implantation in Mondini malformation. Otolaryngol Head Neck Surg 116(1): 104-6.

Papsin BC, Bailey CM, Albert DM, Bellman SC (1996) Otitis media with effusion in paediatric cochlear implantees: the role of peri-implant grommet insertion. Int J Pediatr Otorhinolaryngol 38(1): 13-9.

Phelps PD, Annis JAD, Robinson RJ (1990) Imaging for cochlear implants. Br J Radiol 63: 512-16.

Pikis A, Kavaliotis J, Tsikoulas J, Andrianopoulos P, Venzon D, Manios S (1996) Long-term sequelae of pneumococcal meningitis in children. Clin Pediatr (Phila) 35(2): 72-8.

Rosen NJ (1999) Etiology of hearing loss in children. Pediatr Clin North Am 46 (1): 49-64.

Souliere CR, Quigley SM, Langman AW (1994) Cochlear implants in children. In Isaacson G (ed.) Pediatric Otology. Otolaryngol Clin N Am 27(3): 533-54.

Teissi C, Kremser C, Hochmair ES (1998) Cochlear implants: in vitro investigation of electromagnetic interference in MRI imaging – compatibility and safety aspects. Radiology 208: 700-8.

Tomaski SM, Grundfast KM (1999) A stepwise approach to the diagnosis and treatment of hereditary hearing loss. Pediatr Clin N Am 46(1): 35-48.

Tranebjaerg L (2000) Genetic causes of hearing loss–status and perspectives. Ugeskr Laeger 22; 162(21): 3044-51.

Tucci D et al. (1995) Cochlear implantation in patients with cochlear malformations. Arch Otolaryngol Head Neck Surg 121: 833.

Waltzman SB, Cohen NL, Gomolin RH, Green JE, Shapiro WH, Hoffman RA, Roland JT-Jr (1997) Open-set speech perception in congenitally deaf children using cochlear implants. Am J Otol 18: 342-9.

Waltzman SB, Scalchunes V, Cohen NL (2000) Performance of multiply handicapped children using cochlear implants. Am J Otol 21(3):329-35.

Yune HY, Miyamato RT, Yune ME (1991) Medical imaging in cochlear implant candidates. Am J Otol 12: 11-17.

Chapter 6
Electrophysiological and objective measures

STEVE MASON

Introduction

Cochlear implantation is an effective form of management of profoundly deafened patients who obtain little or no benefit from conventional amplification (House, 1991; O'Donoghue, 1999). In recent years the number of very young children receiving cochlear implants has increased significantly as the efficacy and benefits of early implantation become apparent. The assessment and management of young children requires more specialized skills and test techniques when compared with the implantation of adult patients (Gibbin, 1992; McCormick, 1997). Objective and electrophysiological tests have a valuable role to play in the management of young children both before and after implantation using acoustical and electrical stimulation. The transfer from conventional acoustical stimulation of the cochlea to the electrical modality has led to the development of a wide range of electrically evoked potentials and associated objective measures (Kileny, 1991; Mason, 1997; Shallop, 1997). Many of these techniques have been implemented in the Nottingham Paediatric Cochlear Implant Programme (NPCIP) and will be described in this chapter.

Overview

Historical aspects

The functioning of the auditory system at different levels of the pathway has been extensively investigated in both man and animals from recordings of electrical activity evoked by sounds.

162

The electroencephalogram (EEG) was first recorded from the intact scalp in humans by Berger in 1929, and Berger (1930) described changes in the rhythm of the EEG to loud sounds. P A Davis (1939) and H Davis et al. (1939) subsequently described more specific changes in the EEG. This was the birth of electric response audiometry (ERA). Since that time electrical responses evoked by auditory stimuli have been recorded from the entire length of the auditory pathway (Picton et al., 1974; Abbas, 1988).

In 1957, Djourno and Eyries first reported a device that could directly stimulate the cochlea and, since then, many investigators have studied the electrically generated sensation of hearing. Early studies of evoked potentials to electrical stimulation were reported in guinea pigs (Meikle et al., 1977) and in humans (Starr and Brackmann, 1979). The requirement to have a method of objective evaluation of young children with cochlear implants has led to considerable interest in the application of electrophysiological tests and other associated objective measures in recent years.

Electrophysiological and objective measures

Auditory evoked potentials, similar to those associated with conventional ERA, can be recorded using electrical stimulation. In ascending order through the auditory system these include the electrically evoked compound auditory nerve action potential (ECAP), auditory brainstem response (EABR), middle latency response (EMLR), auditory cortical response (EACR), and event-related potentials (EERP) (Miyamoto, 1986; Pelizzone et al., 1989; Shallop et al., 1990; Kileny, 1991; Mason, 1993). It is common convention to introduce a leading 'E' for electrical stimulation to denote electrically evoked responses (for example EABR for ABR) and to use 'e' to label an electrically evoked component (for example eV for wave V of the ABR). This form of terminology will be used throughout this chapter.

In addition to these electrophysiological responses, there are other important objective measures that form part of the test battery for implanted young children. The electrically evoked stapedius reflex (ESR) (Battmer et al., 1990; Stephan et al., 1991), back-telemetry measurements of device function (BT), and the integrity test (IT) (Almqvist et al., 1993; Mahoney and Proctor, 1994; Mason et al., 1997; Shallop, 1997). The presence of the ESR confirms an intact reflex pathway in the peripheral and lower brainstem pathways and its response threshold provides an indication of the maximum comfortable levels of electrical stimulation that the patient might experience from the implant. Monitoring of device function is achieved objectively through application of BT and IT measurements.

Clinical application

Many of the advantages and drawbacks that affect the selection and application of a particular auditory evoked potential are similar for both acoustical and electrical stimulation. The auditory brainstem response (ABR), and the auditory nerve action potential (AP) are therefore widely employed in young children, as described later. Conventional ERA techniques, such as the ABR and electrocochleography (ECochG), can provide objective confirmation of a profound hearing loss as part of the overall audiological assessment prior to implantation. The EABR can also be recorded in the pre-operative stage using electrical stimulation presented at the promontory or round window (Kileny et al., 1994; Mason et al., 1997). This technique in conjunction with MRI imaging can provide valuable information regarding the presence of intact auditory neurones and the suitability of a child for cochlear implantation. When a child has been implanted, a battery of electrically evoked potentials and other objective measures can be used to assess the functioning of the implant. In young children, the intra-operative stage is a valuable time to implement some of these tests that can then be used to assist with the initial fitting of the device a few weeks after surgery (Mason et al., 1995a). Post-operative measures are also an integral part of the management of a young child when problems of device function and difficulties with tuning arise.

Electric response audiometry before implantation

Electric response audiometry (ERA) with acoustical stimulation is a valuable – and in some children an essential – tool in the assessment of suitability for cochlear implantation. In the early years of the NPCIP, ERA was performed on all children in order to confirm the presence of a profound bilateral hearing loss. However, as our experience and knowledge of assessing children for implantation grew it became apparent that routine ERA in every case was not an efficient or appropriate protocol. An audit of our early results confirmed this situation and led to our current protocol where ERA is used in selected cases such as very young children, complex cases, or where there is any doubt about the reliability of behavioural testing.

Electric response audiometry (ERA)

Auditory evoked potentials in ERA can be subdivided into those arising from the cochlea and auditory nerve (electrocochleography, ECochG), brainstem pathways (auditory brainstem response, ABR), thalamus and primary auditory cortex (middle latency response, MLR), and primary and secondary auditory cortices and frontal association cortex (auditory cortical response, ACR). The ABR and ECochG are the techniques normally employed for objective audiological assessment in young children. They are resilient to the effects of adaptation and habituation, and are not affected significantly by sleep, sedation or anaesthesia. In contrast the MLR and ACR can be very variable and unreliable in young children (Stapells et al., 1988; Hall, 1992).

For routine objective audiometry in young children, the ABR is generally preferred to ECochG because placement of either a trans-tympanic or extra-tympanic ECochG electrode will require a general anaesthetic (Davis, 1976; Mason et al., 1988). The ABR test technique only requires the use of surface scalp electrodes and has largely superseded the routine use of ECochG. Nevertheless, there is still a role for ECochG in selected and complex cases as described later.

However, the disadvantage of both the ABR and ECochG is the limited information they can provide about hearing loss at specific frequencies of sound, particularly when using a click stimulus. Application of tone-pip stimuli (Stapells and Oates, 1997) improves the frequency specificity of the test and is employed in the NPCIP. More recently, steady-state potentials have been proposed as an alternative method of recording objective frequency specific thresholds (Rance et al., 1998; John and Picton, 2000).

Auditory brainstem response (ABR)

The electrical activity evoked in the ascending auditory nerve and brainstem pathways by an auditory stimulus is known as the auditory brainstem response (ABR). The first definitive description of the ABR in humans was reported by Jewett and Williston in 1971, although Sohmer and Feinmesser first recorded these neurogenic responses in 1967. The generator sites of the classic seven waves (I to VII), arising in the first 10 ms after the click stimulus, have been extensively documented (Hall, 1992; Möller, 1999). Wave I is known to be the compound action potential of the auditory nerve and is the far field equivalent of the AP component in ECochG. Wave II is thought to arise predominantly from proximal regions of the auditory nerve and wave III from the cochlear nucleus. The superior olivary complex is considered to be the main source of wave IV and the lateral lemniscus wave V. Waves VI and VII are thought to arise mainly from the inferior colliculus. The typical click-evoked ABR waveform is shown in Figure 6.1.

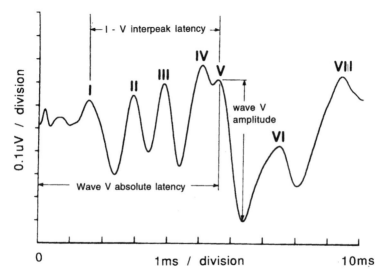

Figure 6.1. The typical waveform of the normal oto-neurological ABR (NABR) evoked by acoustical click stimulation showing measurements of the amplitude and latency of waves I and V.

As well as these fast individual waves of the ABR, there is a slow wave associated with wave V and a negative component at a latency of about 10 ms. This slow negative response is often termed SN10 after Davis and Hirsh (1979) and is thought to originate in the mid-brain probably representing post-synaptic activity within the inferior colliculus (Hashimoto, 1982). These slow components can be identified reliably with stimulus levels very close to hearing threshold as shown in Figure 6.2.

The stimulus and recording parameters for the ABR are selected to optimize the response characteristics and test procedure for either audiological application (slow waves) or as an

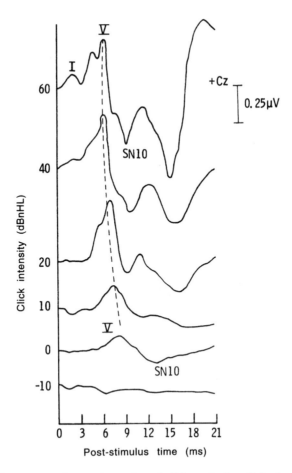

Figure 6.2. A typical intensity series of click-evoked audiological ABR (TABR) waveforms in normal hearing.

oto-neurological investigation (fast waves). The methodology is well documented in the literature (Jacobson, 1985; Thornton, 1987; Mason, 1993; Hall, 1992; Lightfoot et al., 2000; Stevens et al., 1999). Typical test parameters employed in the NPCIP for the audiological ABR (TABR) are as follows:

Electrode configuration:	Active = vertex (Cz) or high forehead
	Reference = ipsilateral mastoid
	Guard = forehead or contralateral mastoid
Amplifier sensitivity:	10μV per display division
Artefact rejection level:	+/– 25μV peak amplitude (referred to input)
On-line signal display	+/– 25μV full scale
Filter bandwidth:	20 Hz (or 30 Hz) to 1 kHz (or 3 kHz)
Stimulus type:	Click and tone-pips (for example 1 kHz)
Stimulus polarity:	Alternating phase

Repetition rate:	31 pps
Sweep time:	20 ms
Averaging sweeps:	2,000
Averaged display:	+/- 0.5 µV full scale
Plotter output:	0.2 µV per cm

The stimulus is often presented to the child through standard headphones. Ideally these are electrically and magnetically screened with mu-metal enclosures in order to reduce the effects of artefacts arising from high intensity stimuli. In the NPCIP the ABR is also recorded using stimuli presented through the child's own hearing aid (aided-ABR). The aided technique is more difficult to implement than unaided stimulation, both from a technical and interpretation point of view. Nevertheless, this technique has proven to be particularly valuable in young children and complex cases in order to support the results of aided behavioural testing (Garnham et al., 2000a). This mode of stimulus presentation has also been described by other workers (Mahoney, 1985; Picton et al., 1998). Bone conduction stimuli are of limited use in the pre-implant assessment since the maximum intensity levels available are insufficient to assess the severe to profound sensorineural hearing losses that normally exist.

Occasionally, there may be significant residual response activity present and in this situation it is particularly valuable to record the ABR as an oto-neurological investigation (NABR). If a normal I-V inter-peak latency can be established then this strongly suggests a cochlear loss rather than a retrocochlear deafness. A recording of the NABR requires the following changes in four of the TABR test parameters:

- filter bandwidth: 100 Hz to 3 kHz;
- stimulus type: click only; alternating phase (occasionally single phase);
- click repetition rate: 11 pps;
- sweep time: 12 ms.

These changes enhance the identification of the faster waveform components (waves I, III and V) and improve the accuracy of the latency measurements, which are essential for the NABR.

Electrocochleography (ECochG)

Three response components are recorded in ECochG; cochlear microphonics (CM), summating potential (SP) and the compound auditory nerve action potential (AP). The CM and SP are predominantly receptor potentials, and reflect the functional status of the hair cells. The AP is the first neurogenic response originating from nerve fibres close to the cochlea. The AP is the only component in ECochG that has good threshold sensitivity and can be used for assessment of hearing threshold. Typical recordings of the different components in ECochG are shown in Figure 6.3.

Electrocochleography can be recorded using either a trans-tympanic (invasive) or extra-tympanic (non-invasive) technique. The trans-tympanic method, first described by Portmann et al. in 1967, involves placing a needle electrode through the tympanic membrane coming to rest on the promontory in the middle ear. With the extra-tympanic technique, which is often employed in

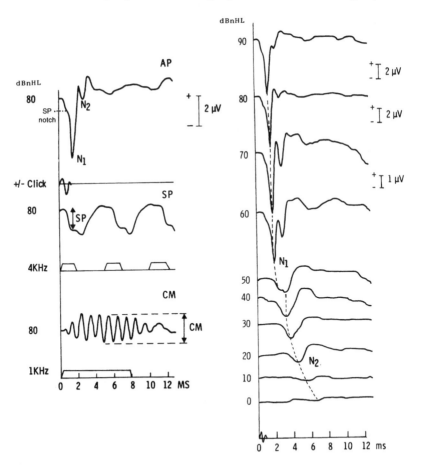

Figure 6.3. Extra-tympanic electrocochleography in the normal ear showing the three response components; the compound auditory nerve action potential (AP), summating potential (SP) and cochlear microphonics (CM). Only the AP (N1 and N2 components) can be recorded reliably with stimulus levels close to threshold.

Nottingham, an electrode is positioned on the surface of the posterior-inferior wall of the external auditory meatus close to the tympanic membrane (Mason et al., 1980). Tests in young children with either of these techniques require a general anaesthetic. Details of these test techniques have been described previously (Gibson, 1978; Abramovich, 1990).

Typical stimulus and recording parameters employed in the NPCIP are as follows:

Electrode configuration:	Active = (a) ear canal for extra-tympanic (XECochG)
	(b) promontory for trans-tympanic (TECochG)
	Reference = ipsilateral earlobe
	Guard/common = forehead
Amplifier sensitivity:	10 µV or 20 µV per display division
Artefact rejection level:	+/- 50 µV peak amplitude (referred to input)
On-line signal display:	+/- 50 µV full scale
Filter bandwidth:	5 Hz to 3 kHz
Stimulus type:	Click and tone-pip (for example 1 kHz) via a mu-metal screened headphone
Stimulus polarity:	Single phase with waveform subtraction for the CM Alternating phase for the SP/AP waveform
Repetition rate:	11 pps
Sweep time:	12 ms
Averaging sweeps:	2,000 (XECochG), 500 (TECochG)
Averaged display:	+/- 1 µV full scale (XECochG), +/-10 µV full scale (TECochG)
Plotter output:	0.2 µV per cm (XECochG), 2 µV per cm (TECochG)

Frequency specificity

In the NPCIP, one of the following audiological criteria needs to be met depending on the configuration of the hearing loss (see Chapter 4 for more detail) before a child is referred for cochlear implantation.

• audiometric thresholds at 2 kHz and 4 kHz are 105 dB HL or more;
• averaged thresholds for 500 Hz, 1 kHz and 2 kHz are 90 dB or more and the threshold at 4 kHz is 95 dB or more;
• aided thresholds at 2 kHz and 4 kHz are greater than 50 dBA.

The click stimulus is widely used in ERA and provides valuable information regarding hearing in the 2 kHz to 4 kHz region of the audiogram (Drift et al., 1987). The unaided and aided modes of presentation of the stimulus are valuable in this application. However, more specific frequencies of hearing can be targeted using tone-pip stimuli. For example, lower frequency hearing can be assessed with the ABR using tone-pip stimuli (typically 1 kHz or 500 Hz) which may assist with the management of a young child.

Use of tone-pip stimuli for the ABR requires appropriate expertise and very good recording conditions. The tone-pip response, particularly for mid to low tones, is not as easily identified as the click-evoked waveform and has a different morphology. Frequency specificity is still limited, particularly with high-intensity stimuli, due to spread of energy in the cochlea away from the nominal tone frequency (Stapells et al., 1997). This can be improved using ipsilateral masking noise (high pass or notched noise). Use of the tone-pip, with or without ipsilateral masking, is a valuable asset in helping to identify residual cochlear activity.

Short latency component (SLC)

In addition to the conventional ABR waves, some recordings using high-intensity click stimuli (100 dB nHL or more) exhibit a negative component at a latency of about 3 ms (Mason et al., 1996; Kato et al., 1998). This response has been called a short latency component (SLC) or N3 and can be clearly identified when there is no obvious response from the auditory sensory pathway, as in the case of profound hearing loss (Figure 6.4). The presence of the SLC appears to be unrelated to the conventional ABR since it is present both with and without a wave V component. It believed to arise from stimulation of the vestibular system with the response arising primarily from the vestibular nuclei in the brainstem. A similar component to the SLC has also been observed on the electrical auditory brainstem response waveform evoked by electrical stimulation at the promontory.

In our studies (Mason et al., 1996) we showed that the SLC was present in 26% of children being assessed for cochlear implantation in the NPCIP and its incidence was significantly higher in congenitally deaf children (48%) compared with post-meningitic deafness (6%). Specific damage to receptors in the peripheral vestibular apparatus might be an explanation as to why the component is rarely seen in post-meningitic deafness. When the SLC was first observed during the pre-implant assessments there was concern that this might represent a retro-cochlear pathology (an early component in the ABR recording with no wave V). However we now know that the presence of the SLC is not a contraindication for proceeding with cochlear implantation.

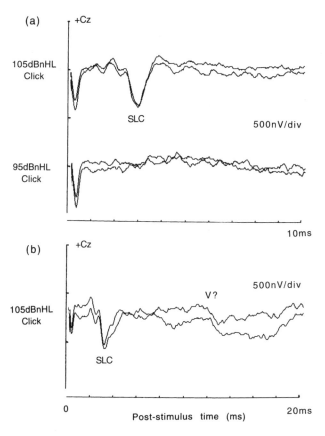

Figure 6.4. An example of the short latency component (SLC) in profound hearing loss using data collection parameters for the NABR (a) and the TABR (b).

Clinical application

In the NPCIP, ERA (normally ABR) is employed in very young children, complex cases, or where there is any doubt about the reliability of behavioural testing. Electrocochleography is available for those children where detailed examination of response activity of the cochlea (hair cells) and peripheral auditory nerve is required. The frequency of use of ERA and the approach adopted varies between different implant centres being influenced to some extent by the facilities and expertise that are available locally.

Test protocol

The NPCIP test protocol for pre-implant ERA assessment includes both click and tone-pip stimuli with a choice of unaided and aided stimulus presentation, testing both ears. A decision as to whether a child requires ERA is reached at the time of the audiological assessment and is based on factors such as age, reliability of the behavioural testing, or complexity of the case. The aided ABR testing (Garnham et al., 2000a) is generally performed in conjunction with the unaided stimulus presentation. Thus, the standard pre-implant test protocol, in order of priority, is as follows:

Unaided	Click TABR
	4 kHz tone-pip TABR
	1 kHz tone-pip TABR
	Click NABR (omitted if no response on unaided click TABR)
Aided	Click TABR
	4 kHz TABR (omitted if no response on aided click TABR)
	1 kHz TABR (included with borderline criteria or unexpected responses present)
	Tympanometry

Sedation is necessary in many of the young children in order to achieve reliable identification of small residual responses. The child is sedated and tested in a quiet side room on the ENT ward. Maximum stimulus intensities are 105 dB nHL for unaided stimuli and 80 dB nHL free field for aided presentation, and are limited by the effects of saturation and distortion by the transducer. The standard test protocol may be modified due to (i) referral information, (ii) previous testing (for example, unaided), (iii) auditory neuropathy and (iv) time constraints (for example, when the child is difficult to sedate).

Tympanograms are recorded at the time of the ERA investigation in order to check for normal middle ear function and to exclude any underlying conductive loss. Exclusion and management of middle ear pathology is essential in the pre-implant assessment prior to both audiological and ERA testing. In the NPCIP, all children are seen by their local ENT and audiology department (including tympanometry) a week before their assessment date. If there is any evidence of significant middle ear problems at that stage then their appointment date is rearranged as necessary.

In a child with persistent conductive hearing loss, undergoing a general anaesthetic for aspiration of glue/fluid and insertion of grommets, it is tempting to take the opportunity of performing ERA immediately after surgery while the child is still anaesthetized. Unfortunately, the outcome of the test is complicated in some of these cases due to transient threshold shift originating from the surgical procedure (Mason et al., 1995b). A cautious approach to interpretation of pre-implant ERA in this situation should be adopted.

Electrocochleography is available in the NPCIP test battery for special cases:

- investigation of ambiguity between the behavioural findings and ABR assessment using the action potential (AP);
- recording the cochlear microphonics (CM) to investigate the presence of an evoked otoacoustic emission and hence the possibility of some cochlear function in suspected cases of auditory neuropathy;
- using the summating potential (SP) component to assess the presence of endolymphatic hydrops that might be associated with a fluctuating loss, although the presence of a response probably means that the child is outside the audiological criteria for a cochlear implant;
- assistance with the differential diagnosis of cochlear and retrocochlear deafness using the AP and CM. If there is good cochlear function but an atrophic or damaged auditory nerve then the effectiveness of the implant will be severely or totally impaired.

Typical outcome

The most likely outcome on ERA is an absence of the majority of response components because of a profound bilateral cochlear loss. Occasionally some residual or more positive response activity is observed and this requires more detailed examination. In a series of 70 children in the NPCIP, pre-implant ERA exhibited some residual ABR activity (either click or tone-pip related) in 30 children (43%) and a click-evoked SLC was observed in 18 children (25%). The SLC was present in 15 of the 31 congenitally deaf children but in only 2 of 33 children deafened after meningitis. These results are likely to change in the future as children with more residual hearing are considered for cochlear implantation.

Examples of ABR recordings using unaided and aided stimulus presentations are shown in Figures 6.5 and 6.6 respectively. Identification of significant levels of response activity on one or both ears is important because this may influence the decision regarding which ear to implant or, in some cases, may suggest further audiological assessment before proceeding with implantation. Some children will have acquired a profound

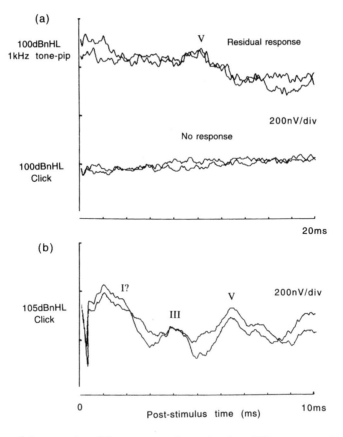

Figure 6.5. Examples of the outcome of a pre-implant ABR assessment in a case of severe to profound hearing loss using data collection parameters for the TABR (a) and the NABR (b). A no response condition is typical with the occasional presence of a residual response. Small wave I, III and V components are indicated in (b) which are just within the limits of the normal range for a young child.

hearing loss following meningitis. Occasionally, in these cases there can be some recovery of hearing (McCormick et al., 1993). It may be necessary to monitor this recovery using ERA techniques in addition to behavioural testing.

In children where a clearly defined TABR waveform is recorded the threshold of the response must be measured. The NABR should also be recorded in order to measure the absolute latency and inter-peak latencies of waves I, III and V. Abnormal wave I-III and I-V intervals will suggest the possibility of retrocochlear pathology. An absence of all response components on the ABR waveform (including wave I) is consistent with cochlear hearing loss but cannot exclude the possibility of retrocochlear pathology or neural damage.

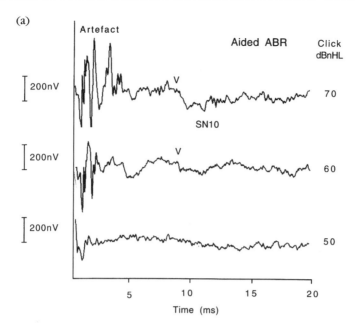

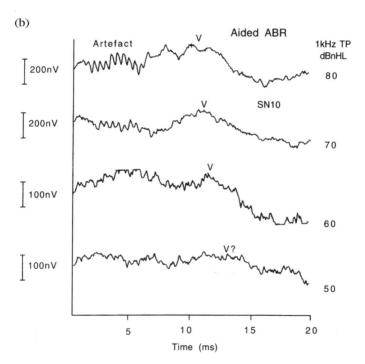

Figure 6.6. Example waveforms of the aided ABR using a click stimulus (a) and a 1 kHz tone-pip; (b) Aided thresholds were around 55 dB in both cases, which is at the lower limit of the NPCIP criteria for candidacy for implantation.

Investigations based on electrical stimulation

The change in stimulus modality from acoustical to electrical has led to the development of a wide range of electrophysiological and associated objective measures that have proven to be useful in the management of young children both before and after cochlear implantation (Kileny, 1991; Mason et al., 1997; Shallop, 1997). These measures have been applied to assess neuronal survival before implantation and to monitor the functioning and performance of the implant both during and after surgery.

However, the change from acoustical to electrical stimulation increases the problem of stimulus artefact particularly for the early latency responses and with high levels of stimulation. These artefacts arise from the electrical component of the stimulus as well as the RF transcutaneous transmission signals which are employed in the majority of commercially available implant devices. Addressing this problem requires some modifications to the methodology of data collection, as described later.

Electrically evoked potentials

Electrical stimulation of the peripheral auditory nerve evokes neural activity in the ascending auditory pathway, which can be recorded using techniques similar to those employed in conventional acoustical ERA. Electrically evoked responses arise from similar generator sites as with acoustical stimulation (Pelizzone et al., 1989) and for this reason factors such as sleep, sedation and anaesthesia affect the responses in a similar way. It is not surprising therefore that the ECAP and EABR have received the widest development and application in the paediatric population, analogous to the ECochG and ABR in acoustical ERA. These responses are very robust and suitable for use in young children. The complete range of electrically evoked responses will be described in this section with particular emphasis on the ECAP and EABR.

Electrical compound action potential (ECAP)

Intra-cochlear recordings of the ECAP in humans was reported by Brown and Abbas (1990) using individual electrodes of an Ineraid intra-cochlear electrode array. One electrode was used for electrical stimulation and an adjacent electrode for recording the electrically evoked response. A subtraction technique was used to extract the response component from the large stimulus artefact. The success of this technique was dependent on having direct access to the intra-cochlear electrodes through the percutaneous connector of the Ineraid device. The ECAP waveform, described by Brown et al. was relatively large (up to 2 mV) and consisted of a predominantly negative deflection (N1) at approximately 0.2 to 0.4 ms after onset of the current stimulus. They postulate that the peripheral ECAP response may be more directly related to neuronal survival than the more centrally derived EABR.

More recently the ECAP has been recorded from within the cochlea using the back (reverse) telemetry technique known as neural response telemetry (NRT), which is available on the Nucleus range of cochlear implants currently supplied by the Cochlear Corporation (Carter et al., 1994; Abbas et al., 1999). The basic principles of the stimulation and recording techniques for NRT are similar to that described by Brown and Abbas (1990). A probe stimulus pulse is presented on a selected electrode of the 22-channel array and the response recorded from an adjacent electrode. The ball electrode on the temporalis muscle (MP1) and the electrodes on the body of the implant (MP2) are used as the reference electrodes for stimulating and recording respectively. A subtraction technique is used to extract the ECAP from the stimulus artefact that takes advantage of the refractory properties of the auditory nerve. Recordings are performed with and without a masker pulse which precedes the probe stimulus and this process enables subtraction of the stimulus artefact. Figure 6.7 shows a schematic diagram of the set-up for NRT and a detailed description of the test parameters are presented in the NRT 'cookbook' published by Cochlear AG. A summary of typical test parameters is as follows:

- stimulating electrode (n); recording electrode (n + 2); where n is the selected electrode;
- probe pulse width = 25 μs; pulse rate = 80 Hz;
- full subtraction paradigm = A-(B - (C - D)) as documented in the NRT cookbook;
- analysis window = 1.5 ms in high resolution mode (32 data points);
- amplifier gain = 40 or 60 dB;
- sampling delay = 50 μs;

- number of averaging sweeps = 100 or 200 for amplifier gains of 60 dB and 40 dB respectively;
- masker advance = 500 µs; masker pulse width = 25 µs.

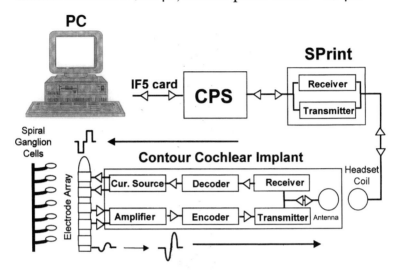

Figure 6.7. A schematic diagram of the set-up for recording the ECAP using NRT (adapted from Cochlear AG).

Typical ECAP waveforms recorded intra-operatively from a young child in the NPCIP are shown in Figure 6.8. The N1 and P2 components are clearly identifiable. There have been extensive studies of post-operative recordings of the ECAP in adult implantees, as part of a European multi-centre trial of NRT co-ordinated by Cochlear AG and also from reports in the US (Brown et al., 2000). Results from these studies have been disseminated at regular NRT workshop meetings. The aim of these studies has been to establish the optimum stimulus and recording parameters for acquiring reliable recordings of the ECAP using NRT and to examine potential clinical applications. More recently, these studies have been extended to children both intra-operatively and post-operatively (Hughes et al., 2000; Cullington, 2000; Mason et al., 2001).

Electrical auditory brainstem response (EABR)

The EABR is normally evoked by a biphasic electrical pulse stimulus delivered either through a single channel of an intra-cochlear electrode array (using the implant system) or in the case of pre-implant assessment with an extra-cochlear electrode positioned on the promontory or round window. Intra-cochlear

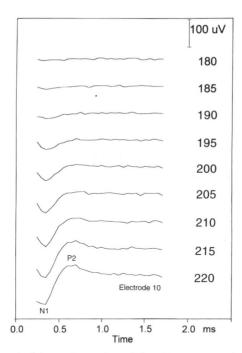

Figure 6.8. A typical intensity series of the ECAP (N1 and P2 components) recorded intra-operatively using NRT. Threshold of the response is 185 stimulus units.

stimulation usually evokes an EABR that has more clearly defined waveform characteristics compared with the response from an extra-cochlear stimulus. An electrical pulse stimulus has a very fast rise and fall time, and short duration, which is very similar to the acoustical click stimulus. It evokes a very high level of synchronization of neural activity that is optimum for eliciting the EABR. A train of individual pulses is required in order to record an averaged waveform consisting of 1,000 or 2,000 sweeps. Relatively high stimulus rates can be employed (typically 85 pps) since there is minimal adaptation of the individual waves of the EABR with electrical stimulation compared with the acoustical ABR (Mason et al., 1993). The adaptive mechanisms in the cochlea involved with generation of the acoustical ABR are bypassed with electrical stimulation. Fast stimulus rates enable shorter test times, which is particularly valuable for young children.

A conventional evoked potential (EP) recording system is used to acquire the data. The stimulus system and EP equipment must be accurately linked in time using a trigger pulse so that data collection is synchronized with onset of the stimulus. Most implant systems now have a trigger pulse available for this purpose, which can be applied to an external trigger input on the EP system. The programming software on many implant systems has now been customized for EABR measurements, including appropriate stimulus repetition rates and alternately inverted biphasic pulses for cancellation of stimulus artefact.

Typical stimulus and recording parameters for the EABR are as follows:

Electrode configuration:	Active = vertex (Cz)
	Reference = contralateral mastoid
	Guard = forehead
Amplifier sensitivity:	10 µV or 20 µV per display division
Artefact rejection level:	+/-25 µV peak amplitude (referred to input signal)
Online signal display:	+/-25 µV full scale
Filter bandwidth:	100 Hz to 3 kHz
Stimulus type:	Biphasic electrical pulse
Stimulus pulse duration:	In the range 25 µs to 400 µs per phase
Stimulus polarity:	Ideally alternating onset phase to reduce stimulus artefact
Pulse rate:	Typically 85 pps
Sweep time:	10 ms
Averaging sweeps:	2,000 (1,000 with high supra-threshold stimuli)
Averaged display:	+/-1 µV full scale (+/-5 µV with high supra-threshold stimuli)
Plotter output:	0.2 µV per cm (1 µV with high supra-threshold)

The EABR is recording from surface scalp electrodes in a similar way to the acoustical ABR. Aspects of the methodology specific to the EABR include disabling the amplitude artefact rejection across the time period of the stimulus artefact (typically 0 ms to 2 ms) otherwise there will be rejection of the signal. Occasionally a low amplifier sensitivity (50 µV or 100 µV) is needed to avoid saturation of the signal amplifier caused by a large stimulus artefact and hence poor quality or unreliable recordings. This artefact arises from the RF transmission signal and the electrical pulse stimulus. The RF component of the artefact can be reduced by placing a passive RF filter in line with the electrode leads (Game et al., 1990; Mason et al., 1993). The electrical artefact in the averaged waveform can be reduced by presenting a train of stimulus pulses with the polarity of the pulse alternately inverted during the averaging process. This is analogous to the alternately inverted polarity of the acoustical click stimulus.

Stimulus artefact must not adversely affect the performance of the signal amplifier in the EP equipment. There should be relatively quick recovery from any saturation at the onset of each sweep. Recording the signal with a very low cut-off frequency (typically 1 Hz) on the filter bandwidth can be helpful in reducing the spread of a large artefact across the EABR waveform. Some workers have employed a signal blanking circuit across the time period of the stimulus artefact (Millard et al., 1992). The electrical component of the artefact is generally larger when either the stimulating or reference electrode is extra-cochlear due to the effects of current spread.

A typical intensity series for the EABR evoked by the cochlear implant is shown in Figure 6.9. Although the general characteristics of the EABR waveform are similar to the acoustical ABR, there are some notable differences. The slow components normally associated with wave V and SN10 of the ABR are usually absent in the EABR. A low cut-off frequency of 100 Hz is

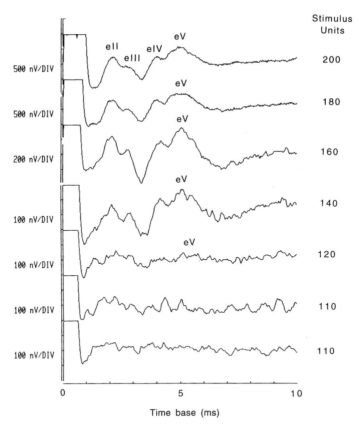

Figure 6.9. A typical intensity series of the EABR evoked by presentation of a biphasic pulse stimulus on one electrode of the cochlear implant. Threshold of the response is 120 stimulus units.

normally employed for the EABR, as there is no advantage in extending this down to 20 Hz or 30 Hz as used for the TABR (Mason, 1984). The latencies of the individual components of the EABR arise at 1.0 to 1.5 ms earlier compared with the ABR (Allum et al., 1990) and exhibit only a small increase in latency with reduced stimulus intensity. Absolute latency of wave eV arises at around 4.0 ms to 4.5 ms compared with 5.5 ms to 6.0 ms for the acoustical wave V. Wave eV is usually the component identified for estimation of response threshold although in some implanted patients waves II and III are equally dominant close to threshold. The amplitude of wave eV is determined in a similar way to the acoustical ABR using a peak-to-trough measurement.

The earlier latencies of the EABR, compared with the ABR, are of the result of the electrical stimulus bypassing the mechanics of the middle ear and cochlea. There is no travelling wave along the basilar membrane that would normally influence generation of activity in the auditory nerve and brainstem pathways. These shorter latencies mean that a post-stimulus epoch of 10 ms is sufficient to capture the response waveform. Using high suprathreshold stimuli, the EABR often exhibits all the individual waves normally seen on the ABR, except for wave eI, which is usually obscured by the stimulus artefact.

In addition to the neurogenic components of the EABR a compound muscle action potential (CMAP) is occasionally seen in some patients particularly with extra-cochlear stimulation (Figure 6.10). Excessive spread in current can cause direct stimulation of other neural pathways such as the facial nerve (Maxwell et al., 1999). These muscle responses are typically large biphasic or triphasic waveforms having different characteristics to the EABR.

Electrical middle latency response (EMLR)

Electrically evoked activity in the thalamic auditory pathway and primary auditory cortex is known as the electrical middle latency response (EMLR). The most prominent components of the EMLR are eNa, ePa and eNb and can be recorded reliably in adult subjects (Kileny, 1991). These three components arise in the latency period from about 25 ms to 35 ms and are slightly earlier than their acoustical counterpart (Kileny et al., 1989). One advantage of recording these response components compared with the EABR is that there is minimal spread of stimulus artefact into this later time period.

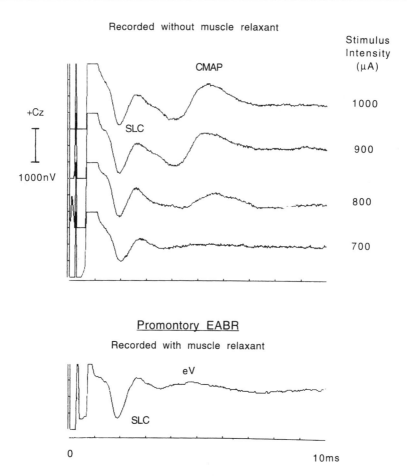

Figure 6.10. An example of the compound muscle action potential (CMAP) waveform evoked by electrical stimulation at the promontory. A small wave eV can be observed when the CMAP is removed by administration of muscle relaxant.

The reliability of the EMLR in young children, however, depends on the effects of maturation and psychological state, in the same way as the acoustical MLR (McGee and Kraus, 1996). Application of this response is therefore difficult in young children, particularly during sedation and general anaesthesia. Early attempts at recording electrically evoked potentials were targeted at the later EMLR rather than the EABR (Shallop et al., 1990) because of the adverse effects of stimulus artefact. However, as recording techniques for the EABR were developed and improved this response became the established tool for objective assessment of the auditory pathway in young children in much the same way as the acoustical ABR.

Electrical auditory cortical response (EACR)

Electrical stimulation of the peripheral auditory will evoke activity in the auditory pathway, which subsequently generates a response at cortical level (Brix and Gedlicka, 1991). This response is known as the electrical auditory cortical response (EACR) and has similar characteristics to the acoustical ACR. In the adult response, the eN1 and eP2 are the most prominent components with latencies of about 100 ms and 150 ms to 200 ms respectively. The integrity of the whole auditory pathway is assessed using the EACR and problems of contamination of the signal baseline with stimulus artefact are minimal because of the long latency response components. Recording the EACR in young children is very difficult because of its inconsistency, which is exacerbated during sleep, sedation and general anaesthesia. However, in awake older children (aged six years or more) and adults the EACR becomes more reliable and is a potentially valuable clinical tool.

Ponton et al. (1996) studied the effects of maturation of the EACR with respect to the age at implantation and duration of post-implantation experience. They showed that, during the period of deafness before implantation, maturation of cortical function does not progress. However, at least some if not all maturational processes resume after stimulation is reintroduced. The EACR is therefore a valuable objective research tool for investigation of processing activity at cortical level.

Electrical event-related potentials (EERP)

Beyond the evoked potentials that register sensory input are the endogenous potentials that reflect higher level processing such as perceptual and cognitive function. The term event-related potential (ERP) is used to distinguish them from sensory evoked potentials. Two auditory ERP responses, the mismatch negativity (MMN) and the P300, sometimes referred to as the P3, can be used to assess objectively how well an individual is able to discriminate and attach meaning to different sounds. These responses are typically evoked by presenting a train of standard stimuli, such as a 1 kHz tone burst or speech sound, interspersed with an occasional deviant stimulus, which could have a difference in frequency content, intensity, and so forth. This is often called an 'oddball stimulus paradigm'.

Recordings of the MMN and P300 in both adults and children have been reported extensively in the literature (Näätänen,

1990; Taylor, 1991; Kraus et al., 1992; Cheour et al., 2000), including a special issue on MMN in *Ear and Hearing* prefaced by Picton (1995). The MMN consists of an enhanced negative potential occurring at about 200 ms following presentation of the rare stimulus. It is a passive response and does not require active attention to the stimuli. The P300 or P3 is a multicomponent positive response with a latency of 300 ms to 400 ms depending on the type of stimulus. Generation of this response requires the subject to attend to the rare (target) stimuli. There is therefore considerable interest in application of the MMN in children because of its passive characteristics. The MMN and P300 responses arise as a result of the activation of separate systems, deviance detection and shifts in attention respectively, and as such are evoked from different regions of the brain (Sussman et al., 1999; Alho et al., 1998).

The MMN and P300 can be elicited by electrical stimulation in patients with cochlear implants (Oviatt and Kileny, 1991; Kraus et al., 1993; Ponton and Don, 1995). An example of response waveforms is shown in Figure 6.11 and they are reported as being remarkably similar to responses recorded in normally hearing subjects (Kraus et al., 1993). Both the MMN

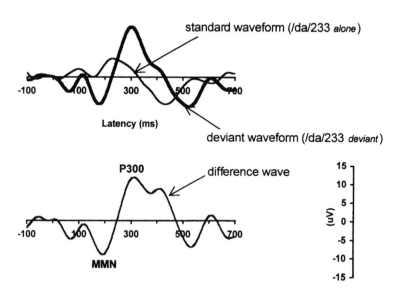

difference wave = deviant stimulus responses - stimulus alone responses

Figure 6.11. Typical mismatch negativity (MMN) and P300 response components exhibited in the difference in response to deviant (rare) and standard (common) speech sounds.

and P300, recorded from cochlear implant recipients show considerable promise as objective measures of discrimination ability, and for the study of central auditory processing.

Electrical stapedius reflex (ESR)

A reflex response from the stapedius muscle in the middle ear can be elicited by a high suprathreshold electrical stimulus presented through one of the channels of a cochlear implant. The ESR can be recorded using a conventional acoustic imped-ance meter, or detected by visual observation of movement of the muscle and tendon during implant surgery. The presence of a response confirms that the implant is functioning and that the neural pathways of the peripheral auditory nerve and lower regions of the brainstem are intact. The threshold of the ESR (ESRT) can provide guidance towards the comfort level of elec-trical stimulation experienced by patients (Battmer et al., 1990).

Stimulus

A one-second burst of biphasic stimulus pulses (250 pps) is typi-cally used to evoke the ESR. Most implant systems have this mode of stimulus presentation available as an option within the standard software package, for example in WinDPS for the Nucleus Contour device. For implant systems employing analogue stimulation, a burst of a low frequency sine wave electrical stimulus can be used (Stephan et al., 1991).

Visual observation of the response

The contraction and movement of the stapedius muscle and tendon, which constitutes the ESR, can be observed through the operating microscope by the surgeon before closure of the middle ear during implant surgery (Sheppard et al., 1992). The lowest level of the stimulus, which initiates a response, is recorded as the ESRT. Detection of this small response often relies on observation of a minute change in the reflected light from the surface of the muscle and tendon, rather than observ-ing the movement directly. There can be hysteresis associated with the ESRT when measurements from both ascending and descending stimulus protocols are compared. A slightly lower threshold is often observed when a descending stimulus is employed since this protocol helps the visual tracking of the response at it approaches threshold.

Acoustic impedance measurements

The ESR can be recorded using acoustic impedance techniques on the contra-lateral side to the implanted ear (Spivak and Chute, 1994). This measurement can be performed either during surgery or post-operatively. A train of 5 or 10 stimulus bursts, with a repetition rate of around one per second, will assist detection of the reflex response.

Integrity testing (IT)

The electrical biphasic pulse stimulus, generated by the implant inside the cochlea, can be recorded from surface scalp electrodes using data collection techniques similar to those employed for recording the EABR. A small amount of signal averaging is employed for data collection in order to improve the signal to noise ratio and for this reason the resultant waveform is often called the averaged electrode voltage (AEV) (Mahoney and Proctor, 1994; Shallop, 1997; Cullington and Clarke, 1997). The AEV is a far field representation of the electrical pulse stimulus that is often referred to as the stimulus artefact in the EABR. The term stimulogram has also been used to describe a set of AEV recordings from all 22 electrodes of the Nucleus cochlear implant (Almquist et al., 1993). A special stimulation scheme, where the AEV from all combinations of active and reference electrodes of the Nucleus 22 electrode array are represented by an E-E map, has been described by Mens et al. (1994a). In its various forms, recording of the AEV to objectively check the functioning of the implant is known as integrity testing (IT). It is an essential tool for the management of young children and particularly for patients where back-telemetry function tests are not available on their device.

Typical stimulus and recording parameters for IT are as follows:

Electrode configuration:	Active = ipsi-lateral mastoid (or jaw)
	Reference = contra-lateral mastoid
	Guard = forehead
Amplifier sensitivity:	100 µV per display division
Artefact rejection level:	+/- 25 µV peak, excluding the timeframe of the AEV
On-line signal display:	+/- 50 µV full scale
Filter bandwidth:	1 Hz (or 100 Hz) to 3 kHz (or higher if equipment settings allow)
Stimulus type:	Biphasic electrical pulse (single polarity)
Stimulus mode:	Monopolar, bipolar, and common ground
Pulse rate:	85 pps (or higher if data collection parameters allow)
Sweep time:	10 ms (or shorter if equipment settings allow)

| Averaging sweeps: | 100 (or 200 with an active signal baseline) |
| Averaged display/plot | In the range +/- 4µV to +/- 400µV full scale |

Several methodological factors affect the configuration of the AEV, including the site of the scalp recording electrodes, the mode of presentation of the stimulus, the filter bandwidth of the signal amplifier, and whether there has been full insertion of the electrode array. Moreover, the way in which the current is conducted from the inside of the cochlea to the outside will affect the pattern of the response. Mens et al. (1994b) have suggested two types of current flow:

• through the fluid along the scala and not through the dense cochlear bone, leaving the cochlea only at the basally located opening;
• through the very permeable cochlear bone in the case of otosclerosis.

Using a specified data collection protocol the amplitude and shape of the AEV can be characterized across different electrode channels and any malfunction in one or more channels will disturb this configuration. Typical examples of normal AEVs recorded in pseudo-monopolar (MP1), bipolar (BP+1) and common ground (CG) modes for a fully inserted Nucleus CI22 electrode array are shown in Figure 6.12. In MP1 mode the AEV has the same phase across the electrode array and amplitude is generally stable except for a reduction towards the basal end of the array. In bipolar modes there is a progressive change in the amplitude and phase of the stimulus artefact from basal to apical electrode channels. Common ground exhibits a slightly more complex picture with a relatively large AEV at the basal end of the array (electrode 1). This amplitude falls rapidly to a nodal point at around electrodes 5 to 7 whereupon it changes phase and amplitude rises more slowly towards the apex of the array. These profiles of the AEV for both intra-operative and post-operative measurements have been documented by Garnham et al. (2001).

Back telemetry (BT) measurements

All commercially available cochlear implant systems now have the capability to check the functioning of the internal implant and the integrity of the electrode array using a feature known as back telemetry (or reverse telemetry). This technique enables

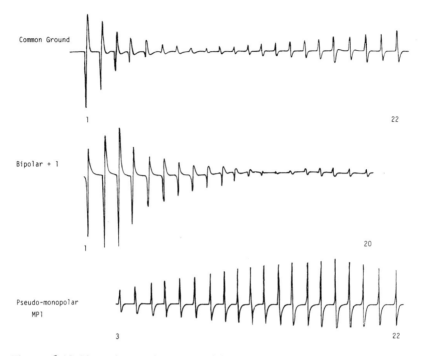

Figure 6.12. Typical normal patterns of the AEV across the 22 electrodes of the array for the CI22 cochlear implant using common ground, bipolar +1, and psuedo-monopolar stimulation modes.

data, transmitted from the implant, to be picked up by the coil on the outside of the head. This direction of transmission is opposite to the way that the implant functions when stimulating.

Typical tests available using BT are:

- function check of the internal circuitry;
- measurement of impedance of the electrode-tissue interface;
- electric field distribution along the electrode array;
- compliance of the delivered stimulus;
- recording the ECAP using neural response telemetry (NRT).

Back telemetry is a valuable tool in the routine clinic and measurement of electrode impedance is probably the single most important test. It is simple and quick to implement across all electrodes on the array and values of impedance enable the detection of possible broken wires (high impedance) and shorting electrodes (very low impedance). An example of impedance values recorded intra-operatively with the Nucleus CI24M cochlear implant is shown in Figure 6.13.

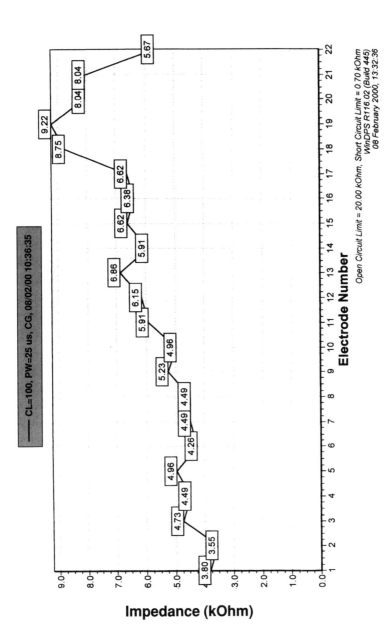

Figure 6.13. An example of the range of values of electrode impedance recorded intra-operatively using BT with the CI24M implant. The normal range is 700Ω to 20kΩ. Values outside this range suggest either a short circuit or open circuit respectively.

Electrical stimulation before implantation

The suitability of a cochlear implant as a means of hearing re-habilitation depends on the availability of electrically excitable auditory neurones that will subsequently result in auditory sensation and perception. Pre-operative assessment of the level of this neuronal survival can be approached through the use of imaging, and whether extra-cochlear electrical stimulation results in either auditory sensation or the generation of an evoked potential such as the EABR.

Presentation of the stimulus

The current spread from an electrical stimulus is not constrained by the mechanics of the middle ear and cochlea and it is therefore possible to apply a stimulus in the ear canal, at the promontory, or on the round window. The closer that the site of stimulation is to the cochlea the more effective is the stimulus. Electrical stimulation with a ball electrode at the round window is considered to be more sensitive than the promontory. However, placement of the electrode at the round window requires some visualization of landmarks on the medial wall of the middle ear via a small tympanotomy or tympano-meatal flap procedure. For this reason stimulation at the promontory is a popular technique, being minimally invasive whilst still main-taining an effective stimulus.

In a young child the promontory or round window electrode techniques require the use of a general anaesthetic. Since evalu-ation of a child for implantation may already involve investiga-tions requiring a general anaesthetic or sedation, such as ERA and imaging (CT, MRI), implementation of an additional session for electrical testing must be fully justified regarding manage-ment of the child. We have examined the possibility of combin-ing the electrical testing with imaging under the same general anaesthetic session but the logistics of implementing this are very complicated.

Behavioural stimulation testing

When an electrical stimulus is applied to the promontory in the middle ear using a trans-tympanic needle electrode, many patients will experience some degree of auditory sensation. This is a feasi-ble technique in co-operative adults and older children but is not a practical option in young children. Alternative objective methods of testing young children under a general anaesthetic, such as the EABR, are therefore required.

In the early days of adult cochlear implantation behavioural promontory testing was widely employed (Gray and Baguley, 1990). An absence of any acoustic sensation with the pre-operative promontory (and round window) stimulus was taken as a contraindication for cochlear implantation (Kileny et al., 1992). However, the value of routine behavioural testing with electrical stimulation as a predictor of outcome has been questioned and many implant centres now use the technique only on selected complex adult patients. Gantz et al. (1993) reported considerable variability in the ability of pre-operative tests to predict audiological performance with multi-channel cochlear implants.

Pre-implant EABR

The electrical auditory brainstem response (EABR) can be evoked by presentation of an extra-cochlear electrical stimulus at the promontory or round window (Kileny et al., 1994). The methodology of the technique and characteristics of the response will be described.

Methodology

In the NPCIP a battery-powered, custom-built stimulator is used to present the biphasic charge-balanced pulse stimulus because commercial stimulators are not readily available. It has constant current output so as to overcome changes in contact impedance of the stimulating electrode. Problems of stimulus artefact are exacerbated with extra-cochlear stimulation compared with intra-cochlear stimulation by the implant (Kasper et al., 1991). Some of these problems can be addressed using stimulus and data collection parameters that minimize the effects of the stimulus artefact on the signal, as described earlier in this chapter and in Mason et al. (1997).

The Prom-EABR waveform

The characteristics of the Prom-EABR are similar to those evoked by stimulation with the cochlear implant, except that the amplitude and definition of waves eII, eIII and eIV are generally reduced. Figure 6.14 shows some typical waveforms where (a) individual waves are well defined, (b) there is only a small wave eV present, and (c) the electrically evoked SLC is clearly

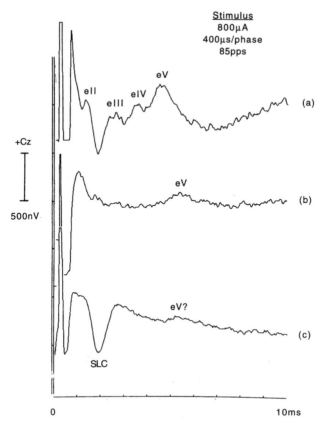

Figure 6.14. Examples of Prom-EABR waveforms showing (a) well-defined individual waves, (b) a small wave eV component only, and (c) a large and clearly defined SLC.

identifiable. An intensity series for a well-defined Prom-EABR is shown in Figure 6.15. The SLC threshold in this case is clearly more sensitive than threshold of the wave eV.

A compound muscle action potential (CMAP) can also be recorded on the Prom-EABR waveform that can hinder the interpretation of the wave eV component. This arises as a result of current spread from the promontory stimulating the facial nerve. However, since testing is often performed under a general anaesthetic, a muscle relaxant can be administered that inhibits the CMAP. Examples of recordings performed with and without muscle relaxant are shown in Figure 6.10.

Predicting peripheral neuronal survival and outcome

There is evidence from animal studies that suggest that the amplitude input/output (I/O) function of the EABR can predict

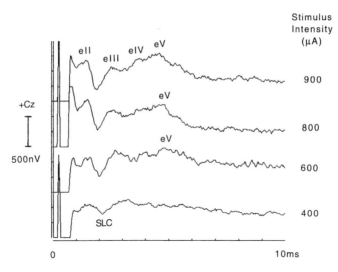

Figure 6.15. An intensity series of well-defined Prom-EABR waveforms that also exhibit the SLC.

neuronal survival (Smith and Simmons, 1983). An analysis of the EABR waveforms should therefore include measurements of these characteristics (Nikolopoulos et al., 1997). In the NPCIP, the technique of recording the EABR evoked by promontory stimulation (Prom-EABR) is available in the test battery. For several years the technique was used routinely in the peri-operative stage (immediately before implantation) to assist with selection of the ear for implantation (Mason et al., 1997). The ear with the 'best' EABR was chosen providing there were no other factors influencing the decision, such as ossification of the cochlea or MRI imaging of the nerve bundles in the internal auditory canal. In a study of 25 children (Mason et al., 1997), the Prom-EABR influenced the decision of which ear to implant in 20 cases (80%). A reliable response was recorded in 40 (80%) of the 50 ears tested. There are a number of explanations for the absence of a response: status of the auditory nerve, lack of sensitivity of the test technique, positioning of the needle electrode, poor recording conditions in which interpretation of the waveform was hindered by a large stimulus artefact. The incidence of absent responses is also significantly higher in children deafened after meningitis compared with congenitally deaf children (Nikolopoulos et al., 1999).

Recent experiences in the NPCIP have shown that children with no pre-operative Prom-EABR (wave eV) still receive significant benefit from a cochlear implant. A study of 47 implanted children (Nikolopoulos et al., 2000) showed that children with no Prom-EABR waveform (12 cases) performed as well as children with well-defined responses (35 cases). Speech perception and speech intelligibility were assessed annually up to three years after implantation using the IOWA sentence test, Connected Discourse Tracking (CDT), Categories of Auditory Performance (CAP) and Speech Intelligibility Rating (SIR). There was no statistically significant difference ($p > 0.05$) between the two groups of children using these outcome measures. Further analysis revealed that the outcome measures had not been affected by possible confounding factors (age at implantation, duration of deafness, etiology of deafness and number of inserted electrodes). This study shows that the prognostic value of the Prom-EABR is limited and absence of a prom-EABR is not, in itself, a contraindication for cochlear implantation. However, in selected cases (cochlear malformations, suspected cochlear nerve aplasia, narrow internal auditory canals and so forth) the presence of a Prom-EABR is a positive finding in the assessment of candidates for cochlear implantation as it confirms the existence of intact auditory neurones.

In view of the results from the study by Nikolopoulos et al. (2000) the Prom-EABR is no longer employed routinely to guide the selection of the ear for implantation. It is nevertheless maintained as a diagnostic tool for complex cases and provides valuable guidance regarding the decision of whether to proceed with implantation.

Assessment of central auditory pathways

The EABR will only assess the integrity of the auditory pathway up to the level of around the lateral lemniscus in the brainstem pathways, whereas other electrically evoked potentials, the EMLR and EACR, will examine more central pathways. Reliable recordings of the EMLR and EACR are possible in co-operative awake adults and older children but the effects of sedation and general anaesthesia, which are necessary for implementation of promontory stimulation in very young children, restrict their use in this situation.

An alternative approach to examine the central auditory pathways is through the use of functional MRI imaging of the auditory cortex following electrical stimulation at the promontory. Practical aspects of this technique in adults have been reported recently by Obler et al. (1999). This method of assessment is also currently undergoing investigation in Nottingham. The technique should enable a more complete objective assessment of candidates for cochlear implantation and might provide some guidance as to the level of performance that will be achieved post-operatively with the implant.

Investigations during surgery

Electrophysiological and objective measures at the time of implant surgery can confirm that the cochlear implant is functioning correctly and that the peripheral auditory nerve fibres are being stimulated effectively. This information provides valuable reassurance to both parents and professionals immediately after surgery, particularly when implanting a young child. Results of intra-operative recordings of the EABR, ESR and ECAP can be used in the initial fitting session to guide the selection of appropriate levels of electrical stimulation for a particular child. This can greatly assist progress in an initial fitting session, particularly with a child who is difficult to assess behaviourally.

Application of these techniques at the time of surgery takes advantage of the child already being anaesthetized for implant surgery. In this situation, the test conditions are good because the recording baseline will be free of movement and myogenic activity, a situation that cannot always be easily achieved post-operatively. Intra-operative testing is therefore popular in young children in many implant centres. The range of tests performed varies depending on the facilities and expertise available. In the NPCIP, the current protocol includes a wide range of investigations and has always been an important part of the management of children at the time of implant surgery.

Stimulus characteristics

The electrical pulse stimulus is usually delivered on a single channel of the electrode array in the scala tympani. The intensity or loudness of the stimulus perceived by the patient depends on the electric charge, which is related to the amplitude of the current (or voltage) and the duration of the stimulus (for example, pulse width). In some implant systems, stimulus intensity is expressed in arbitrary units, such as 'stimulus units' (0 to 255) for the Nucleus Contour implant, or in direct measures of current and pulse width as in the Clarion CII device (Advanced Bionics) and the Combi 40+ (MED-EL). For an intra-cochlear electrode the delivered charge is typically in the range of 10 to 200 nano-coloumbs for most implant users, which is equivalant to 50 μA to 1 mA for a pulse duration of 200 μs. Some aspects of the stimulus characteristics for objective measures (such as pulse rate and polarity, and stimulus train) are different to those required for behavioural tuning. For this reason, programming packages for most cochlear implant systems now have customized menus for application of objective measures that enable presentation of an appropriate stimulus.

The NPCIP protocol in the operating theatre

The cochlear implant programming system (for example, the clinical programming system (CPS) and associated hardware for the Nucleus Contour Device) and the evoked potential recording equipment are positioned in the operating theatre before the start of surgery. Attachment of scalp recording electrodes is performed in theatre immediately after administration of the general anaesthetic and before the child is prepared for surgery. Electrode leads are colour coded for future reference as access to the scalp is not practical during the operation. After implantation of the electrode array and receiver, the transmitter coil and lead are placed in a sterile clear plastic sheath (40 mm wide by 1 m in length) and positioned over the receiver in the wound.

The routine intra-operative monitoring protocol is as follows:

- Back telemetry measurements of electrode impedance in common ground (CG) and monopolar 1 (MP1) modes across all 22 electrodes.
- Threshold of the electrically evoked stapedius reflex on at least one electrode (typically e11) recorded from microscopic observation of the stapedius muscle and tendon.
- Recordings of average electrode voltages (integrity testing) across all 22 electrodes in CG mode.
- Threshold of the electrical auditory brainstem response (EABR) on one electrode (typically e11).
- Back telemetry measurements of electrode impedance across all 22 electrodes in all available modes (CG, MP1, MP2 and MP1+2).
- Recordings of the ECAP threshold using NRT on odd numbered electrodes, suprathreshold recordings on even numbered electrodes.

The initial BT measurements and ESR are performed before the surgeon closes the middle ear. The remaining tests, which take about 25 minutes to complete, are carried out during closure of the wound and suturing of the skin flap. Implementation of this protocol therefore requires very little additional time in the operating theatre.

Confirmation of the functioning of the implant

Back telemetry measurement of implant function is a simple and quick tool in the operating theatre and should always be performed at the time of implantation in both children and adults. These measurements can be performed with the electrodes dry, in sterile saline, or immediately after implantation. The recommended procedure varies depending on the implant supplier. In the NPCIP the BT measurements with the Nucleus Contour device are only performed when the implant has been positioned in the cochlea.

An interesting example of values of electrode impedance in a NPCIP child where there was partial insertion of the electrode array is shown in Figure 6.16. Immediately after insertion of the electrode array, electrodes outside the cochlea were not in contact with fluid or tissue and exhibited high impedance. Later in the procedure, however, these electrodes become bathed in fluid and subsequently showed values of impedance within the normal range (0.7 kΩ to 20 kΩ). Another example of abnormal intra-operative electrode impedance that is not the result of electrode

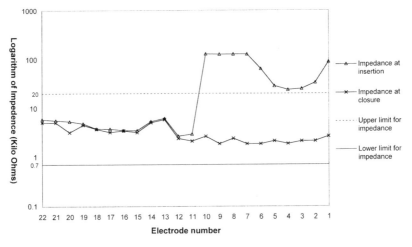

Figure 6.16. Values of electrode impedance across the array in a case of partial insertion (12 electrodes) with the Nucleus CI24M cochlear implant.

malfunction is in a case of Mondini dysplasia (French, 1999). Very low impedances were recorded, which were thought to be caused by an excessive amount of fluid surrounding the electrode array.

In addition to BT, integrity testing (IT) can also be used to confirm the status of the implant. The availability of BT and IT at the time of surgery should eliminate the risk of implanting a faulty device. If significant faults are identified then the backup implant should be used and an immediate reimplantation performed. Although this situation arises very infrequently, a standard procedure should be in place to manage it. Issues that need to be addressed are:

- what constitutes a significant fault;
- selection of tests to confirm the malfunction of the device;
- contact with the manufacturer at the time of surgery regarding the decision and warranty.

Intra-operative electrophysiological and objective measures are valuable tools for monitoring either immediate reimplantation with the backup device or later reimplantation due to implant failure (Mason et al., 2000).

Stimulation of the auditory pathway

The presence of an EABR, ESR, or ECAP waveform confirms that the auditory nerve fibres are receiving and reacting to electrical stimulation, and response activity is being generated in the peripheral nerve pathways (ECAP) and the brainstem pathways (EABR and ESR). Any one of these techniques is therefore an effective check of the functioning of the implant system and the physiological status of the auditory pathway. An absent response in association with an abnormal electrode impedance and/or AEV (identified by BT and/or IT) is suggestive of a malfunctioning electrode. A well-defined EABR waveform with a steep amplitude I/O function is thought to suggest good neuronal survival (Smith and Simmons, 1983; Hall, 1990). The presence of these characteristics on the EABR is therefore desirable but their absence is not necessarily an indicator of poor performance by the implant user. Abbas and Brown (1991) were unable to demonstrate a significant correlation between the amplitude I/O function of the EABR and overall performance. More recently Gallégo et al. (1998) have suggested a relationship between the latency measures of the EABR and outcome measures.

Assistance with fitting

The EABR and the ESR are used extensively by many implant centres to assist with fitting of the implant (Brown et al., 1994; Mason et al., 1994; Spivak and Chute, 1994). Thresholds of these responses can guide the audiologist towards the levels of electrical stimulation that are appropriate for a child. This information can be extremely valuable at the initial fitting session in a young child after implantation and therefore intra-operative recordings of the EABR and ESR can play an important role in management. More recently the value of ECAP in the fitting process, recorded using the technique of NRT, has been reported by Hughes et al. (2000).

Prediction of threshold level: EABR

There are many reports from the last few years that have investigated the use of both intra-operative and post-operative EABR to predict behavioural threshold levels of electrical stimulation. The accuracy of the prediction depends on applying appropriate correction factors (Shallop et al., 1991; Mason et al., 1994). The threshold of the intra-operative EABR is generally less sensitive than the first reliable behavioural threshold level (T level) obtained at around four weeks after surgery. This offset is the result of a number of factors:

- effects of temporal summation due to different pulse rates employed for each test (typically 31 to 85 pps for the EABR and 250 pps or higher for the T level);
- difficulties in the identification of a small EABR close to threshold;
- change in the effective level of stimulation post-operatively.

A typical example of this offset is described in Mason et al. (1994) for the Nucleus CI22 implant. In common ground (CG) stimulation mode this offset was typically around 35 units and when this value was simply subtracted from the EABR threshold on all electrodes resulted in 80% of the corrected thresholds being within 30 stimulus units of the T level, and 58% within 20 units. A significant improvement in this relationship was achieved when offsets specific to a particular electrode were taken into consideration. This resulted in 98% of EABR thresholds being within 30 stimulus units of T level and 78% within 20 units.

Although many of the published reports on the application of the EABR are based on cochlear implants that have subsequently been superseded, the methods of analysis of the data are similar. However, it is vital that correction factors applied to the EABR threshold in order to predict behavioural thresholds are valid for the type of implant currently in use. For example, the Nucleus CI22 has been superseded by the CI24M and the Contour device. As a result of this, the default stimulus mode has changed from common ground to monopolar where an extra-cochlear ball electrode is now used as a reference for the return current. Experience has shown that this transition in the stimulus mode significantly increases the problems of stimulus artefact on the recorded waveform due to an increase in current spread.

Prediction of threshold level: ECAP

In the NPCIP, we use the relationship between the intra-operative recordings of the ECAP and early post-operative behavioural thresholds to assist with management of the children. Results show that there is a statistically significant relationship between the two measures when inter-subject variations in the offset between the two measurements have been taken into consideration. This offset is different between subjects but is similar across all the electrodes within the same subject. In other words the ECAP thresholds follow the pattern of the T levels across the electrode array in any one subject.

In practice, a correction for the offset can be implemented by measuring the behavioural threshold reliably on one electrode on each individual subject at the initial tuning session (electrode 10 for example) as described by Hughes et al. (2000). The difference between this behavioural threshold and the intra-operative ECAP threshold (offset correction) is then subtracted from the absolute ECAP thresholds on all other electrodes. Figure 6.17 shows the high level of agreement that exists once this correction has been applied (Mason et al., 2001). This limited amount of behavioural data enables the ECAP to become a valuable predictor of behavioural threshold levels of electrical stimulation.

Recordings of the ECAP using NRT have the potential to complement or possibly replace the EABR. The NRT technique is simple and quick to implement and does not require the use of surface scalp electrodes. These are valuable attributes in the operating theatre. In straightforward cases undergoing implantation then the argument for ECAP taking priority over of the

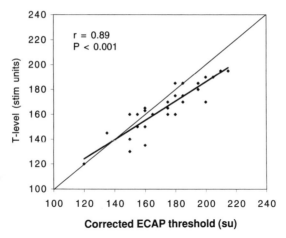

Figure 6.17. The relationship between the intra-operative corrected ECAP threshold and the early behavioural threshold (T) level recorded from electrodes 5, 15 and 20 (30 data points in 14 children). The correction for the ECAP has been derived from the offset in thresholds on electrode 10. A line representing equal values is shown and a linear regression based on these data.

EABR is strong, however in complex cases the EABR should be retained as it provides valuable information about the integrity and functioning of brainstem pathways. There is further discussion of the issue of the ECAP versus EABR later in the chapter.

Prediction of comfort level: ESR

The most popular technique for recording the ESR intra-operatively is from visual observation of the response (Sheppard et al., 1992). In a study of 19 children by Van den Borne et al. (1996), an ESR was detected in all the congenitally deaf children but was absent in 30% of the post-meningitic children. A similar finding has been reported by Spivak and Shute (1994). Possible explanations for the absence of a response include inadequate current levels, insufficient number of surviving neurones and lack of sensitivity of the response detection. Absence of a reflex should be interpreted with caution since children still receive significant benefit from an implant in this situation.

It is generally reported that there is a weak relationship between the threshold of the ESR and the behavioural comfort level (Stephan et al., 1991; Van den Borne et al., 1996; Spivak and Chute, 1994). This relationship is not as strong as the correlation between the threshold of the EABR and behavioural threshold of electrical stimulation. In young children, the intra-operative ESR threshold is generally higher than the early post-operative comfort levels of stimulation. In Sheppard et al. (1992) the early comfort levels were in the range of 45% to 90% of the ESR threshold (mean = 74%). In later post-operative tuning sessions the comfort levels increased and became closer to the intra-operative ESR thresholds.

Effects of anaesthesia on the ESR

When the ESR is recorded intra-operatively, either by visual detection or acoustic impedance methods, it is important to be aware of the possible effects of the anaesthetic procedure (Van den Borne et al., 1996). Administration of muscle relaxants will inhibit the ESR, use of volatile anaesthetic agents can affect the threshold, and nitrous oxide can change the middle-ear pressure on the contra-lateral side thereby influencing acoustic imped-ance measurements. The anaesthetic regime should be carefully controlled in order to achieve reliable and repeatable results.

Dynamic range

Threshold and comfort levels for electrical stimulation define the upper and lower limits of the dynamic range. An objective prediction of the dynamic range can be derived from the corrected thresholds of the EABR, ECAP and ESR. In patients with a wide dynamic range the clinical value of this prediction will be affected to a lesser extent by any inaccuracy in the objec-tive measures compared with patients with a very narrow dynamic range. Additional care must therefore be exercised in applying objective predictions when the difference between the corrected thresholds of the EABR or ECAP and ESR is small.

Assessments after implantation

Objective measures provide valuable support in the manage-ment of children after implantation, particularly those who present with difficult behavioural tuning, possible device fail-ure, or faults with electrodes. In addition, electrophysiological measures enable the research and development of issues such as maturation and survival of the auditory pathways and the assess-ment and optimization of performance.

Objective monitoring of implant function

The majority of children implanted in the last two or three years will have received an implant that has back telemetry (BT).

Using BT, every child attending for tuning should have an assessment of implant function and electrode impedance, whether or not there is any suspicion of malfunction of the device. In addition, if there are specific concerns about the functioning of the device, either on behavioural tests and/or BT, then integrity testing (IT) is desirable. Objective monitoring of implant function in children with older devices, where BT is not available, will rely exclusively on the use of IT. To assist the monitoring process it is valuable to have objective measures performed at the time of surgery, because these provide a valuable source of reference data, enabling any subtle changes in the functioning of the implant to be detected.

Faults with the implant can be divided into two categories. First, complete failure of the device probably arising from internal component failure, a damaged antenna, or broken electrode array. Second, malfunction of individual electrodes as a result of broken wires, electrode weld failures, and loss of insulation on electrode wires. In complete failure, BT may or may not be operable, and there will be no AEV observed on IT. In some cases a residual RF artefact may be observed. Faults with individual electrodes will manifest themselves in different ways. A broken wire (open circuit) will show high impedance on BT and there will be no AEV present. Interpretation of short circuits or partial shorts is more complicated and is affected by the origin of the short, whether it is to another electrode and or to some other structure in the implant. As the number of faulty electrodes increases this significantly complicates the picture. For example, if one of these faulty electrodes is used as a reference for the return current then this will affect the configuration of the AEV. This is particularly evident in bipolar modes where an increase or decrease in amplitude of the AEV, combined with an associated change in phase, can be observed depending on the electrodes involved in the shorting process. In the NPCIP, a summary table for IT results has been developed which assists interpretation of the AEV across the electrode array using different stimulus modes. An example of this table is shown in Figure 6.18.

In addition to children being referred for IT on a case-by-case basis, all children in the NPCIP have a routine investigation carried out five years after implantation as part of the standard protocol. An audit of the results of these tests in 30 children showed that it affected the management of 30% of the children

COCHLEAR IMPLANT - INTEGRITY MAP

Name **I. ABNORMAL**

D.O.B. **5 - 5 - 91**

Investigation No. **IT 00696**

Date **5 - 5 - 96**

No. of electrodes inserted **22 + 3**   Procedure: Intraoperative / Postoperative

Right / Left ear

ELECTRODE CHANNELS

STIMULUS DETAILS				1	2	3	4	5	6	7	8	9	10	11	12	13	14	15	16	17	18	19	20	21	22	COMMENTS
MODE eg. CG	**S or C**	**Pulse Width (µs)**	**Stim. Units**																							
CG	S	–	100	+	+	+	ND	ND	+	+	+	?.	–	–	?.	?.	+	+	+	+	–	+	+	+	+	AEV CHARACTERISTICS:
MPI	C	204	50	/	/	+	+	+	+	+	+	?.	–	?.	?.	+	+	+	+	–	+	+	+	+	OPEN CIRCUITS /
BP+3	C	204	50	+	+	+	+	?.	?.	?.	+	–	–	–	?.	?.	+	+	ND ND	+	/	/	/	/	SHORT CIRCUITS
OVERALL OUTCOME				+	+	+	+	+	+	+	+	–	–	–	–	?.	+	+	+	–	+	+	+	+	

Additional Information:

EXAMPLE : ELECTRODE MALFUNCTION

KEY:
- **+** Normal Function
- **?** Questionable
- **–** Faulty
- **ND** Non diagnostic

Evoked Potentials Clinic, Medical Physics, Q.M.C., NOTTINGHAM.   Ext.43382

CAJ/1995

Figure 6.18. An example of results of integrity testing presented in a summary table as used in the NPCIP.

(Garnham et al., 2000b). Electrodes have either been identified as being faulty or there has been clarification of the function of electrodes that have previously been suspected as faulty on behavioural testing. These findings have subsequently resulted in a change in the electrode map.

Assistance with tuning

The EABR and ESR can be recorded to investigate any unexpected changes in the dynamic range of electrical stimulation. This information can be used to support the results of behavioural assessments in difficult-to-test children, which might include the very young and complex cases. However, implementation of these recordings post-operatively, particularly in a young child, is more difficult than intra-operative testing under general anaesthesia. It may be necessary to use sedation, or even a general anaesthetic, in order to achieve sufficiently reliable test conditions particularly for the EABR. This situation obviously restricts application of the technique to those children in urgent need of the support of objective measures.

ECAP versus EABR

A potential alternative to the EABR for post-operative testing is the ECAP using the technique of NRT. It has the following attractions over the EABR:

- scalp recording electrodes are not required;
- the recordings are not affected by external electrical interference;
- the child only has to sit playing, rather than be very quiet or sedated;
- short set-up and recording time enables measurements on many electrodes.

However, there are the following drawbacks:

- ECAP only represents activity in the peripheral auditory system (equivalent to wave I on ABR);
- careful selection of data collection parameters is needed for reliable recordings;
- limited relationship between the ECAP and behavioural measures;

- small amounts of reliable behavioural data are required for prediction of electrical threshold.

Evoked stapedius reflex

In the post-operative stage, acoustic impedance techniques can be employed for measurement of the ESR. The reported success of ESR in young children is variable and the absence of a response should not be automatically reported as suggesting major problems with tuning. Studies on adults and children have demonstrated significant numbers of subjects with no response; 24% (Battmer et al., 1990), 48% (Stephan et al., 1991); 31% (Spivak and Chute, 1994). In young children the main difficulties appear to be prevalence of middle-ear pathology and ossification of the cochlea. When an ESR is present it has a weak relationship with comfort levels of stimulation, as discussed previously.

Assessment of central auditory processing and maturation

Maturation of the human auditory nervous system is early in life in the periphery but is much slower and later at cortical level. Some auditory related cortical potentials, such as the MMN, which originate from the reticular system, may mature as early as the ABR whereas other potentials, such as the P1 and N1 of the ACR, mature much slower. The EACR has been investigated in implanted children and young adults from the age of five years to 19 years by Ponton et al. (1999). From these data and earlier studies they proposed the following model for the resumption and maintenance of auditory maturation of the auditory cortex after prolonged deafness with post-natal onset:

- The state of cortical maturation at the time of deafness is 'frozen' and is unaffected by substantial periods of deafness.
- An immature state of the auditory cortex may require a period of up to six months after the start of stimulation with a cochlear implant before maturation recommences.
- Ongoing stimulation with the cochlear implant causes cortical maturation to proceed at the same rate as in a normal-hearing subject, but may show a maturational asymptote at a sub-adult or adult level. The final level of maturity will be dependent on the age of the subject and the duration of deafness.

- Continued cortical plasticity is expected to happen well into adulthood. While this may not be expressed in the P1 and N1 components, evidence of adult plasticity may be apparent in other responses such as the MMN (Tremblay et al., 1998).

The clinical implication of the report by Ponton et al. (1999) is that the shorter the period of deafness before implantation and in younger children, the better is the prospect for normal cortical maturation and likely adequate development of verbal language and communication skills.

Assessment of central processing and maturation using evoked potentials, such as the EACR, MMN, and P300 might help to explain why some cochlear implant users communicate better than others for no obvious clinical reason. Subtle discrimination between sounds is central to speech perception. These objective measures are potentially valuable in young implanted children where behavioural tests of discrimination are not always easy to implement reliably.

Future developments

Advances over the last few years in the development and application of electrophysiological and other objective measures has significantly influenced the management of young implanted children. As more children with complex problems are implanted, the value of objective measures will be further enhanced. Over the next few years we will experience further change and development leading to a greater understanding of data and performance, particularly in the post-operative period. Two areas that are ripe for this development are recordings of the ECAP and ERP.

In closing this chapter we should, in the future, look to move forward on the following issues:

- Standardization of protocols for the use of electrophysiological and objective measures in the management of young children.
- Demonstration of improved performance on outcome measures to justify techniques that are employed for selection of patients or ears for implantation.
- Use of objective measures to assess function and performance with respect to neuronal survival, maturation and central processing capabilities.

- Increased accuracy and reliability of objective predictors of dynamic range of electrical stimulation for individual electrodes and different implant devices.
- Greater understanding and improved interpretation of the relationship of integrity testing and back telemetry impedance measurements.

Acknowledgements

The author would like to acknowledge specific contributions to this chapter by Dr Joanne Garnham (Aided ABRs and Integrity Testing) and Sharon Wallace (Event Related Potentials). This work is also dependent on the valuable support of the technical and scientific staff of the Evoked Potentials Clinic in the Medical Physics Department at Nottingham's Queen's Medical Centre.

References

Abbas PJ (1988) Electrophysiology of the auditory system. Clinical Physics and Physiological Measurement 9: 1-31.

Abbas PJ, Brown CJ (1991) Electrically evoked auditory brainstem response: growth of response with current level. Hearing Research 51:123-38.

Abbas PJ, Brown CJ, Shallop JK, Hughes ML, Hong SH, Staller SJ (1999) Summary of results using the Nucleus CI24M implant to record the electrically evoked compound action potential. Ear & Hearing 20: 45-59.

Abramovich, S (1990) Electric Response Audiometry in Clinical Practice. Edinburgh, Churchill Livingstone.

Alho K, Winkler I, Escera C, Houtilainen M, Virtanen J, Jääskeläinen IP, Pekkonen E, Ilmoniemi RJ (1998) Processing of novel sounds and frequency changes in the human auditory cortex: magnetoencephalographic recordings. Psychophysiology 35: 211-24.

Allum JHJ, Shallop JK, Hotz M, Pfaltz CR (1990) Characteristics of electrically evoked 'auditory' brainstem responses elicited with the Nucleus 22-electrode intracochlear implant. Scandinavian Audiology 19: 263-7.

Almqvist B, Harris H, Jonsson K-E (1993) The stimulogram. Presented at the Third International Cochlear Implant Conference, Innsbruck, Austria, 4-7 April.

Battmer R-D, Laszig R, Lehnhardt E (1990) Electrically elicited stapedius reflex in cochlear implant patients. Ear and Hearing 11: 370-4.

Berger H (1929) and (1930) On the electroencephalogram of man. In Gloor P (ed.) Hans Berger on the electroencephalogram of man. Electroencephalography and Clinical Neurophysiology, Suppl. 28, 37, Elsevier, 1969.

Brix R, Gedlicka W (1991) Late cortical auditory potentials evoked by electrostimulation in deaf and cochlear implant patients. European Archives of Oto-Rhino-Laryngology 248: 442-4.

Brown CJ, Abbas PJ (1990) Electrically evoked whole-nerve action potentials: data from human cochlear implant users. Journal of the Acoustical Society of America 88: 1385-91.

Brown CJ, Abbas PJ, Fryauf-Bertschy H, Kelsay D, Gantz BJ (1994) Intra-operative and post-operative electrically evoked auditory brainstem responses in Nucleus cochlear implant users: implications for the fitting process. Ear and Hearing 15: 168-76.

Brown CJ, Hughes ML, Luk B, Abbas PJ, Wolaver A, Gervais J (2000) The relationship between EAP and EABR thresholds and levels used to program the Nucleus CI24M speech processor. Ear and Hearing 21: 151-63.

Carter PM, Fisher AR, Nygard TM, Swanson BA, Sheppard RK, Tykocinski M, Brown M (1994) Monitoring the electrically evoked compound action potential by means of a new telemetry system. International Cochlear Implant, Speech and Hearing Symposium 48-51.

Cheour M, Leppänen PHT, Kraus N (2000) Mismatch negativity (MMN) as a tool for investigating auditory discrimination and sensory memory in infants and children. Clinical Neurophysiology 111: 4-16.

Cullington HE, Clarke GP (1997) Integrity testing of cochlear implants in the awake child. British Journal of Audiology 31: 247-56.

Cullington HE (2000) Preliminary neural response telemetry results. British Journal of Audiology 34: 131-40.

Davis H (1976) Brainstem and other responses in electrical response audiometry. Annals of Otology 85: 3-14.

Davis H, Davis PA, Loomis AL, Harvey EN, Hobart G (1939) Electrical reactions of the human brain to auditory stimulation during sleep. Journal of Neurophysiology 2: 500-14.

Davis H, Hirsh SK (1979) A slow brainstem response for low-frequency audiometry. Audiology 18: 445-61.

Davis PA (1939) Effects of acoustic stimuli on the waking human brain. Journal of Neurophysiology 2: 494-9.

Djourno A, Eyries C (1957) Prosthese auditive par excitation electrique a distance du nerf sensoriel a l'aide d'un bobinage inclus a demeure. Presse Med 35: 14-17.

Drift van der JFC, Brocaar MP, Van Zanten GA (1987) The relation between the pure tone audiogram and the click auditory brainstem response threshold in cochlear hearing loss. Audiology 26: 1-10.

French ML (1999) Electrical impedance measurements with the CI24M cochlear implant for a child with Mondini dysplasia. British Journal of Audiology 33: 61-6.

Gallégo S, Frachet B, Micheyl C, Truy E, Collet L (1998) Cochlear implant performance and electrically-evoked auditory brain-stem response characteristics. Electroencephalography and Clinical Neurophysiology 108: 521-5.

Game CJA, Thomson DR, Gibson WPR (1990) Measurement of auditory brainstem responses evoked by electrical stimulation with a cochlear implant. British Journal of Audiology 24: 145-9.

Gantz BJ, Woodworth GG, Knutson JF, Abbas PJ, Tyler RS (1993) Multivariate predictors of success with cochlear implants. Advances in Oto-Rhino-Laryngology 48: 153-67.

Garnham J, Cope Y, Durst C, McCormick B, Mason SM (2000a) Assessment of aided ABR thresholds before cochlear implantation. British Journal of Audiology 34: 267-78.

Garnham J, Cope Y, Mason SM (2000b) Audit of five-year post-implantation routine integrity tests performed on paediatric cochlear implantees. British Journal of Audiology 34: 285-92.

Garnham J, Marsden J, Mason SM (2001) Profiles of AEVs for intra- and post-operative integrity test measurements in young children with the Nucleus mini 22 cochlear implant. British Journal of Audiology 35: 31–42.

Gibbin KP (1992) Paediatric cochlear implantation. Archives of Disease in Childhood 67: 669–71.

Gibson WPR (1978) Essentials of Clinical Electric Response Audiometry. London: Churchill Livingstone.

Gray RF, Baguley DM (1990) Electrical stimulation of the round window: a selection procedure for single-channel cochlear implantation. Clinical Otolaryngology 15: 29–34.

Hall RD (1990) Estimation of surviving spiral ganglion cells in the deaf rat using the electrically evoked auditory brainstem response. Hearing Research 45: 123–36.

Hall J (1992) Handbook of Auditory Evoked Responses.Boston, MA: Allyn & Bacon

Hashimoto I (1982) Auditory evoked potentials from the human midbrain: slow brain stem responses. Electroencephalography and Clinical Neurophysiology 53: 652–7.

House WF (1991) Cochlear implants in children: past and present perspectives. American Journal of Otology 12: 1–2.

Hughes ML, Brown CJ, Abbas PJ, Wolaver AA, Gervais JP (2000) Comparison of EAP thresholds with MAP levels in the Nucleus 24 cochlear implant: data from children. Ear and Hearing 21: 164–74.

Jacobson JT (1985) The Auditory Brainstem Response. San Diego, CA: College-Hill Press.

Jewett DL, Williston JS (1971) Auditory-evoked far fields averaged from the scalp of humans. Brain 94: 681–96.

John MS, Picton TW (2000) Master: a Windows program for recording multiple auditory steady-state responses. Computer Methods and Programs in Biomedicine 61: 125–50.

Kasper A, Pelizzone M, Montandon P (1991). Intracochlear potential distribution with intracochlear and extracochlear electrical stimulation in humans. Annals of Otology, Rhinology and Laryngology 100: 812–16.

Kato T, Shiraishi K, Eura Y, Shibata K, Sakata T, Morizono T, Soda T (1998) A'Neural' response with 3-ms latency evoked by loud sound in profoundly deaf patients. Audiol Neurootol 3: 253–64.

Kileny P, Kemink JL, Miller JM (1989) An intrasubject comparison of electric and acoustic middle latency responses. American Journal of Otology 10: 23–7.

Kileny PR (1991) Use of electrophysiologic measures in the management of children with cochlear implants: brainstem, middle latency, and cognitive (P300) responses. American Journal of Otology 12: 37–42.

Kileny PR, Zwolan T, Zimmerman-Phillips S, Kemink J (1992) A comparison of round-window and transtympanic promontory electric stimulation in cochlear implant candidates. Ear and Hearing 13: 294–9.

Kileny PR, Zwolan TA, Zimmerman-Phillips S, Telian SA (1994) Electrically evoked auditory brain-stem response in paediatric patients with cochlear implants. Archives of Otolaryngology, Head and Neck Surgery 120: 1083–90

Kraus N, McGee T, Sharma A, Carrell T, Nicol T (1992) Mismatch negativity event-related potential elicited by speech stimuli. Ear and Hearing 13: 158–64.

Kraus N, Micco AG, Koch DB, McGee T, Carrell T, Sharma A, Wiet RJ, Weingarten CZ (1993) The mismatch negativity cortical evoked potential elicited by speech in cochlear implant users. Hearing Research 65: 118–24.

Lightfoot GR, Mason S, Stevens JC (2000) Electric response audiometry and otoacoustic emissions: principles, techniques and clinical applications. Course notes from the Harrogate ERA Course, UK.

Mahoney JM (1985) Auditory brainstem response hearing aid applications. In Jacobson JT (ed.) The Auditory Brainstem Response. San Diego, CA: College-Hill Press, pp. 349-70.

Mahoney JM, Proctor LAR (1994) The use of averaged electrode voltages to assess the function of Nucleus internal cochlear implant devices in children. Ear and Hearing 15: 177-83

Mason JDT, Mason SM, Gibbin KP (1995b) Raised ABR threshold after suction aspiration of glue from the middle ear: three case studies. The Journal of Laryngology and Otology 109: 726-8.

Mason SM (1984) Effects of high-pass filtering on the detection of the auditory brainstem response. British Journal of Audiology 18: 155-61.

Mason SM (1993) Electric Response Audiometry. In McCormick B (ed.) Paediatric Audiology 0-5 years. London: Whurr, pp 187-249.

Mason SM (1997) Objective Measures. American Journal of Otology 18: S84-S87.

Mason SM, Singh CB, Brown PM (1980) Assessment of non-invasive electrocochleography. Journal of Laryngology and Otology 94: 707-18.

Mason SM, McCormick B, Wood S (1988) Auditory brainstem response in paediatric audiology. Archives of Disease in Childhood 63: 465-7.

Mason SM, Sheppard S, Garnham CW, Lutman ME, O'Donoghue GM, Gibbin KP (1993) Application of intraoperative recordings of electrically evoked ABRs in a paediatric cochlear implant programme. Advances in Oto-Rhino-Laryngology 48: 136-41.

Mason SM, Sheppard S, Garnham CW, Lutman ME, O'Donoghue GM, Gibbin KP (1994) Improving the relationship of intraoperative EABR threshold to T-level in young children receiving the Nucleus cochlear implant. In Hochmair-Desoyer IJ, Hochmair ES (eds) Advances in Cochlear Implants. Manz: Wein, pp 44-9.

Mason SM, Garnham CW, Sheppard S, O'Donoghue GM, Gibbin KP (1995a) An intraoperative test protocol for objective assessment of the Nucleus 22-channel cochlear implant. In Uziel AS, Mondain M (eds) Cochlear Implants in Children, Advances in Otorhinolaryngology. Basel: Karger, 50: 38-44.

Mason SM, Garnham CW, Hudson B (1996) Electric response audiometry in young children prior to cochlear implantation: a short latency component. Ear and Hearing 17: 537-43.

Mason SM, O'Donoghue GM, Gibbin KP, Garnham CW, Jowett CA (1997) Perioperative electrical auditory brainstem response in candidates for pediatric cochlear implantation. American Journal of Otology 18: 466-71.

Mason SM, Dodd M, Gibbin KP, O'Donoghue GM (2000) Assessment of the functioning of peripheral auditory pathways after cochlear re-implantation in young children using intra-operative objective measures. British Journal of Audiology 34: 179-86.

Mason SM, Cope Y, Garnham J, O'Donoghue GM, Gibbin KP (2001) Intra-operative recordings of electrically evoked auditory nerve action potentials in young children by use of neural response telemetry with the Nucleus CI24M cochlear implant. British Journal of Audiology 35: 225-35.

Maxwell A, Mason SM, O'Donoghue GM (1999) Cochlear nerve aplasia: its importance in cochlear implantation. American Journal of Otology 20: 335-7.

McCormick B (1997) Paediatric audiology and cochlear implantation in the UK: taking off in the fast lane. British Journal of Audiology 31: 303-7.

McCormick B, Gibbin KP, Lutman ME, O'Donoghue GM (1993) Late partial recovery from meningitis deafness after cochlear implantation: a case study. American Journal of Otology 14: 1-3.

McGee T, Kraus N (1996) Auditory development reflected by middle latency response. Ear and Hearing 17: 419–29.

Meikle MB, Gillette RG, Godfrey FA (1977) Comparison of electrically and acoustically evoked responses in the auditory cortex of the guinea pig: Implications for a cochlear prosthesis. Transactions of the American Academy of Ophthalmology and Otology 84: 183–92.

Mens LHM, Oostendorp T, Van den Broek P (1994a) Identifying electrode failures with cochlear implant generated surface potentials. Ear and Hearing 15: 330–8.

Mens LHM, Oostendorp T, Van den Broek P (1994b) Cochlear implant generated surface potentials: current spread and side effects. Ear and Hearing 15: 339–45.

Millard RE, McAnally KI, Clark GM (1992) A gated differential amplifier for recording physiological responses to electrical stimulation. Journal of Neuroscience Methods 44: 81–4.

Miyamoto RT (1986) Electrically evoked potentials in cochlear implants. Laryngoscope 96: 178–85.

Möller AR (1999) Neural mechanisms of BAEP. Electroencephalography and Clinical Neurophysiology Supplement 49: 27–35.

Näätänen R (1990) The role of attention in auditory information processing as revealed by event-related potentials and other brain measures of cognitive function. Behavioral and Brain Sciences 13: 201–88.

Nikolopoulos TP, Mason SM, O'Donoghue GM, Gibbin KP (1997) Electric auditory brain stem response in paediatric patients with cochlear implants. American Journal of Otology 18: S120–1.

Nikolopoulos TP, Mason SM, O'Donoghue GM, Gibbin KP (1999) Integrity of the auditory pathway in young children with congenital and post-meningitic deafness. Annals of Otology, Rhinology and Laryngology 108: 327–30.

Nikolopoulos TP, Mason SM, Gibbin KP, O'Donoghue GM (2000) The prognostic value of promontory electric auditory brainstem response in pediatric cochlear implantation. Ear and Hearing 21: 236–41.

Obler R, Köstler H, Weber B-P, Mack KF, Becker H (1999) Safe electrical stimulation of the cochlear nerve at the promontory during functional magnetic resonance imaging. Magnetic Resonance in Medicine 42: 371–8.

O'Donoghue GM (1999) Hearing with our ears: do cochlear implants work in children? British Medical Journal 318(7176): 72–3.

Oviatt DL, Kileny PR (1991) Auditory event-related potentials elicited from cochlear implant recipients and hearing subjects. American Journal of Audiology 1: 48–55.

Pelizzone M, Kasper K, Montandon P (1989) Electrically evoked responses in cochlear implant patients. Audiology 28: 230–8.

Picton TW (1995) The neurophysiological evaluation of auditory discrimination. Ear and Hearing 16: 1–5.

Picton TW, Hillyard SA, Krausz HI, Galambos R (1974) Human auditory evoked potentials. I. Evaluation of components, Electroencephalography and Clinical Neurophysiology 36: 179–90.

Picton TW, Durieux-Smith A, Champagne SC, Whittingham J, Moran LM, Giguere C, Beauregard Y (1998) Objective evaluation of aided thresholds using auditory steady state responses. Journal of the American Academy of Audiology 9: 315–31.

Ponton CW, Don M (1995) The mismatch negativity in cochlear implant users. Ear and Hearing 16: 131–46.

Ponton CW, Don M, Eggermont JJ, Waring MD, Masuda A (1996) Maturation of human cortical auditory function: differences between normal-hearing and children with cochlear implants. Ear and Hearing 17: 430-7.

Ponton CW, Moore JK, Eggermont JJ (1999) Prolonged deafness limits auditory system developmental plasticity: evidence from an evoked potentials study in children with cochlear implants. Scandinavian Audiology 28: 13-22.

Portmann M, Lebert G, Aran J-M (1967) Potentiels cochleares obtenus chez l'homme en dehors de toute intervention chirurgicale. Revue de Laryngologie 88: 157-64.

Rance G, Dowell RC, Rickards FW, Beer DE, Clark GM (1998) Steady-state evoked potential and behavioural hearing thresholds in a group of children with absent click-evoked auditory brainstem response. Ear and Hearing 19: 48-60.

Shallop JK, Beiter AL, Goin DW, Mischke RE (1990) Electrically evoked auditory brainstem response (EABR) and middle latency responses (EMLR) obtained from patients with the Nucleus multichannel cochlear implant. Ear and Hearing 11: 5-15.

Shallop JK, VanDyke L, Goin DW, Mischke RE (1991) Prediction of behavioural threshold and comfort values for Nucleus 22-channel implant patients from electrical auditory brain stem response test results. Annals of Otology, Rhinology and Laryngology 100: 896-8.

Shallop JK (1997) Objective measurements and the audiological management of cochlear implant patients. In Alford BR, Jerger J, Jenkins HA (eds) Electrophysiological Evaluation in Otolaryngology. Advances in Otorhinolaryngology. Basel: Karger 53: pp85-111.

Sheppard S, Mason,SM, Lutman ME, Gibbin KP, O'Donoghue GM (1992) Intraoperative electrical stapedial reflex measurements in young children receiving cochlear implants. Presented at the First European Symposium on Paediatric Cochlear Implantation, Nottingham, September 1992.

Smith L, Simmons FB (1983) Estimating eighth nerve survival by electrical stimulation. Annals of Otology, Rhinology and Laryngology 92: 19-25.

Sohmer H, Feinmesser M (1967) Cochlear action potentials recorded from the external ear in man. Annals of Otology, Rhinology and Laryngology 76: 427-35.

Spivak LG, Chute PM (1994) The relationship between electrical acoustic reflex thresholds and behavioral comfort levels in children and adult cochlear implant patients. Ear and Hearing 15: 184-92.

Stapells DR, Galambos R, Costello JA, Makeig S (1988) Inconsistency of auditory middle latency and steady-state responses in infants. Electroencephalography and Clinical Neurophysiology 71: 289-95.

Stapells DR, Oates P (1997) Estimation of the pure-tone audiogram by the auditory brainstem response: a review. Audiology and Neuro-otology 2: 257-80.

Starr A, Brackmann DE (1979) Brainstem potentials evoked by electrical stimulation of the cochlea in human subjects. Annals of Otology, Rhinology and Laryngology 88: 550-6.

Stephan K, Welzl-Muller K, Stiglbrunner H (1991) Acoustic reflex in patients with cochlear implants (analog stimulation). The American Journal of Otology 12: 48-51.

Stevens J, Elliott C, Lightfoot G, Mason S, Parker D, Stapells D, Sutton G, Vidler M (1999) Click auditory brainstem response testing in babies – a recommended test protocol. BSA News: Issue 28.

Sussman E, Ritter W, Vaughan HG Jr (1999) Attention affects the organisation of auditory input associated with the mismatch negativity system. Brain Research 789: 130-8.

Taylor MJ (1991) EPs and ERPs in paediatrics. In Barber C, Taylor M (eds) Evoked Potentials Review No.4, Nottingham: IEPS Publications, pp 1-14.

Thornton ARD (1987) Electrophysiological measures of hearing function in hearing disorders, British Medical Bulletin 43: 926-39.

Tremblay K, Kraus N, McGee T (1998) The time course of auditory perceptual learning: neurophysiological changes during speech-sound training. Neuroreport 9: 3557-60.

Van den Borne B, Snik AFM, Mens LHM, Brokx JPL, Van den Broek P (1996) Stapedius reflex measurements during surgery for cochlear implantation in children. The American Journal of Otology 17: 554-8.

Chapter 7
Fitting and programming the external system

Yvonne Cope, Catherine L Totten

Introduction

Irrespective of the cochlear implant system, mode of stimulation and speech processing strategy used, all speech processors and implanted components function by converting acoustic signals into electrical currents. This current is then used to produce an auditory percept by stimulating the remaining auditory nerve fibres, via the implanted electrode array. The signal processing and mode of stimulation used determine how the incoming acoustic signals are converted into electrical patterns and delivered to the implanted electrodes. In order to maximize the speech information received by the recipient, the speech processor requires programming. In the most simplistic form this involves establishing which electrodes produce a useful sensation of hearing and then measuring the dynamic range for electrical stimulation on each electrode. The dynamic range is obtained by measuring the behavioural threshold and either the most comfortable loudness level or the uncomfortable loudness level, then setting the latter at a comfortable level. With infants and very young children, the information obtained in the initial stages of programming may be limited and will need refining and verifying over a number of additional sessions. The values of the psychophysical measures and speech processing strategy used are stored within the speech processor and used to create a programme or map. Each cochlear implantee's map is unique to them. When optimal, it enables speech and other sounds to be presented at a level that is both audible and comfortable.

In this chapter we provide an introduction to the concepts involved in cochlear implant tuning and the techniques used for speech processor fitting. The reader is guided from initial stimulation through to map optimization. Fitting verification methods and the identification and management of changes in device function are also discussed. Techniques used for children who do not have the perceptual development to undertake modified adult tasks are presented. Basic programming concepts specific to mode of stimulation and speech processing strategies are discussed.

Speech processors

All speech processors, whether they are body-worn or worn at ear level comprise the same basic components, as illustrated in Figures 7.1 and 7.2.

The microphone is worn at ear level, either integral to the speech processor as with the ear-level device or as a separate

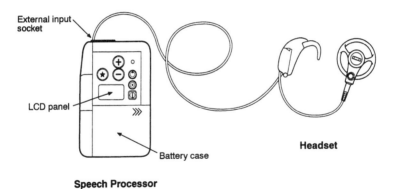

Figure 7.1. Diagram of the externally worn components of a Nucleus CI24M SPRint body-worn speech processor. (Adapted from Cochlear user manual for the SPRint speech processor and accessories 1998.)

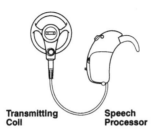

Figure 7.2. Diagram of the externally worn components of a Nucleus CI24M ESPrit ear-level speech processor. (Adapted from Cochlear user manual for the ESPrit speech processor and accessories 1997.)

component as with body-worn devices. The sound received by the microphone is delivered to the speech processor, which selects and codes the useful components and in turn sends them to the transmitting coil. The coil is held in place by a magnet, which aligns with the magnet located in the implanted receiver/stimulator. The transmitting coil conveys via radio frequency waves, this specific code to the receiver/stimulator where it is converted into electrical signals. The electrical signals are then sent to the implanted electrodes.

Equipment required for programming and clinic set up

Programming an individual's speech processor, requires connecting it to a computer controlled interface unit. The connection may be direct or via a fly cable. An example of the set up of a programming system can be seen in Figure 7.3.

Stimuli are presented either by using the computer keyboard or a hand-held stimulus attenuator, known as the control knob. Psychophysical measurements are obtained by the methods discussed later. Specialized computer software, specific to individual devices, controls the stimulus parameters. The programming software is designed to be flexible, to ensure that the parameters can be altered by the clinician to ensure all implantees are fitted optimally. These parameters include choice of speech processing strategy and mode of stimulation, together with the facility to adjust certain features of the stimulus itself.

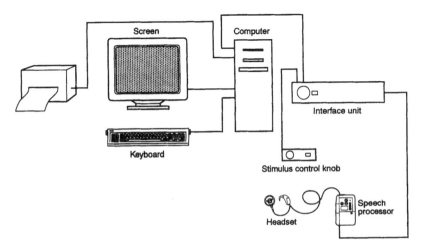

Figure 7.3. Diagram of the Nucleus CI24M programming equipment.

It is usual for programming systems to be located in a clinical setting. However, in the future with the greater availability of portable versions, an outreach service may be the preferred option. A typical layout of a clinic is shown in Figure 7.4.

In this clinic, when programming young children, the computer and interface unit are located in an observation room and the child's speech processor is connected by a fly cable. The processor and fly cable are fed through into the adjacent sound-proofed clinic where the child is located. This serves to mini-mize visual distractions and thus focus the child's attention on the task in hand. Two clinicians are involved in the tuning of the cochlear implant: one controlling the computer and stimulus delivery; the other working with the child. The clinician in the observation room is able to monitor the tuning session by observing the child through a one-way observation window. With older children, often one clinician is involved in the tuning of the device and the complete programming system is located in the same room as the child.

Speech processor tuning schedule

Following cochlear implantation each usable electrode requires tuning. The softest levels that can be detected, the threshold (T) level and the loudest levels that can be tolerated, the comfort

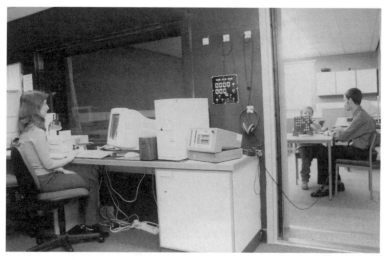

Figure 7.4. The clinic layout for speech processor programming with a child. In this situation there are facilities for the tester working with the programming equipment to observe, via a one-way observation window, the tester working with the child in the adjacent room.

(C) levels, must be measured for each electrode. Electrophysiological measures obtained intra-operatively provide a useful guide to initial stimulation levels. Once a selection of threshold and comfort levels has been established an individual programme or map can be created and programmed into the implantee's speech processor. The minimum tuning schedule for Nottingham is detailed in Table 7.1. A half-day period is allocated for each tuning session. Intermediate sessions are arranged when further tuning is indicated. The British Cochlear Implant Group and the National Deaf Children's Society have set out guidelines for the programming of the speech processor in their Quality Standards for Paediatric Cochlear Implantation document (1999).

Table 7.1. Minimum tuning schedule for Nottingham. Initial stimulation is undertaken over a two-day period. A half-day period is allocated for subsequent sessions Tuning schedule

Initial stimulation	
Post initial stimulation -	3 weeks
	6 weeks
	3 months
	6 months
	1 year
	1 year 6 months
	2 years
	2 years 6 months
	3 years
	Annually thereafter

Preparing the child for initial stimulation

Following surgery and discharge from hospital a member of the cochlear implant teacher of the deaf team arranges to visit the child and their family at home. A factor in how well children accept their speech processor, whether it is a body-worn or an ear-level device, is their familiarity with the system. For this reason it is essential, irrespective of their age, that prior to initial stimulation they have been introduced to the externally worn equipment in the form of a dummy speech processor and headset. At this stage, decisions can be made with regard to where the speech processor will be worn. The child can also be shown pictorial information, photographs of other children wearing their speech processor and perhaps meet existing users.

During this period the children should be encouraged to continue to wear their acoustic hearing aid in their non-implanted ear. This is particularly important for infants or very young children and those with a strong will. In certain cases parents may have experienced difficulties in establishing consistent hearing aid use and without action at this stage it can be anticipated that problems could occur with the acceptance of the implant system.

The procedure involved in the initial stimulation of the implant and the speech processor fitting should be conveyed to those children who developmentally have the perceptual skills to comprehend the process. This may take the form of pictorial representation, videos, explanation with signing where necessary and if possible meeting with other children who have been through the process. The time interval between surgery and initial stimulation is variable: two to six weeks dependent on the device used (Roberts in Cooper, 1991; Cowen and Clark in Clark, Cowan and Dowell, 1997). In Nottingham, it is usual to allow a period of three to four weeks before initial stimulation. During this time the wound will heal and any swelling around the transmitter coil and receiver/stimulator site will subside. A medical consultation is advisable prior to the initial stimulation.

Planning the initial stimulation session – objective measurements and medical reports

Objective measurement techniques are well established with regards to their use with cochlear implant recipients before, during and after surgery (see Chapter 6). Threshold measures such as the electrically evoked auditory brainstem response and the electrically evoked stapedial reflex, performed either intra-operatively or post-operatively have been the subject of numerous studies looking specifically at their usefulness for behavioural threshold and comfort level prediction respectively (Battmer, Laszig and Lehnhardt, 1990; Shallop et al., 1990; Stephan, Welzl-Muller and Stiglbrunner, 1991; Van den Borne et al., 1994; Brown et al., 1994; Spivak and Chute, 1994; Shallop and Ash, 1995; Hodges, 1997; Kileny et al., 1997; Lindstrom and Bredberg, 1997; Mason, 1997).

The electrical auditory brainstem response threshold typically correlates with the behavioural threshold when the same stimuli are used. Shallop (1993) reports that the electrical auditory brainstem response threshold levels will be higher than the thresholds measured via the speech processor as a consequence of the temporal integration functions for electrical stimuli. The actual auditory brainstem response threshold provides the clinician with a stimulus level at which the child may be conditioned, with the reassurance that it will be audible and at a level that is not uncomfortably loud. The presence of this response is confirmation that the auditory nerve fibres are receiving and reacting to electrical stimuli, thus providing reassurance that the implanted device is functioning and the stimulus is being delivered effectively.

A comparison of intra-operatively measured electrical stapedial reflex thresholds and most comfortable listening level with three different cochlear implant devices has been made and reported by Opie, Allum and Probst (1997). In Medel and Clarion subjects the thresholds were higher than the most comfortable level; in Nucleus subjects the thresholds were more variable, being both below and above the most comfortable level. This difference was thought to be due to the different stimulation modes used by the different devices. Thus, when an electrical stapedial reflex is elicited it will provide the clinician with the reassurance that the individual electrodes can elicit an auditory response. The levels, however, at which the response is measured are much higher than could be tolerated by the child in the initial stages of stimulation and should therefore not be exceeded. It is not always possible to elicit this response (Battmer, Laszig and Lehnhardt, 1990; Stephan, Welzl-Muller and Stiglbrunner, 1991; Sheppard et al., 1992). Factors that may affect the ability to record the electrical stapedial reflex threshold may be related to the current level, the pathological status of the recording middle ear and primarily whether the reflex is intact. When recorded intra-operatively, the reflex may be influenced by anaesthetic agents. Better estimates of the behavioural comfort level have been reported when the effect of the concentration of the anaesthetic used has been taken into account (Makhdoum et al., 1998). Absence of the reflex must therefore be treated with caution.

More recently, the advent of Neural Response Telemetry specific to the Nucleus CI24M device has proven promising with regards to its application in assisting with the setting of levels at initial stimulation. The neural response arises from the stimulation of the implant, which causes nerve fibres in the spiral ganglion to fire, which in turn generates an action potential. A technique for recording the whole nerve action potential was initially described by Brown, Abbas and Gantz (1990). Telemetry is the method by which these action potentials are recorded via the implant by a process involving the amplification of the signals from the intra-cochlear electrodes. These action potentials have been recorded reliably in children. They appear stable over time, occur at levels that are audible and tend to lie within the dynamic range at later post-operative intervals (Hughes et al., 2000).

Measurement of the averaged electrode voltages provide a further method of verifying the operation of the internal receiver/stimulator and electrode integrity. This integrity test is of use both intra-operatively and post-operatively if a device function change is suspected (Mason, 1997; Stephan and Welzl-Muller, 1997).

In conjunction with the electrophysiological report, particularly integrity testing, the surgical report and post-operative X-ray will provide the clinician with information regarding the number of usable intra-cochlear electrodes. This information is useful in determining the number of channels that are available for speech processing and selecting the most appropriate mode of stimulation, as discussed later. In cases where it has not been possible to achieve a full electrode insertion or the supporting ring/active electrode interface is at the intra-cochlear/extra-cochlear boundary, extreme caution should be taken to avoid stimulating the most basal electrodes.

Any electrode that is suspected of functioning less than optimally should remain deactivated during the initial phases. Investigation at a later stage is advisable when an accurate picture of the well-functioning electrodes has been established. Stimulation of electrodes with a less-than-optimal function may result in a painful sensation. This must be avoided with children and the tuning session should be as playful and enjoyable as possible if their co-operation is to be maintained.

Initial stimulation

The initial tuning phase is undertaken over a two-day period. The behavioural approach adopted for the measurement of threshold and either comfortable loudness or uncomfortable loudness level depends on the cognitive ability of the child. Although a period of time will have passed between assessment and the initial stimulation, an indication of the child's capabilities will have been gained during the pre-implant assessment phase. The post-implant activities of the teacher of the deaf should have already familiarized the child with the externally worn equipment. The appropriate colour of lead and coil, the correct length of connecting leads and correct strength of magnet should all be selected prior to initial stimulation. Incorrect length of lead or strength of transmitting coil magnet may result in poor headset fit which in turn may interfere with the child's concentration. Valuable time will be saved if a few minutes can be devoted to these points of detail prior to the initial tuning session.

Behavioural measurements

The fundamental process in the tuning and fitting of the speech processor to the child involves the determination of the dynamic range for electrical stimulation for each individual electrode. Normal acoustic hearing can process sounds over a range of 120 dB, with speech sounds in normal conversation falling between 40-65 dB. The dynamic range for electrical stimulation is considerably narrower: 6-30 dB (Clark and Tong, 1982; Patrick et al. in Clark, Tong and Patrick, 1990). The speech processor accommodates for this difference by compressing the larger range of acoustic amplitude variation into the much narrower range of electrical stimulation. The achieved transformation allows for the preservation of the intensity relationships between phonetic elements. Accurate determination of the threshold and comfort levels is essential to enable this function to be achieved. The information from the objective electrophysiological measures and surgical report allow the clinician to plan the programming strategy in terms of which electrodes to stimulate, the starting level for threshold determination and the levels to avoid when investigating comfort levels particularly in the initial phases. When the cochlear implant device allows for a choice of stimulation mode and speech processing strategy the results from the electrophysiological investigations may assist the clinician with their choice, particularly in cases of partial insertion or limited usable electrodes. Behavioural techniques, however, are essential to the optimal setting of the speech processor.

Determination of threshold for very young or complex cases

The procedure involved in establishing threshold level should be explained to the child's parent/carer. Initial stimulation can be an anxious and emotional time. It is therefore essential that any concerns of adult observers are allayed, particularly in cases where a child is taking a long time to show an initial response. If the clinic is equipped with the facility for the clinician working with the child to have an audible feedback to coincide with the stimulus presentation and to assist with judging response reliability, then the child's parents/carers will be aware that a stimulus is being presented but that the child may not always be responding. A simple explanation at the beginning of the session regarding the procedure for establishing threshold will help to minimize any anxiety that may arise as a result of the child not always responding when a stimulus is presented.

The approach adopted for the measurement of threshold depends on the developmental age of the child. For those children developmentally able to undertake formal assessment then well-established techniques such as visual reinforcement audiometry and performance testing may be used. Visual reinforcement audiometry, as described by Bamford and McSporran in McCormick (1993) can be successful in establishing threshold levels in infants as young as six months of age. One factor that must be considered is the potentially greater number of sound presentation trials and responses when using this technique to establish electrical threshold level for individual electrodes, compared with establishing acoustic hearing threshold. With the Nucleus CI24M device, dependent on the mode of stimulation and speech processing strategy, up to 22 electrical thresholds may need to be measured, which is significantly more than when compared with establishing acoustic threshold for a selection of frequencies across the speech frequency range. A study by Moore, Thompson and Thompson (1975) on children, aged between 12–18 months, looked at their response behaviour as a function of different reinforcement conditions. They showed that habituation behaviour was observed as the number of sound trials was increased and that habituation was more rapid with less complex reinforcement. Thus, arrangements that allow the tester to vary the reinforcer between simple and complex and having the facility to change the reinforcer in each category may help to increase the number of responses before habituation.

Performance testing, where the child is conditioned to wait for a stimulus and respond by performing a simple play activity such as placing a peg in a board or a piece in a puzzle, is usually successful with children who have developmental ages of 2.5 years and above. The principle involved is described fully by McCormick in McCormick (1993) and in Chapter 4 of this volume. As children are likely to undergo repeated assessments using the same technique, maintaining their co-operation, concentration and the novelty factor is of prime importance. This will require a wide range of materials and resourcefulness. The activity selected should be matched to the child's ability. A complex task may capitalize the child's attention, such that they are no longer in an optimal state for listening for the stimulus at threshold levels. Equally a task that has been used with the child on several previous occasions may hold little interest for him or her. Both situations may result in responses at supra-threshold levels. Careful consideration should therefore be given to the choice of activity.

For those individuals who are developmentally not ready for formal assessment, behavioural observation should be employed. The child's attention can be engaged in a simple activity and his or her response or change in behaviour to stimulus presentation observed. This may take the form of stilling, a change in facial expression, such as widening of the eyes or looking up, touching the headset, tensing of the body, moving towards the parent/carer or an adverse reaction. It is desirable that children's attention does not become too fixated on the activity as this may affect their overall level of responsiveness. Assessing children's responsiveness and observing their reaction to a stimulus that is known to elicit awareness, for example, a warble tone with a strong vibrotactile component, may assist the clinician both in assessing children's state of alertness as well as observing their response pattern.

Individual children's reactions to initial stimulation are varied. To avoid adverse reaction it is wise to be extremely cautious with the starting level. If electrical auditory brainstem thresholds or neural response telemetry have been recorded, they can be used as a guide. It is advisable to select an electrode on which these measures have been undertaken and to present the initial stimulus to this electrode at a level below the electrophysiological threshold level. If no such measures are available it may be necessary to start at the lowest level of stimulation.

Where the programming software permits, the stimulus duration should be selected to be of a sufficient length to give the
child time to note its presence and react. Stimuli of 1 s duration
are used by the clinic in Nottingham. The facility to vary the
length of time between presentations, rather than presenting a
continuous train of pulses, is also an advantage. This will enable
the clinician to present the stimulus at an optimal time, dependent on the child's attention state. It will also facilitate in assessing the response reliability. Varying the pause interval by up to
10 seconds will reduce the possibility of false positive responses
due to anticipation and impulsive behaviour.

It may prove difficult to keep infants and very young children
on task for the required duration, their attention state may vary,
which as a consequence may also affect their responsiveness to
the stimuli. If a child starts to give varying responses and the
clinician is unsure as to whether this is as a result of varying
attention state or a non-optimally functioning electrode, the situation may be clarified by presenting a stimulus to an electrode
that has been stimulated already and at a level that is known to
elicit a positive response. If the child still fails to show a
response then a change in attention state may be the reason.

Once the child has conditioned to the stimulus or a reliable
response pattern has been established, it may be useful to
measure levels on a selection of electrodes at widely spaced
intervals across the electrode array, rather than concentrating on
adjacent electrodes. If a particular mode of stimulation is known
to produce a typical response pattern it may be possible to inter-
polate levels when necessary. It is important, however, that electrodes are activated or included in maps only if they have been
stimulated, both at the threshold level and comfort level and the
child's behavioural response observed. This is essential to
observe any adverse reaction to stimulation and ensure that no
unpleasant sensations are experienced.

Comfort level assessment for very young or complex cases

There are two main approaches to the measurement or setting
of comfort levels in infants and young children. For the very
young child who has little or no concept of loudness growth,
then typically a method of behavioural observation is used. The
child is engaged in a simple play activity, whilst the stimulus
level is gradually increased up to the point where loudness
discomfort is observed. Responses such as changes in facial

expression, the presence of the aural palpebral reflex, cessation of a play activity, seeking comfort from the parent/carer, stilling or removal of the headset may all be elicited in response to an uncomfortably loud stimulation level.

For older children, who are able to comprehend the concept of loudness, it may be possible to use a simple graduated scale to assist them with their judgement of stimulus intensity. Staller, Beiter and Brimacombe in Cooper (1991) have documented their use of pictorial representation, such as faces with changing expressions. Lynch, Craddock and Crocker (1999) describe a technique called the Child-Directed Comfort Level. This method uses a column of 10 visual reinforcement audiometry type reinforcers operated by a hand-held pre-select switch. The child is taught to press a button to request an increase in loudness. In response to the push of the button, the child sees a further chamber in the column illuminated revealing a different toy.

We have introduced children as young as five years old to the concept of loudness by using increasing sizes of the same objects such as cars of the same colour or animals of the same species. These objects can be hidden under boxes of increasing size to correspond to the increase in loudness. The child is then trained to point to the smallest box in response to a stimulus presented at a level just above threshold level, as the stimulus level is increased they are instructed to point to larger boxes and therefore reveal larger hidden objects. An appropriate written scale can also be placed alongside the boxes for those children who are able to read. As the child may need to undertake this task several times, novelty is of great importance. It is useful therefore to change the hidden object as many times as resources permit, to both encourage and prolong co-operation. The graduations in loudness may be simplified to as few as two steps – for example, quiet and loud – or there may be several depending on the child's ability. An end point, to prompt and allow children to request no further stimulation on an individual electrode is important and can be provided by allowing them to push a button to signify 'stop'. This method has proven useful in assessing for the presence of loudness growth on individual channels and also whether the loudness growth on a selection of channels is comparable. If the child never reaches the 'stop' or 'too loud' level and the maximum level of stimulation has been reached, then this approach has been useful in determining when stimulus parameters need to be changed or in identifying when an electrode has less than optimal function. It is essential that in any activity that involves an element of surprise the child's reliability is assessed as they may just be interested in revealing the hidden object as quickly as possible. It is useful, therefore, to present a few stimulus levels in a random sequence, for example, quiet, loud, quiet and observe if the child responds appropriately.

It is usual in the initial stages, for those children who are unable to give an indication of relative loudness level, to set the comfort level very low – well below the level of the electrical stapedial reflex threshold. The map will therefore be conservative with a small dynamic range. Even for those children in whom it has been possible to gain a measure of loudness growth, the range is still likely to be conservative as it is usual for tolerance of the stimulus to increase with time.

Creating a speech processor map or programme

Once a selection of threshold and comfort levels have been measured it is possible to create a map and programme it into the speech processor. The reaction to the first map tested may differ from one child to another. It is important that the map is introduced gradually by slowly increasing the sensitivity of the microphone or raising the volume setting over a period of time. The reaction to single channel stimulation may be quite different to the reaction to a number of channels being activated together (Rance and Dowell in Clark, Cowen and Dowell, 1997). The latter may produce a more pronounced reaction. Soundfield stimuli in the form of speech, noise makers, warble tones and narrow band noise, can be introduced whilst gradually increasing the sensitivity or volume. It is important to observe the child's reactions very carefully for any signs of loudness discomfort and to make further fine adjustments if necessary. In cases where the loudness discomfort level has been measured, the comfort level for each channel should be set a standard percentage of the dynamic range below this level (typically 30%) to ensure that the map is at a comfortable level .

Follow-up tuning sessions and map optimization

Following the initial stimulation phase, additional programming sessions will be necessary in order:

- to verify previous measurements (particularly threshold levels);
- to increase the dynamic range by further investigation of the comfort levels;
- to introduce more electrodes in cases where not all electrodes were activated during the initial tuning phase.

Changes over time in adult implantees' electrical thresholds have been reported by a number of investigators, including Waltzman, Cohen and Shapiro (1991) and Skinner et al. (1995). Changes in electrical threshold are also evident in children. Shapiro and Waltzman (1995) suggested that factors such as increasing reliability and consistency in responses and the physiological stabilization of threshold might be attributed to this. The fact that the threshold can change is an indication for frequent tuning sessions particularly in the early stages to enable map optimization to occur as soon as possible. At the point where there are no further changes in the threshold level or increases in the comfort level, the assumption can be made that the map is stable. Factors that may affect how long it takes to reach map stability are the age of the child, the ease of programming and the occurrence of electrode faults.

Once a map is considered to be stable, depending on the maturity of the child, it may be possible to undertake more complex psychophysical tasks such as loudness balancing between electrodes or loudness scaling, if not previously undertaken for the measurement of comfort level and pitch ranking.

The concept of providing a signal that is loudness balanced across the frequency range is not new. A number of hearing aid prescription procedures aim to provide all frequency bands of speech at an equal loudness level – for example Byrne and Tonnison (1976). A map with balanced electrodes will ensure that the relative loudness of the incoming signal is accurately represented by the implant. The effect of loudness imbalance between electrodes in the maps of cochlear implant users has been described by Dawson, Skok and Clark (1997). They simulated unbalanced maps with varying degrees of imbalance between electrodes. They concluded that for the majority of subjects tested, performance in noise was poorer when their comfort levels were unbalanced. In very young children loudness balancing between adjacent electrodes is an impossible task to undertake. If an older child can comprehend the meaning of same and different then loudness balancing should be attempted. If however, the procedure used for the measurement of a child's comfort or discomfort level has been the same on each electrode measured and there have been no indications of a change in the child's criteria during the measurement, it can be assumed that the electrodes are fairly equally balanced for loudness. Dawson, Skok and Clark (1997) recommend that if children's communication development and speech perception performance with their implant is failing to progress at the expected rate, then one factor that should be considered and investigated is loudness imbalance between electrodes.

With multichannel cochlear implant systems, the electrode array is designed to follow the tonotopicity of the normal cochlea. A study by Nelson et al. (1995) has shown this to be the case. Stimulation of electrodes in the more basal areas of the cochlea resulted in higher perceived pitches and stimulation of electrodes closer to the apex resulted in lower perceived pitches. Pitch ranking will establish whether the implantee perceives this even range of pitch. Roberts in Cooper (1991) described a simple way of evaluating this, which involves sweeping through the electrodes in order, either from a basal to apical or apical to basal direction. The implantee is then asked to judge whether the sounds are presented in either an increasing or decreasing pitch. In the event of any channel sounding very different from the others, Roberts in Cooper (1991) advises that it should be excluded from stimulation, rather than an attempt made to place it in another position in the stimulation order. As with loudness balancing, place pitch discrimination is a difficult concept to convey, even for adults and particularly so for those with little experience with their implant.

Modes of stimulation and processing strategies – the choices available

A decision needs to be made at initial stimulation with regards to which mode of stimulation and processing strategy to use. The choice available depends on the cochlear implant system. Factors such as the number of electrodes available for stimulation, the type of speech processor being fitted and the strategies it is able to support and current clinical practice may all contribute to the decision. However, as the programming progresses, it may also become apparent that a different mode or strategy to that chosen originally may be more suited to the implantee. The factors that affect initial choice and the decision to change at a later stage are presented in the following section.

Modes of stimulation

To achieve a sensation of hearing there needs to be a current flow across the implanted electrodes. The current flow occurs between an active electrode and a reference electrode. The choice of reference electrode defines the mode of stimulation. The most widely used modes of stimulation are common ground, bipolar and monopolar (see Figure 7.5).

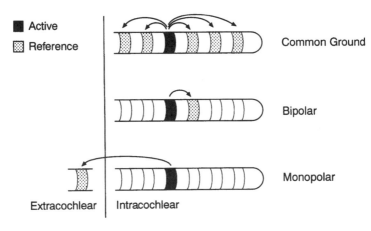

Figure 7.5. Diagram illustrating the most widely used modes of stimulation with the Nucleus cochlear implant systems. In each case the active electrode, reference electrode/s and the direction of current flow are shown.

Examples of stimulation modes

Common Ground mode of stimulation

At initial stimulation, the mode used with children with a full electrode insertion of a Nucleus CI22M device is the common ground mode. With this mode of stimulation all the electrodes, with the exception of the active electrode, are joined together to form the reference electrode (see Figure 7.5).

In this mode, the dynamic range of the electrode array has a characteristic shape with smaller dynamic ranges for electrodes at the basal and apical ends of the array (see Figure 7.6). This allows for interpolation and for extrapolation of threshold levels where necessary. This is an invaluable tool when programming infants and young children, where information obtained in the

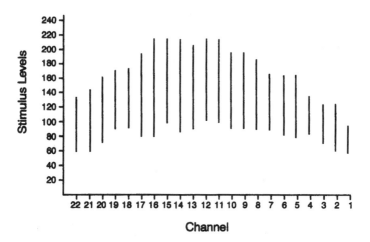

Figure 7.6. The characteristic bell shape of a typical map using the common ground mode of stimulation with the Nucleus CI22M cochlear implant.

initial stages may be limited. Measurements may have been investigated on a range of electrodes only, due to factors such as short or variable attention span. It is possible to estimate the comfort level using similar methods, but it is advisable to determine the comfort level behaviourally to ensure that appropriate levels of stimulation are introduced in the first map. The common ground mode allows for easier identification of faults on specific electrodes, and this is an extremely useful feature when the implantee is young. The method of identification and the nature of electrode faults will be discussed in more detail later in this chapter.

For children who have a partial insertion of the electrode array the bipolar mode of stimulation has an advantage over the common ground mode. With the common ground mode of stimulation there can be a small amount of current flow to electrodes outside the cochlea, even when they are deactivated and this may cause unpleasant non-auditory sensation that in turn may lead to rejection of the cochlear implant system.

Bipolar mode of stimulation

The bipolar mode is used in the Nucleus CI22M and Clarion cochlear implant systems. As discussed above, this is the preferred mode of stimulation for children with partial insertions and also for all adult implantees with the Nucleus CI22M device. With this mode of stimulation the current flows between a pair of electrodes and the active electrode has just one reference electrode.

The physical distance between the electrode pair affects the distribution of electrical current, which, in turn, influences the amount of current needed to elicit a response. The closer the pair of electrodes, the smaller is the spread of electrical current and fewer ganglion cells will be stimulated. More current will be needed to elicit a response. In fact, with narrower bipolar modes, the electrode pairs may be so close as to be unable to induce a perception of loudness even at the maximum stimulation levels produced by the programming system. That is, the comfort level cannot be obtained at the maximum level of stimulation. The active electrode is described as 'topping out'. This is overcome by increasing the distance between the electrodes. In the Nucleus CI22M device this is achieved by choosing the bipolar +1 mode of stimulation which has one electrode in-between the active and reference electrode (see Figure 7.5). In the Clarion device, the enhanced bipolar mode of simulation is chosen. The reference electrode is the next but one lateral electrode rather than the adjacent lateral electrode.

The distance between the electrodes can be increased further should this be necessary. For example in the bipolar +2 mode, there are two electrodes separating the active and reference electrode (see Figure 7.7). The optimal bipolar mode of stimulation will be the lowest bipolar mode where the full dynamic range is achievable with each of the active electrodes.

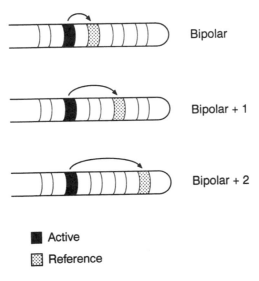

Figure 7.7. Diagram illustrating the active electrode, reference electrode and the direction of current flow in different bipolar modes of stimulation for the Nucleus cochlear implant systems.

Each patient's map will be unique depending on the psychophysics and on the position of the implanted device. It is reported by Rance and Dowell in Clark, Cowen and Dowell (1997) that the higher bipolar modes are mainly needed for those patients who have malformed cochleae. This has been the authors' experience with a child who has Mondini's dysplasia.

In theory, the bipolar mode, with its more discrete distribution of electrical current between a pair of intra-cochlear electrodes, should give greater frequency specificity than that of the common ground mode, or other modes with a widely spaced active and reference electrode. Lim, Tong and Clark (1989) were not able to confirm this frequency-related feature. It may be that the common ground mode of stimulation has a large enough amount of current directed to the active electrode, relative to the surrounding reference electrodes to ensure good frequency specificity (Rance and Dowell in Clark, Cowen and Dowell, 1997).

Identification of faulty electrodes in the bipolar modes of stimulation for the Nucleus CI22M device is difficult. It is, however, easier to identify extra-cochlear electrodes in bipolar modes because sudden increases in threshold and comfort levels are recorded for those outside the cochlea (Rance and Dowell in Clark, Cowen and Dowell, 1997).

Monopolar mode of stimulation

The monopolar mode of stimulation is used in the Nucleus CI24M, Clarion and Medel Combi 40+ cochlear implant devices when using particular speech processing strategies. The extra-cochlear reference electrode can be a separate ball electrode placed in the temporalis muscle or it can be housed in the receiver/stimulator package. With the Nucleus CI24M device, both types of extra-cochlear electrodes are available and it is possible to combine them to form the reference electrode known as Monopolar 1+2. This increases the relative size of the reference electrode compared with the active electrode, thereby reducing the current levels needed to establish a dynamic range. The reduction in current level has two advantages: it allows speech processing strategies to run faster; and potentially reduces power consumption. The latter requirement is of particular importance for ear-level speech processors.

Monopolar stimulation is often used with children who have a Nucleus CI24M device. The authors' programme is currently using the Monopolar 1+2 stimulation mode as routine. It, too, has a predictable map configuration (see Figure 7.8), allowing interpolation and/or extrapolation of threshold levels. Estimation of comfort levels can be made, but should be undertaken with extreme caution. Behavioural measurement of comfort level for each electrode is essential in our experience to ensure that the first stimulation of a map is acceptable to the child. Despite the conceptual differences between bipolar and monopolar stimulation modes implantees seem to show similar levels of functioning. Waltzman, Cohen and Roland (1999) indicate no significant difference in word and sentence perception at the three-month interval when comparing CI22M implantees using a bipolar mode of stimulation with CI24M implantees using a monopolar mode of stimulation. Pilot data even suggested a trend towards better scores in the monopolar mode over a longer period of use.

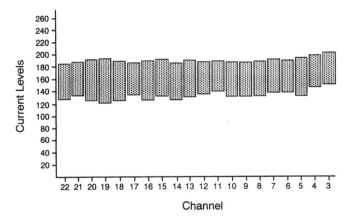

Figure 7.8. A map created using the pseudomonopolar mode of stimulation for a patient with Mondini defect, implanted with the CI22M cochlear implant.

Recognizing electrode faults from behavioural measurements alone is more difficult in the monopolar mode of stimulation than in common ground and bipolar modes of stimulation but the use of back telemetry (described in Chapter 6) in conjunction with the threshold and comfort level measurements should assist identification of such faults.

As with the other modes of stimulation, it is possible to reach maximum stimulation levels and still be unable to obtain a satisfactory perception of loudness on individual electrodes. The electrode may be reported as 'out of compliance'. In these cases, alterations to the stimulus parameters, particularly with regards to pulse width, will resolve the problem. Information on non-standard methods of programming can be obtained from the manufacturers.

For those Nucleus CI22M device users, where loudness perception is unobtainable in the highest bipolar mode of stimulation, the bipolar +5 stimulation mode, it is possible to mimic the monopolar mode of stimulation and its properties. This is known as the pseudomonopolar mode of stimulation. Instead of using an extracochlear electrode, as the reference electrode, either the most basal or the most apical electrode is assigned. The following case study illustrates its use.

Case study

Onset of deafness (years):	0
Age at implantation (years):	4
Aetiology:	Mondini defect

Background information: full insertion of a Nucleus CI22M multichannel cochlear implant. Intra-operative integrity testing indicated all electrodes to be functioning.

Initial stimulation: 18 electrodes were activated in the common ground mode of stimulation. High threshold levels were measured and comfort level testing indicated all electrodes to be 'topping out'.

Tuning reviews: at the following tuning session measurements were made in the bipolar +2 stimulation mode. High threshold levels again were recorded. At the six-week post-stimulation tuning session, bipolar +5 stimulation mode was investigated. Comfort level investigation revealed most electrodes to be 'topping out'. Increases in threshold level were measured at subsequent tuning sessions on all electrodes. All electrodes, with the exception of the three most basal ones, 'topped out'. Pseudomonopolar stimulation mode was investigated. Threshold levels and comfort levels were investigated with electrode 1, the most basal electrode, assigned as the reference electrode. Comfort levels were obtained on all electrodes with the exception of 3 to 6 inclusive. Figure 7.9 is a representation of the map

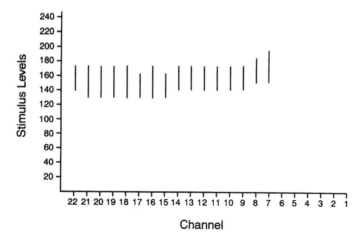

Figure 7.9. A typical map using the monopolar 1+2 mode of stimulation with the Nucleus CI24M cochlear implant.

created in this mode. Table 7.2 shows the improvement in aided soundfield warble tone measurements with change in stimulation mode.

Conclusion

A device with the flexibility of different programming modes allowed for an optimum dynamic range to be achieved. In this case the pseudomonopolar mode of stimulation resulted in a significant improvement in aided soundfield detection levels, giving better access to the speech frequency range.

Table 7.2. Aided soundfield warble tone responses (dB (A)) for the different modes of stimulation with the speech processor set to optimum sensitivity

	500 Hz	1000 Hz	2000 Hz	4000 Hz
Bipolar +2	60/65		60	45/50
Bipolar +5	>78	65	50	40
Pseudomonopolar	44	42	44	36

Changing modes

The outcome of research, and the increased experience of clinicians using different cochlear implant devices, provides a greater understanding of programming concepts. This information may lead to changes in practice, particularly with regard to preferred mode. In Nottingham, experience has shown that changing modes of stimulation may affect a child's performance in the short term. In the majority of cases, however, performance soon returns to at least that previously achieved, if not better. Notable improvements in performance have also been reported by other UK cochlear implant programmes, in particular for children using the Nucleus CI22M cochlear implant (Ajayi, Jamieson and Khan, 1998). For the small number of implantees who may experience a deterioration in performance following a change in stimulation mode, even when a period of adjustment and acclimatization has been allowed for, they may return to their original stimulation mode. Older children who are long-term users may find it too difficult to acclimatize to changes and may actually prefer to stay with their original stimulation mode.

Changes in mode of stimulation may also be advised for children who are experiencing problems with device function. For children with the Nucleus CI22M device, programmed in one of the bipolar modes of stimulation, a return to the common ground mode of stimulation is advisable, particularly if the problems are intermittent in nature.

Speech processing strategies

It will be recalled that the speech processor's function is to convert the incoming sound into electrical signals. How the sound is processed and the most salient information delivered to the implanted electrode array is determined by the speech processing strategy. The speech processing strategies differ across the different cochlear implant systems. They can be rich in temporal information, such as with the Continuous Interleaved Sampling (CIS) or CIS-like strategies, or rich in spectral information, such as with the SPEAK strategy used with the Nucleus devices, or the 'n of m' strategy used with the MEDEL Combi 40+. Even within the same device there are numerous options available to the clinician. Speech processing strategies have been discussed in greater detail in Chapter 1.

The wide diversity of speech processing strategies gives greater flexibility to the clinician, but the decision as to which one to use can be complex. To assist with the choice the manufacturers publish the results from clinical trials detailing the potential benefits of each strategy. Further information can be obtained from independent studies and seminars. The studies usually compare within system strategies (Osberger and Fisher,

1999; Battmer et al., 1999) or compare strategies across the different systems (Young et al., 1999). Loeb (1997) cautions that the present speech processing strategies are not specifically designed for young implantees with the developing nervous system. The majority of strategies have been designed using psychophysical data from adult post-lingually deafened implantees. In the paediatric cochlear implant population, the majority will be pre-lingually deaf. Neurophysiological experiments on animals indicate that the developing nervous system has greater plasticity and differs from the mature nervous system in its ability to adapt more readily to new stimulation.

Manufacturers' clinical trials can also identify specific cases where one strategy is preferable to another. For instance, with the Nucleus CI24M device, where the implantee has less than 12 active electrodes, the recommended strategy is CIS (European Custom Sound Outcomes Seminar – Sintra, 1999). When a limited number of active electrodes are available, SPEAK and Advanced Combination Encoders (ACE) speech processing strategies will not operate optimally. A reduction in the number of usable electrodes may occur following a partial insertion of the electrode array, as a consequence of ossification or unusual anatomy. Another possibility is that the electrode array may be fully inserted, but lying either in an atypical position within the cochlea or there may be kinking of the array. This could lead to interaction between electrodes that are lying in close proximity to each other resulting in unusual pitch perception or short-circuiting should they be activated.

With any speech processing strategy there is a wide range of performance outcomes for both children and adults. The clinician may be presented with a number of choices, but with no clear-cut evidence that one speech processing strategy is better than another; the decision with regard to which speech processing strategy to use may therefore be a difficult one. A study comparing the performance of children with the Nucleus CI22M device using the Multipeak and the (then) newly developed SPEAK speech processing strategy, provided substantial evidence that the majority of users in the study benefited from changing to the SPEAK strategy (Cowan et al., 1995). In this case, the decision to change strategy was not a difficult one. A more recent study by Arndt et al. (1999) compared the performance of SPEAK, CIS and ACE speech processing strategies for use with the Nucleus CI24M cochlear implant. This indicated possible benefits for speech recognition in noise with the ACE strategy relative to the CIS and SPEAK. However, they also reported inter-subject variation with regard to user preference. In this instance, when children are the subjects, the decision is more difficult and may need to be made in conjunction with informed parents/carers. However, technological advances have eased the decision-making process.

Many speech processors now have multiple programme locations, enabling storage of maps using different speech processing strategies in the different programme locations. The Nucleus CI24M Sprint speech processor has this feature and has allowed the authors' clinic to place maps using up to two strategies in different programme locations. When a child's speech processing strategy is changed, for example from SPEAK to the more recently developed ACE, this feature enables parents/carers to easily access the child's previous speech processing strategy should they experience problems with their new one. Older, more experienced implantees may value having the choice of strategy for different listening situations, for example, for the appreciation of music (Anft et al., 1999).

Another consideration that the clinician may take into account when deciding whether to change to a different strategy is whether the current map is optimal. This is evident when there are no significant changes in threshold and comfort-level measurements over a number of successive tuning sessions. Map optimization will allow for a more valid comparison of performance to be made between the two strategies. It is important to remember that changing strategies often involves investigating all behavioural measurements again. Obtaining a complete set of measurements with a very young child may take more than one tuning session and further sessions may be needed to verify that the new map is optimal.

There have been numerous recent advances in the development of new speech processing strategies and the clinicians must constantly re-evaluate their current approach. A greater understanding of the central processing strategies of the brain will lead to further advances and to the likelihood that more options will be available across the different implant systems. Objective measurements may contribute to the decision process. A study by Battmer et al. (1999) reported that, for those adult Clarion users who preferred using the Simultaneous Analog Stimulation (SAS) speech processing strategy, higher electrode impedance values were recorded than for those who preferred the CIS speech processing strategy.

Diagnosis and management of changes in device function

The cochlear implant is not immune to breakdown – either partial, total, internal or external. A change in the function of the externally worn equipment is relatively easy to identify and rectify. Malfunction of the implanted components can manifest in varying forms and to differing extents. There may be a change in one or more of the active electrodes, on either a permanent or an intermittent basis, or there may be a total device failure. By the very nature of their occurrence, intermittent device problems are more difficult to identify. Changes in electrode function can manifest in such diverse ways, as reports of pain, a reluctance or refusal to wear the device, or a change in the child's performance. Regular and ongoing tuning sessions, once the map has stabilized, are essential in order to monitor device function and recognize any change as early as possible. The facility to see a child at short notice, should there be concern about their progress or use of the device, is advisable.

If a parent/carer or professional suspects a change in the child's performance with their implant, or the child reports a problem, it is useful to work through a series of steps to try to determine the source of the problem. Initially, the externally worn equipment should be checked at a local level, where possible, to avoid unnecessary travel. This should be undertaken by the child's parent/carer or the teacher if more appropriate. It is useful, for this reason, to provide the child's family and teacher with a spare set of connecting cables. The external equipment should be replaced in a logical order and then, after each replacement, the function of the speech processor checked again. The connecting cables should always be inspected for cuts or kinks as these can cause an intermittent transmission. The transmitting coil may break but the breakage point may be difficult to see without careful inspection. Some devices such as the Nucleus CI22M and the CI24M speech processors have the facility for a normally hearing individual to listen to the sound quality of the microphone. If dealing with all the external equipment that can be checked and replaced at a local level has not solved the problem, then the speech processor itself should be replaced. If this does not return the child to his or her previous level of performance, then the child should be seen in clinic for a full behavioural assessment with objective assessment of the internal device if indicated.

The rate of cochlear implant failures in adults and children is different. The failure rate in children is recognized as being greater than in adults. Cochlear Limited, the company who develop the Nucleus cochlear implant systems, has recently published data on their reliability. In March 1999, of the 3,400 individuals who had received their CI24M system, the cumulative survival percentage at 18 months of implant use was 99.6% for adults and 97.9% for children. For the CI22M system, the cumulative survival percentage at 12 years of implant use was 97% for adults and 92.5% for children. In the authors' clinic, out of a total of 310 implantees we have experienced 12 failures requiring device reimplantation.

Several authors have identified a number of risk factors associated with failure. Parisier, Chute and Popp (1996) suggest the following as risk factors for implant failure in children: fluctuating threshold and comfort levels in conventional psychophysical testing; a lack of performance not commensurate with the child's age; reports of sudden extraneous noises and negative stimulation; the loss of function of one or more electrodes over time; and frequent external equipment changes. Within the authors' programme, investigation into the manifestation of internal device faults in those children who had experienced total device failure was undertaken by Twomey and Archbold (1997). Out of a total of six failures, four were identified in routine tuning sessions. Unlike the Parisier, Chute and Popp (1996) findings none of these children used an unusual number of spare pieces of external equipment before failure but there were reports of discomfort through the device and deterioration in speech production as in their study.

To ensure that faults are identified as quickly as possible it is important to have a close liaison with members of the implant team, as well as with parents/carers and the local professionals working with the child. The ability to respond quickly and take appropriate action when a device problem is suspected is also very important. Device failures are very difficult to deal with both for the implantee and their family. Twomey and Archbold (1997) delivered a retrospective questionnaire to the parents of those children who had experienced an implant failure. They reported that, during this time of high anxiety, the effects at home and in the work environment may be broad ranging and relationships may become strained.

Fluctuations in threshold or comfort level, and hence in the dynamic range, should be viewed with caution. Rance and Dowell in Clark, Cowen and Dowell (1997) regard the threshold to be the most sensitive psychophysical measure to indicate a change in function of the system. Threshold levels are well-defined whereas comfort levels are based on subjective estimates of loudness, or a behavioural observation, and a change in these may not always reflect a change in device function. They recommend that, for the Nucleus device, changes in dynamic range of greater than 20% should be regarded as abnormal.

Electrode faults may be classed as definite or suspect. In any event, if there are suspicions about the function of a particular electrode it should remain deactivated until behavioural, objective or both investigations have clarified the situation. Definite electrode faults such as open circuits and short circuits show a characteristic pattern of response on stimulation. An open circuit arises when the wire leading to a particular electrode breaks, then, regardless of the stimulus amplitude, there will be no sensation and hence no response. Short circuits between two active electrodes occur when the insulation coating surrounding a number of electrodes is damaged, but the actual electrode wire itself remains intact. Stimulation will produce an auditory sensation, but the current distribution will be unusual and dependent on the mode of stimulation used. Identification of this type of malfunction is often difficult in the bipolar modes of stimulation because more than one channel will be involved. In common ground mode only those channels with the short will be affected and typically the fault manifests by showing a high threshold level with no comfort level, as there will be no loudness growth. It is also possible for a short circuit to occur between an active electrode and one of the supporting rings. This may produce a tactile sensation on stimulation as a result of current flow from the active intra-cochlear electrode to a non-active electrode, which may be at the boundary of the cochlea or outside the cochlea.

In addition to an electrode fault, non-auditory stimulation may occur as a result of stimulating a functioning electrode. This may take the form of a tactile sensation, tingling of the tongue or twitching of the face or eye. Kelsall et al. (1997) looked specifically at facial nerve stimulation. They identified a prevalence of 7% in their clinic population. Young children may not be able to report this sensation and it is, therefore, extremely important to observe any behavioural signs very carefully. Eye twitching may be obvious but a tactile sensation in another part of the face is much more difficult to identify. Occasionally children have been observed to point to their mouth or their neck if a non-auditory sensation has occurred. Questioning children, if possible, about what they perceive may help to clarify the situation. In addition to these observations or reports, an electrode that produces a non-auditory sensation on stimulation is likely to have a very narrow dynamic range because small increases in stimulation level, above threshold, usually produce an adverse reaction.

Any electrode that exhibits an atypical threshold or comfort level response pattern should be deactivated and then investigated objectively by measuring the averaged electrode voltages as described in Chapter 6. An electrode, however, that has an atypical threshold level when compared with surrounding electrodes is not necessarily faulty: it may be exhibiting a 'T-tail'. An electrode is described as having a 'T-tail' when there is no perceived increase in loudness with increasing level of stimulation up to a given point, known as the knee point. Above the knee point the electrode behaves like a normally functioning electrode, such that increases in the level of stimulation produce associated increases in loudness. These electrodes have an identifiable pattern. The threshold level is significantly lower than those on surrounding electrodes, whereas the comfort level is in line. The clinician does not need to deactivate the electrode exhibiting the 'T-tail' but can optimize its use by setting the threshold level in the map at the knee point so that there is normal loudness growth when it is stimulated. For the very young child the level may be interpolated from the threshold levels of surrounding electrodes if a typical response pattern for the mode of stimulation is known. Once the child is more mature and familiar with the concepts of loudness and loudness growth, the knee point can be established using the methods of assessment described earlier.

The Nucleus CI24M, the Clarion and the Medel Combi 40+ programming systems all incorporate an objective means of assessing electrode function. These telemetry functions allow for measures of electrode impedance and voltage levels of all active and non-active electrodes in a matter of a few minutes and can be undertaken during the tuning session. This is particularly beneficial for very young children or those individuals who have very little experience with their implant. It does not, however, replace the need for careful behavioural monitoring as device problems do not always manifest on objective assessment, particularly if they are intermittent in nature. Behavioural and objective assessments are complimentary in the identification and verification of device problems.

As a consequence of deactivating a faulty electrode, the number of electrodes available for programming may be reduced. For devices, such as the Nucleus CI22M cochlear implant, this compromises the strategy used. It limits the frequency range of the information sent to the electrode array, particularly with regard to the high frequencies. To overcome this, the frequency band allocated to each electrode may be altered by 'doubling up'. That is, certain electrodes, usually those at the apical end of the array, are allocated two channels, rather than the usual one channel. The frequency bandwidth where the 'doubling up' occurs is thus increased. This is usually considered with older children who can report on the quality of signal they receive.

Electrode faults are quite common. With very young children who may be unable to report a change in device function it is essential to have a system in place to investigate and identify electrode faults. This may be both complex and time consuming but essential to ensure optimum use of the device.

Assessing the benefit and efficacy of programming with a cochlear implant

An integral part of the programming process involves assessing the benefit that implanted children receive from their cochlear implant system in terms of sound detection and speech discrimination. For older children, a range of speech discrimination and perception tests appropriate to the child's language and cognitive development can be used. These are described in detail by Beiter, Staller and Dowell (1991) and also in other chapters of this book. Younger children require a speech discrimination test more appropriate to their linguistic ability, such as the McCormick Toy Discrimination Test described in Chapter 4.

For the pre-lingual/pre-verbal child, sound detection measures offer means of assessing performance in terms of access to sound. Warble tone soundfield detection levels can be obtained across the speech frequency range using similar test techniques to those used in threshold level testing as described in Chapter 4.

The above measurements are particularly useful for demonstrating to parents/carers the range of sounds that children are able to hear through their cochlear implant and for confirming the progress they are making. In everyday situations it is often difficult to appreciate children's responsiveness to quiet sounds. The mean warble tone responses obtained at the 12-month interval post-initial stimulation for a sample group of 100 children implanted at the Nottingham paediatric cochlear implant programme can be seen in Table 7.3. These are obtained with the speech processor at the optimum sensitivity setting and they lie in the region where quiet speech is audible.

Prior to implantation the majority of children are unable to complete the automated version of the McCormick Toy Discrimination test and none are able to perform the test at conversational levels of 65 dB (A) in the ear to be implanted. One year after implantation 8% of the first 200 children implanted at the Nottingham cochlear implant programme obtained the optimum 71% discrimination score at quiet conversational levels of less than 60 dB (A). At three years and five years after implantation, for those who had reached this stage, 45% and 68% respectively were able to complete the test at or below the above detection level. The detection level required to achieve the 71% correct score this test uses compares favourably with those obtained by severely deaf children who are successful hearing aid users (McCormick, Cope and Robinson, 1998).

These assessments have the advantage that they are very quick and, whenever possible, are repeated at each tuning session. They enable any reprogramming to be evaluated and map comparisons to be made. Warble tone measurements can show certain frequencies to be less sensitive than others, thus identifying areas within the map where further investigation and adjustment is necessary. Speech discrimination testing allows

Table 7.3. Mean aided soundfield warble tone responses (dB (A)) of a sample of one hundred children measured at 12 months after initial stimulation

500 Hz	1000 Hz	2000 Hz	4000 Hz
42	41	39	34

comparison with previous performance and assesses current ability. If there is a deterioration in the score obtained, this may indicate that reprogramming has not been beneficial. The results, however, should be interpreted cautiously taking into consideration factors such as when the test was undertaken. For example, following a long tuning session, children's attention state may be poor and this may affect their responsiveness. If a newly created map is significantly different to the previously used one and if it uses a different mode or processing strategy, a period of acclimatization may be needed before a reliable comparison can be made. Should the new map be considered to be less than optimal and the above factors ruled out, children may be given their previous map and a subsequent tuning session arranged. With older children with good linguistic ability, the clinician can also establish from the implantee their perception of sound quality and their opinion on whether reprogramming has been beneficial.

These results are not used in isolation in establishing the efficacy of processor settings. The clinician is reliant on feedback from the implant team's rehabilitation staff and the results they obtain on their performance measures. Reports on the children's performance and listening capabilities from local professionals and the implantees' parents and other family members are also essential.

Assistive listening devices

There are listening situations where the use of a FM radio hearing aid system or a direct connection to the sound source may improve the signal quality received by the implantee. To achieve this the speech processor must be able to accept signals directly through an external input socket. Current body-worn and ear-level speech processors, have this capability. The interface cables that connect the speech processor to the sound source are customized and individual to each implant system. The Nucleus system has a range of cables available, each designed for specific audio equipment – a TV/hi-fi cable for use with the television, hi-fi or other AC powered equipment, and an audio cable, for use with personal stereos.

The use of any assistive device requires feedback from the implantee with regard to optimal setting. Therefore, it is wise to wait until the implantee is capable of giving a qualitative report on the signal before considering issue. The implantee must also understand the concept of loudness, as the sensitivity or volume control on either the speech processor or accessory often needs to be adjusted.

FM radio hearing aid systems

The microphone of the speech processor, like that of a conventional acoustic hearing aid, delivers all sounds that it receives into the speech processor. Hence, the listener receives not only the signal of interest, but any competing background noise as well.

In most educational establishments the listening environment has unfavourable acoustic conditions. For hearing impaired listeners speech discrimination is made difficult by the presence of a number of factors:

- Background noise, competing with the signal of interest.
- The poor location of the speaker relative to the listener. Generally the speaker is neither close to nor at a constant distance from the listener.
- Reverberation effects. The absence of soft furnishings and lack of acoustic treatment to floors, walls and ceilings within most listening environments will serve to enhance the effects of reverberation.

If the signal-to-noise ratio and the reverberation time can be manipulated to give a higher signal-to-noise ratio and a lower reverberation time, it is possible to enhance the intelligibility of speech.

For normally hearing individuals a signal-to-noise ratio of +6 dB is desirable to allow for the receipt of intelligible speech. The hearing impaired individual is more susceptible to the degrading effects of noise on speech intelligibility and therefore requires a more favourable signal-to-noise ratio. Finitzo-Hieber and Tillman (1978) recommend that for persons with any degree of hearing impairment a signal-to-noise ratio of +20 dB is required to facilitate the reception of intelligible speech. Due, however, to noise, reverberation and changes in speaker location the signal-to-noise ratio in an average classroom is much lower than this ideal and in certain situations the noise level may exceed the level of speech (Markides, 1986).

Cochlear implant users will therefore benefit from the use of FM radio hearing aids, particularly in the educational environment. Most of the major cochlear implant manufacturers have developed the facility for their speech processors to interface with a FM radio hearing aid system. The output of the FM receiver is connected to the speech processor by a custom-built interface cable.

Historically, the use of FM radio hearing aids with speech processors has had difficulties. Problems due to the signal cutting in and out and poor interference free range were evident in the early stages of development and trial. This was due mainly to the design of the interface cable and the presence of frequency harmonics, which can be generated by the speech processor and occur in the same region as those frequencies used by some radio hearing aids. Improvements in the design of the interface cable have led to an increase in the interference free transmission range for many systems and the use of radio aids with speech processors now being a viable option. Interference, however, can still be a problem. It is advisable that such systems are introduced only to those children who are capable of giving a reliable qualitative judgement about the signal.

Prior to fitting and trial it is important to ensure that children meet a number of criteria:

- they have had sufficient listening experience with their cochlear implant to give qualitative comparisons of signal between the speech processor alone and the speech processor FM radio aid combination;
- they have been programmed in their optimum mode of stimulation;
- their map is stable and they are not experiencing any device problems.

The later two points are extremely important because when a map is changing, whether it is to a different mode or within the same mode, it can take the child a period of time to adapt to these changes. In our experience this can range from a few days up to two or three weeks. If a FM radio aid is introduced at the same time as the map change and the child fails to progress, the clinician would be unsure as to the cause of the problem. If a map is unstable, or there are problems with the device that are in the process of being solved, introducing a FM radio aid at the same time would potentially serve only to introduce another source of variability. Provision of FM radio aids should not be undertaken without due regard to all of these factors.

Future developments

Technological advancements have resulted in the introduction of a new generation of speech processors. These incorporate features that may improve the quality of life for some implantees. The availability of more than one programme location to give the implantee the choice of using different maps dependent on the listening environment is one such feature. The Nucleus CI24M Sprint body-worn speech processor also has a liquid crystal display facility to identify when a programme is faulty and when battery power is low. This is an improvement on earlier speech processors from the same manufacturer and not only gives the parents/carers of young or inexperienced implantees greater reassurance about the functioning of the speech processor, but also provides independent implantees with useful information about the function/malfunction of their speech processors.

The advent of ear-level speech processors has been long awaited and their recent release has been well received by implantees. The first-generation ear-level speech processors that are currently available may be considered for use with children, but often with caution. In our experience with the Nucleus Esprit 24 ear-level speech processor, there are both benefits, especially cosmetically, and limitations in fitting such a device (Totten, Cope and McCormick, 2000). With this in mind, our protocol has been to fit older children, aged from seven to 16 years, who are experienced listeners with optimal stable maps. Initial fitting with an ear-level speech processor is not recommended because a small percentage of final maps do not convert to the Esprit device, although they run successfully in the Sprint body-worn speech processor. At present, all our children with the Nucleus CI24M cochlear implant are initially fitted with the Sprint speech processor.

Currently, not all ear-level speech processors are capable of supporting the complete range of speech processing strategies available with the body-worn speech processors. This is mainly due to limitations in battery technology. The drain on batteries is far greater for the new faster speech processing strategies, as they require a greater amount of power in order to run effectively.

For this reason, those implantees who are using one of the faster rate strategies in a body-worn speech processor will need to change to a slower rate strategy in order to use an ear-level processor. It is important that the implantee and parents/carers are aware of these issues when considering the option of an ear-level speech processor.

Any future developments by the implant manufacturers must include backward compatibility with earlier cochlear implant systems. Their responsibility to existing cochlear implant users is paramount, especially with the advent of the ear-level speech processor. The option of upgrading to an ear-level device is extremely important as younger recipients approach adolescence. Implant manufacturers appear to be taking these requirements into consideration and we can look forward to new and improved versions of cochlear implants designed specifically for children in the future.

References

Ajayi F, Jamieson L, Khan S (1998) Optimising programming parameters for existing cochlear implant users. Presented at the British Society of Audiology annual conference, University of Hull, September 1998Anft D, Rasinski C, Galow R, Dahl R (1999) Effect of stimulation rate in ACE. Presented at the European Custom Sound outcomes seminar, Sintra, Portugal, June.

Arndt P, Staller S, Arcaroli J, Hines A, Ebinger K (1999) Within-subject Comparison of Advanced Coding Strategies in the Nucleus 24 Cochlear Implant. Cochlear Corporation.

Bamford J, McSporran E (1993) Visual reinforcement audiometry. In McCormick B (ed.) Paediatric Audiology 0–5 Years. London: Whurr, pp.124–54.

Battmer RD, Haake P, Zilberman Y, Lenarz T (1999) Simultaneous Analog Stimulation (SAS)-Continuous Interleaved Sampler (CIS) pilot comparison study in Europe. Annals of Otology, Rhinology and Laryngology 108: 69–73.

Battmer RD, Laszig R, Lehnhardt E (1990) Electrically elicited stapedius reflex in cochlear implant patients. Ear and Hearing 11: 370–4.

Beiter AL, Staller SJ, Dowell RC (1991) Evaluation and device programming in children. Ear and Hearing 12(4) (suppl.): 25S–35S.

British Cochlear Implant Group and National Deaf Children's Society (1999) Quality Standards in Paediatric Audiology. Cochlear Implants for Children. Volume III.

Brown CJ, Abbas PJ, Gantz BJ (1990) Electrically evoked whole nerve action potentials: data from human cochlear implant users. Journal of the Acoustical Society of America 88: 1385–91.

Brown CJ, Abbas PJ, Fryauf-Bertschy H, Kelsay D, Gantz BJ (1994) Intraoperative and postoperative electrically evoked auditory brainstem responses in Nucleus cochlear implant users: implications for the fitting process. Ear and Hearing 15: 168–76.

Byrne D, Tonisson W (1976) Selecting the gain of hearing aids for persons with sensorineural hearing impairments. Scandinavian Journal of Audiology 5: 51-9.

Clark GM, Tong YC (1982) A multiple-channel cochlear implant: a summary of results for two patients. Archives of Otolaryngology 108: 214-17.

Cowan RSC, Brown C, Whitford LA, Galvin KL, Sarant JZ, Barker EJ, Shaw S, King A, Skok M, Seligman PM, Dowell RC, Everingham C, Gibson WPR, Clark GM (1995) Speech perception in children using the advanced SPEAK speech-processing strategy. Annals of Otology, Rhinology and Laryngology 104 (suppl. 166): 318-21.

Cowen RSC, Clark GM (1997) The Melbourne Cochlear Implant Clinic Program. In Clark GM, Cowen RSC, Dowell RC (eds) Cochlear Implantation for Infants and Children. Advances. San Diego, CA: Singular Publishing Group, pp 47-70.

Dawson PW, Skok M, Clark GM (1997) The effect of loudness imbalance between electrodes in cochlear implant users. Ear and Hearing 18: 156-65.

European Custom Sound Outcomes Seminar, Sintra, Portugal (1999). Highlights. Cochlear publication.

Finitzo-Hieber T, Tillman T (1978) Room acoustics effects on monosyllabic word discrimination ability for normal and hearing impaired children. Journal of Speech and Hearing Research 21: 440-58.

Hodges AV, Balkany TJ, Roger RA, Lambert PR, Dolan-Ash S, Schloffman JL (1997) Electrical middle ear muscle reflex: use in cochlear implant programming. Otolaryngology-Head and Neck Surgery 117: 255-61.

Hughes ML, Brown CJ, Abbas PJ, Wolaver AA, Gervais JP (2000) Comparison of EAP thresholds with MAP levels in the Nucleus 24 Cochlear Implant: Data from children. Ear and Hearing 21: 164-75.

Kelsall DC, Shallop JK, Brammeier TG, Prenger EC (1997) Facial nerve stimulation after Nucleus 22-channel cochlear implantation. The American Journal of Otology 18: 336-41.

Kileny PR, Zwolan TA, Boerst A, Teilen SA (1997) Electrically evoked auditory potentials: current applications in children with cochlear implants. The American Journal of Otology 18: (S)90-(S)92.

Lim HH, Tong YC, Clark GM (1989) Forward masking patterns produced by intra-cochlear electrical stimulation of one and two electrode pairs in the human cochlea. Journal of the Acoustical Society of America 86(3): 971-80

Lindstrom B, Bredberg G (1997) Intraoperative electrical stimulation of the stapedius reflex in children. The American Journal of Otology 18: (S)118-(S)119.

Loeb GE (1997) Speech-processing strategies designed for children. American Academy of Otolaryngology-Head and Neck Surgery 117 (3) Part 1: 170-3.

Lynch CA, Craddock C, Crocker SR (1999) Developing a child centred approach for paediatric audiologists: a model in the context of cochlear implant programming. The Ear 1: 10-16.

McCormick B (1993) Behavioural hearing tests 6 months to 3.6 years. In McCormick B (ed.) Paediatric Audiology 0-5 Years. London: Whurr, pp. 102-23.

McCormick B, Cope Y, Robinson K (1998) An audiometric selection criteria for paediatric cochlear implantation. Presented at the 4th European symposium on paediatric cochlear implantation, 's-Hertogenbosch, The Netherlands, June.

Makhdoum MJA, Snik AFM, Stollman MHP, de Grood PMRM, Van den Broek P (1998) The influence of the concentration of volatile anaesthetics on the stapedius reflex determined intraoperatively during cochlear implantation in children. The American Journal of Otology 19: 598-603.

Markides A (1986) Speech levels and speech-to-noise ratios. British Journal of Audiology 20: 84-90.

Mason S (1997) Objective measures. The American Journal of Otology 18: (S)84-(S)87.

Moore JM, Thompson G, Thompson M (1975) Auditory localisation of infants as a function of reinforcement conditions. Journal of Speech and Hearing Disorders 40: 29-34.

Nelson DA, Van Tasell DJ, Schroder AC, Soli S (1995) Electrode ranking of 'place pitch' and speech recognition in electrical hearing. Journal of the Acoustical Society of America 98(4): 1987-99.

Nucleus Cochlear Implant Systems Reliability Update (March 1999).

Opie JM, Allum JHJ, Probst R (1997) Evaluation of electrically elicited stapedius reflex threshold measured through three different cochlear implant systems. The American Journal of Otology 18: (S)107-(S)108.

Osberger MJ, Fisher L (1999) SAS-CIS preference study in postlingually deafened adults implanted with the Clarion cochlear implant. Annals of Otology, Rhinology and Laryngology 108: 74-9.

Patrick JF, Seligman PM, Money DK, Kuzma JA (1990) Engineering. In Clark GM, Tong YC, Patrick JF (eds) Cochlear Prostheses. London: Churchill Livingstone. pp 99-124.

Parisier SC, Chute PM, Popp AL (1996) Cochlear implant: mechanical failures. The American Journal of Otology 17: 730-4.

Rance G, Dowell RC (1997) Speech processor programming. In Clark GM, Cowen RSC, Dowell RC (eds) Cochlear Implantation for Infants and Children. Advances. San Diego, CA: Singular Publishing Group, pp. 141-71.

Roberts S (1991) Speech processor fitting for cochlear implants. In Cooper H (ed.) Cochlear Implants: A Practical Guide. London: Whurr Publishers Ltd. pp 201-218.

Shallop JK, Beiter AL, Goin DW, Mischke RE (1990) Electrically evoked auditory brainstem responses (EABR) and middle latency responses (EMLR) obtained from patients with the Nucleus multichannel cochlear implant. Ear and Hearing 11: 5-15.

Shallop JK (1993) Objective electrophysiological measures from cochlear implant patients. Ear and Hearing 14: 58-63.

Shallop JK, Ash KR (1995) Relationships among comfort levels determined by cochlear implant patients' self-programming, audiologists' programming and electrical stapedius reflex thresholds. Annals of Otology Rhinology and Laryngology 104 (Suppl.166): 175-6.

Shapiro W, Waltzman S (1995) Changes in electrical thresholds over time in young children implanted with the Nucleus cochlear prosthesis. Annals of Otology Rhinology and Laryngology 104 (Suppl.166): 177-8.

Sheppard S, Mason SM, Lutman ME, Gibbin KP, O'Donoghue GM (1992) Intraoperative electrical stapedial reflex measurements in young children receiving cochlear implants. Presented at the first European Symposium on Paediatric Cochlear Implantation, Nottingham, September.

Skinner MW, Holden LK, Demorest ME, Holden TA (1995) Use of test-re-test measures to evaluate performance stability in adult cochlear implant users. Ear and Hearing 16: 187-97.

Spivak LG, Chute PM (1994) The relationship between electrical acoustic reflex thresholds and behavioural comfort levels in children and adult cochlear implant patients. Ear and Hearing 15: 184-92.

Staller SJ, Beiter AL, Brimacombe JA (1991) Children and multichannel cochlear implants. In Cooper H (ed.) Cochlear Implants: A Practical Guide. London: Whurr, pp 283–321.

Stephen K, Welzl-Muller K, Stiglbrunner H (1991) Acoustic reflex in patients with cochlear implants (Analog stimulation). The American Journal of Otology 12: 48–51.

Stephen K, Welzl-Muller K (1997) Assessment of electrostimulation in children supplied with cochlear implants. The American Journal of Otology (S)97–(S)98.

Totten C, Cope Y, McCormick B, Robinson K (2000) Early experience with the Cochlear Esprit ear level speech processor in children. Annals of Otology, Rhinology and Laryngology 109: 73–5.

Twomey T, Archbold A (1997) Electrode and device problems: Manifestation and management. The American Journal of Otology 18 (Suppl.): 99–100.

Van den Borne B, Mens LHM, Snik AFM, Spie TH, Van den Broek P (1994) Stapedius reflex and EABR thresholds in experienced users of the Nucleus cochlear implant. Acta Otolaryngology (Stockh) 114: 141–3.

Waltzman SB, Cohen NL, Shapiro WH (1991) Effects of chronic electrical stimulation on patients using a cochlear prothesis. Otolaryngology – Head and Neck Surgery 105: 797–801.

Waltzman SB, Cohen NL, Roland Jr JT (1999) A comparison of the growth of open-set speech perception between the Nucleus 22 and Nucleus 24 cochlear implant systems. The American Journal of Otology 20: 435–41.

Young NM, Carrasco VN, Grohne KM, Brown C (1999) Speech perception of young children using Nucleus 22-channel or Clarion cochlear implants. Annals of Otology, Rhinology and Laryngology 108: 99–103.

Chapter 8
Facilitating progress after cochlear implantation: rehabilitation – rationale and practice

SUE ARCHBOLD, MARGARET TAIT

Rehabilitation is the word most commonly used to describe the support given to facilitate progress following cochlear implantation with both adults and children, but the form it should take and how it should be delivered are open to debate. Various models of service delivery were discussed in Chapter 3, but this chapter begins by discussing the concept of rehabilitation itself and whether the term is the most appropriate one to use. It then describes briefly the rationale behind some rehabilitation approaches for children with cochlear implants, and goes on to describe practical activities which have been found useful in helping children learn to use the hearing provided by the implant system. Ideas are examined for use with children with little or no spoken language, those who are developing some spoken language skills, and older children with well-established spoken language skills, either before, or following cochlear implantation.

Rehabilitation, habilitation, or . . .?

The purpose of implantation is to provide access to spoken language via audition – access that was not possible for the individual using conventional hearing aids. It seems reasonable, therefore, that, following implantation, support should be provided that promotes this. With deafened adults and older children the aim is to reopen the auditory channel for spoken language, which was the primary means of communication prior to the onset of deafness. With young children, the aim is to develop communication and spoken language skills through the audition provided by the implant.

The word 'habilitate' originates from the Latin *habilitare*, meaning to enable. Rehabilitation is a word we use with caution; its usual meaning is to restore or re-enable the use of a function that has been lost. It is therefore more relevant to working with deafened adults, or older children with progressive losses than when we are talking about young deaf children with cochlear implants.

Rehabilitation has been considered the reacquisition of lost communication skills (Dettman et al., 1996) and habilitation the facilitation of the initial development of spoken language skills (Barker, Dettman and Dowell in Clark, Cowan and Dowell, 1996). The word 'rehabilitation' has also been used to refer to both acquisition and reacquisition (Allum, 1996). However, using either word, rehabilitation or habilitation, can be taken to imply 'doing' something to the child, rather than the child being active in learning. In the case of a hearing child, the usual route by which communication skills, and hence spoken language, is acquired is audition. A great deal of research (see Chapters 9 and 10) has shown us that the child is an active participant in this process of language acquisition and how vitally important the early months and years of life are in the process. A child who is audiologically appropriate for implantation is likely to have relied for communication upon vision, whether by lipreading or signing. In addition, the child may well have received an impoverished linguistic input whether sign language has been used or not, and the development of language skills in the early months and years of life is likely to be significantly delayed (Mellon in Niparko et al., 2000). Implantation can provide useful hearing for many of these children, but they are likely to have missed many of the important language learning experiences of infancy. When audition is provided, the child will need to learn to interpret and integrate the sound signals received into the already established pattern of communication, in order to communicate effectively. Is it enough then to provide useful hearing and let the usual pattern of development take place? For an infant it may be, but for a child who has been without significant audition for some time, one needs to 'make the normal happen' (Tait, 1987); that is, provide the situations that are known to facilitate the development of spoken language in both hearing and deaf children. In order to maximize the benefits from the implant system, the children need:

- the implant system to be worn all waking hours, in good working order;
- the device to be appropriately tuned for the individual;
- good listening conditions, bearing in mind the difficulties of learning to listen in conflicting background noise;
- high expectations of the use of audition in the acquisition of spoken language;
- opportunities for non-linguistic listening experiences;
- opportunities to develop appropriate communication skills in adult/child, child/child and adult/children interactions;
- experience of success in developing listening and communication skills in age-appropriate interactions;
- the co-operation of all involved with the child: parents, siblings, peers, teachers, speech and language therapists and any other carers.

These requirements are not so different from those appropriate for young children who wear conventional acoustic hearing aids. The practical suggestions described later in this chapter are similar to those used with children with hearing aids and are based on ideas developed with such children over many years, which experienced teachers of the deaf and therapists will recognize. However, whilst relying on experiences with children with hearing aids, some differences are worth noting in working with children with cochlear implants:

- the complexity of tuning the implant system;
- the complexity of monitoring device functioning, particularly with very young deaf children;
- the sudden onset of audition after a comparatively long period with little useful auditory input;
- the provision of audition after communication skills may have been established without it;
- the necessity to help the child use audition through the implant system as effectively and as quickly as possible;
- the changing auditory potential of the children over time following implantation and hence the need to be flexible about the nature of support given.

Robbins, in Niparko et al. (2000), stresses that although there are many similarities in children with cochlear implants and those with hearing aids, the major differences are:

- the time course of learning is altered;
- detection is easier with a cochlear implant;
- high-frequency sounds are more accessible with a cochlear implant;
- the potential for incidental learning.

This last point is an important one that has much relevance to this chapter and one which will be developed later: the idea that children with cochlear implants may be able, given the right circumstances, to learn to use the hearing provided by the implant without, necessarily, the use of a didactic approach to rehabilitation. That is, the hearing provided by the implant system can give such a useful signal that the child has the possibility, implanted young and given the right circumstances, of acquiring spoken language through audition in a natural way. A very real challenge for parents and clinicians is to recognize the altered auditory potential of the child and to meet their changing needs over time.

Children receiving implants should already have been receiving specialized support prior to implantation and decisions may already have been made about communication approach and educational placement. After implantation, whilst educational placement and communication styles may initially remain the same, the consensus of opinion is that a strong auditory/oral component is essential to optimize the use of the implant, whatever the communication philosophy (Cooper, 1991; Somers, 1991; Tye-Murray in Tyler, 1993; Dettman et al. in Allum, 1996; Robbins in Niparko et al., 2000). An emphasis on audition may well have been inappropriate prior to implantation, but once more useful hearing has been provided by an implant, then the child needs to be given opportunities to interpret the new auditory information and integrate it into existing communication development. Those children receiving implants are likely to have experienced failure in the use of hearing (Somers, 1991) and must now be placed in a situation where success is not just possible, but likely, to enable the child to develop confidence in new auditory skills as soon as possible.

While the emphasis following implantation is likely to be on the use of audition in the development of spoken language, the child may already have established signing skills prior to implantation; if the child is young, this may be useful in having promoted the development of communication skills and a language base on which to build. Following implantation, one would expect the continuation of the use of signing with the child, while gradually the emphasis changes as the auditory signal becomes more useful to the child. In the experience of the authors, if the adults supporting the child are flexible and aware of the potential of the powerful auditory input provided by the implant over time, and give the child access to rich models of spoken language, the child will gradually show a preference for spoken language in everyday situations, with sign language remaining as an option. However, the older the child at implantation, the less likely this transfer of communication skills. We would be cautious about a child above the age of about five with well-established sign language skills, and little use of audition and spoken language prior to implantation being able to make the transfer, although clearly each child needs individual assessment.

Thus we must recognize the changed auditory potential of the child and attempt to maximize its attainment. Osberger (1990) states: 'there is no question that rehabilitation is an essential part of paediatric implant work'. This statement now needs some qualification. What do we mean by rehabilitation? Does it have a broader meaning than previously thought, when often taken to imply formal auditory training? Robbins, in Niparko et al. (2000), states that rehabilitation is regarded as 'an essential part of the management of these patients'. However, it is still unclear: do we mean the complete programme of support that will enable the child to develop the use of hearing in the development of spoken language skills? Or do we mean a rehabilitation programme of clinic-centred listening activities, which are designed to enable the child to learn specific listening skills in a hierarchical fashion?

We will continue to use the common term 'rehabilitation' in this chapter, but take it to mean the entire programme of support provided for the child by parents, clinic and local professionals to facilitate progress. It includes managing and tuning the system, as described in Chapter 7, and then providing opportunities for the child to use auditory information in everyday learning, whether at home or at school. While the word rehabilitation will continue to be used, as it is in common usage, a more appropriate term might be programme of support, implying flexibility and a total programme of care, rather than the focus being training in the development of listening skills.

This programme of support must be in close liaison with the child's parents and local professionals, who are likely to bear the main responsibility for developing the child's use of the system. With the progress of universal neonatal hearing screening worldwide leading to earlier diagnosis of deafness and the trend towards increasingly young children receiving cochlear implants, it is likely to be the parent or major caregiver who provides the major input to the child, rather than the teacher of the deaf or speech and language therapist. The implant team and local professionals may be providing the support programme through the major caregiver rather than working with the children or infants themselves. This may require a major shift in thinking by those providing the support programme, and one that will necessitate the use of more courses for parents such as the John Tracey correspondence course, or Hanen parent interaction programmes (Hanen, 1994), which help parents to optimize the language learning process for their children. The role of the educator of the deaf may well change to facilitating the parents as the major players in the children's acquisition of spoken language following implantation. This is not an entirely new role for teachers of the deaf: Northcott's (1978) materials for the development of communication and language emphasized the role of parents and the focus of language acquisition being in the home. However, the support provided by the local educator for the child and family should not be at the expense of the other deaf children in the educator's care. It may well be that, following implantation, the child will not receive more input than before, but that the specialist time spent with the child and/or family will have a different focus: the use of audition in the development of communication and spoken language skills. Many of the activities described later in this chapter have been used by parents or other caregivers, and we have developed materials to help parents have confidence in their own ideas.

Approaches to rehabilitation, or the programme of support provided

Having established that these children need rehabilitation, defined as the support programme provided following implantation, what form should it take? Although many of the issues surrounding work with deaf children are old, cochlear implantation opened a new chapter in the saga, with discussion about the most effective way to maximize the use of audition. Techniques used with children with cochlear implants include those with varying emphases on communication approach; and those with a varying emphasis on learning theory. Those with varied emphases on communication approach include those that emphasize a uni-sensory approach, which may be auditory or visual, and those that emphasize a multi-sensory approach, using visual and auditory modalities. Those programmes that vary in approach to learning include those with an emphasis on synthetic or analytical training; unstructured or structured methods, didactic or generalization approaches. These theoretical frameworks are described elsewhere (Eisenburg, 1985; Somers, 1991; Cooper, 1991; Tye-Murray in Tyler, 1993; Dettman et al. in Allum, 1996; Robbins in Niparko et al., 2000); the aim here is not to add to the conflict, but briefly to consider what is known of children's learning, whether deaf or hearing, and how this knowledge can influence rehabilitation in its broadest sense.

The quality of adult/child interaction and the importance of meaning within early language learning experience is vital (Bruner, 1983); the adult must be responsive to the child's attempts at communication, in order to facilitate the development of language, rather than imposing the adult's interests on the child (Webster in Cline, 1992). 'Motherese' or infant-directed speech facilitates language development and emotional development with its specific differences (Mellon in Niparko et al., 2000). This involves the child being active in learning and in acquiring linguistic competence having been given exposure to appropriate models at appropriate times. Deaf children, with delayed diagnosis, may not have received useful auditory or sign input as infants. In order to make up this delay it may be tempting to put into place highly structured programmes of listening activities in order to speed up the process of language acquisition via hearing. However, emphasis on the repetition of the adult's contribution, the correction of the child's own contribution and on adult questioning have been found to be counter productive to the development of communication skills, and hence language, in both hearing and hearing-impaired children (Wood et al., 1986). This theme will be developed further as the acquisition of communication skills in children at the pre-verbal stage is discussed. Highly structured adult-controlled methods of promoting the use of the implant system are contrary to what we know to facilitate communication and linguistic development both in hearing and hearing-impaired children. The emphasis on analytical or didactic rehabilitation relies on training children in specific goals within the clinic, assuming that a skill learned will be generalized into everyday life. The approach we use in Nottingham tends towards the synthetic (or top-down) approach in which children learn to use hearing in natural everyday situations, discovering the rules of communication for themselves, so that they are able to generalize and to use their useful hearing in the development of language. However, it is recognized that a range of approaches may be required, changing over time, and there will be occasions when a more didactic approach may be appropriate. It is also vital that a clinician who works with a child has the hierarchy of development in mind at all times, whether it is made explicit or not.

Bench and Bamford (1992) comment that the deaf child's learning of a first language is rather like that of learning a second language, relying on being taught, rather than acquired. Robbins in Niparko et al. (2000) emphasizes that one of the main differences found with children with cochlear implants is the opportunity that hearing through the implant provides for incidental learning. Cochlear implantation may provide such effective access to audition that learning spoken language once more can rely on the natural processes of language acquisition, rather than being taught; that is, in Robbins' terms, through incidental learning.

The adult's role is not that of a mere observer of the process, however, but that of a vital facilitator of the child's learning. The adult must structure the learning experiences for the child, bearing in mind an overview of the likely sequence of development of auditory skills and leading the child on to the next stage of development (Webster in Cline, 1992). These stages are likely to follow Erber's (1982) levels of detection, discrimination, identification and comprehension. The listening experience and opportunities given to the child should follow these levels, but in subtle, rather than explicit, ways. Thus the child is not being *trained* to listen, but is *learning* to listen, and in fact, learning *through* listening (Nevins and Chute, 1996) . The adult's role is complex: to provide the optimal situations for language learning and to ensure that the process happens. Listening experiences can be built into everyday formats by a skilful teacher, and by intuitive parents. It would be unfortunate if the advent of cochlear implantation, with an emphasis on the use of hearing and the implementation of rehabilitation programmes, returned us to auditory training techniques, developing skills that were not generalizable, at the expense of using hearing in the learning experiences of the whole child. As Robbins in Niparko et al. (2000) states, one of the greatest challenges for educators and therapists following implantation, is to use the power of incidental learning and integrate learning to listen into everyday experiences. Thus opportunities to integrate rehabilitation ideas into everyday life can be taken, rather than viewing rehabilitation as a specific programme of structured activities to be worked through.

Although the approach advocated by the authors emphasizes this natural approach, capitalizing on opportunities for incidental learning, it has proved necessary to provide ideas for use with children after implantation for parents and children, and this chapter describes some of those we have found useful. They may be used to facilitate the use of audition in the development of communication skills and spoken language, and at the same time provide parents and professionals with information on progress. This is vital to inform the tuning process (see Chapter 7) and may help to identify problems with the device or early signs of other processing problems within the child, which must be followed up. It is important that parents and professionals are aware that there are times when assessment must take place and, with young children who are unable to perform formal speech tests, observations based on some of these activities may inform ongoing monitoring of progress. However, they must be set in the context of the entire programme of support for the child, and used within the understanding of child development and learning outlined above. At all times, the development of the use of the cochlear implant system is not an end in itself, but the hearing provided should facilitate the development of communication and linguistic skills, and must be integrated into this process.

However, unless the child is wearing the implant system appropriately and unless it is optimally tuned and functioning, a programme of suitable activities is useless. The programme of support, therefore, begins with the management of the implant system itself.

Managing the implant system

For rehabilitation to be effective the child must be wearing the device adjusted comfortably and at appropriate settings. This implies that the audiological scientist has been able to tune the system optimally, and that the child has accepted the device and the new sensations of sound. In practice this might not be so straightforward, particularly with a young or complex child. The tuning of the system, described fully in Chapter 7, may take some time with a number of visits to the clinic. The child may not accept the new sensation happily, and it may be necessary to progress slowly in small steps until the optimum programme for the system is achieved. This will require the combined skills of the family and the local and implant professionals. Fryauf-Bertschy in Tye-Murray (1992) offers practical advice for parents about preparation for initial tuning, which remains helpful; it is useful if the child has seen others wearing the device, and has tried on the dummy processor and headset. Fryauf-Bertschy also gives practical ideas for wearing the processor, and for encouraging children who reject it. Children may reject the implant system and its signal for many reasons; it may have been inappropriately tuned, but at an experienced centre this should be rare. It may be that the child is disturbed by the new sensation, or it may be that the child realizes that this can be a new manipulative weapon to use!

It is important that parents and local educators realize that, although the vast majority of children accept the implant system happily, adverse reactions are possible and may need to be worked through. It is important that the family has confidence in the implant team and all work together in supporting the use of the system for all the waking hours. The major implant manufacturers provide very useful materials for children and their families to use at initial tuning time. There are a variety of child-friendly pouches, colouring books and toys available to help stimulate children's interest in wearing the system before they have had time to value it for what it offers them (Figure 8.1). In the experience of the authors, many children who have previously rejected wearing hearing aids, quickly become constant wearers of the implant system, having discovered how useful the signal is to them.

The age of the child may lead to different problems in wearing the device, and we shall consider these in turn. We will

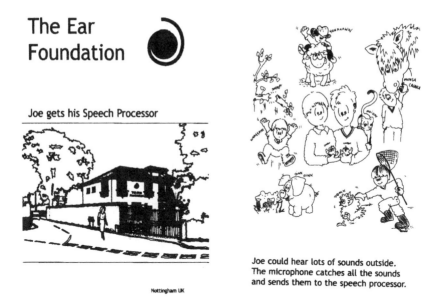

The Ear Foundation

Joe gets his Speech Processor

Nottingham UK

Joe could hear lots of sounds outside. The microphone catches all the sounds and sends them to the speech processor.

Figure 8.1. Toys and books to encourage wearing the system.

consider first the youngest group of children, those under or around the age of two years. With very young infants there are likely to be practical problems in wearing the implant system, many of them similar to those of wearing hearing aids. With ingenuity and care most can be overcome. Beyond the stage of infancy, toddlers are at an age when there are already likely to be several areas that are 'battlegrounds' - feeding, toilet training, bedtime and so on - and wearing the processor and headset can too easily be added to the list. Again, having worn the dummy processor beforehand may help, particularly if all the family pretended to put it on too, but a child who 'sees that wearing the device is yet another opportunity for him to exert control over his parents may simply refuse to put it on' (Nevins and Chute, 1996). As with slightly older children, rewards, praise and distraction may help; otherwise 'negative reinforcement' may be the best strategy (Nevins and Chute, 1996). The device is offered to the child, without the parents insisting or getting upset; if the child refuses, parents indicate that without it there will be no activities, pointing out from time to time what the child is missing by not wearing the device. This is a strategy that several of our parents have found effective. As far as wearing the body-worn processor is concerned, very young children need to wear a harness, or have a pocket on a t-shirt; many parents find the best place for this is on the child's back, but in any case it is best worn under clothing, for extra protection and to be out of the way of small fingers.

With slightly older children, before initial tuning, it is helpful if the child is already made familiar with the appearance of the processor, has seen others wearing it, and has tried on the dummy processor and headset. The child may need to become accustomed to putting on the headset as he or she may remember discomfort in that area and be reluctant to have anyone touch it. Sometimes the dummy processor may be left at home for parents to try on the child so that this difficulty can be overcome before the clinic visit.

At initial tuning, the device will be set at a very conservative level, so that there are no uncomfortable sensations of sound, but the new sensations may still cause distress on the first day. This can usually be overcome by rewards, distraction, praise, and the sort of fun with sound that is described below. It is important that parents and local professionals are supported by, and have confidence in, the implant team, but also that they take responsibility for encouraging the child to wear the device. From the beginning, the child should wear it for the whole day; it may be necessary at first to adjust the controls in noisy conditions – in the car or supermarket, for example – but this is less disruptive for a child of this age than taking the system off and putting it on again. A four-year-old may be happy to wear a harness for the body-worn processor, but as children grow older they are often happier with something like a 'bum bag'. One of our children wears her processor in a shoulder bag (Figure 8.2). Parents in Sweden have developed commercial bags that combine fashion with practicality.

Finally, what about children who are approaching adolescence, or who are already teenagers when implanted? At present, if children this age are implanted it is likely to be because they have had a sudden onset of deafness, or have a deteriorating hearing loss, or because relaxed audiological criteria mean that they are now considered suitable for implantation, despite having some useful residual hearing with hearing aids. These teenagers are likely to be committed to wearing the system. We must not forget the children who were implanted at a young age, and who now are approaching their teenage years too. For most of these children willingness to listen via the implant is not the main difficulty; however, wearing it visibly

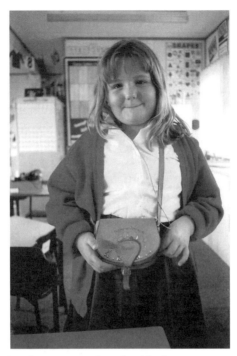

Figure 8.2. Wearing the processor in a shoulder bag.

may be, at an age when appearance is so important. At this age the provision of an ear-level processor may be crucial for the child, but for children for whom this may not be a possibility some thought needs to be given to the positioning of the body-worn processor. Some are happy simply wearing it clipped to a waistband – others prefer it out of sight in a 'bum bag' or something similar.

Constant use of the system is only effective if the device is functioning optimally. Handbooks are produced by the various companies, and at the authors' programme parents and teachers are given a simple trouble-shooting guide and spare leads to keep at home and at school. It is essential that, in addition to carrying out a daily check of the signal through the processor, parents and professionals quickly recognize any changes in the subtle signs that reveal auditory awareness on the part of the child. The rehabilitation ideas in this chapter, in addition to being designed to promote learning through listening in pleasurable ways, are suitable for providing situations in which an observant parent or professional can monitor the device's functioning. Intermittent faults with the system can be particularly difficult to pinpoint and may only be noticed when a child appears confused in a listening activity within his capabilities. The listening activities which are described in this chapter follow a hierarchy of developing skills, and are described under the following headings:

- Working with young children and infants at the pre-verbal stage.
- Working with older children with developing communication skills.
- Working with older children with functional language.
- Working with adolescents.

Working with young children and infants at the pre-verbal stage

The aim with young children and infants at the pre-verbal stage, is to work with parents and clinicians to facilitate the use of audition in the development of communication. Once children have been fitted with the external parts of the system, they will be in a similar position to that of acoustic hearing aid wearers – that is with the potential of using hearing. However, before they begin to understand what is said to them, and to use speech themselves, there needs to be the development of the pre-verbal skills of appropriate eye contact, turn taking, auditory processing and meaningful vocalizations (see Chapter 9 for a fuller discussion).

Increasingly, infants in the first two years of life are being considered for implantation. The younger the child, the more likely it is that provision of a cochlear implant, together with appropriate management, will lead to a 'normal' pattern of development of the understanding and use of spoken language, even if delayed. What do we mean by 'appropriate'? The use of infant directed speech – 'motherese' – as has already been mentioned. Contingent behaviour is another important element and is part of 'motherese': contingent behaviour follows the child's line of gaze and comments on what he is attending to. That is, the adult comments on what is in the child's mind rather than the adult's (Figure 8.3); this is a vital factor in facilitating the acquisition of the meaning of language. Clearly with an infant (Figure 8.4) the people most crucially involved are the parents, and much of the work of rehabilitation professionals needs to be via these key people who, as far as this child is concerned, are the real experts.

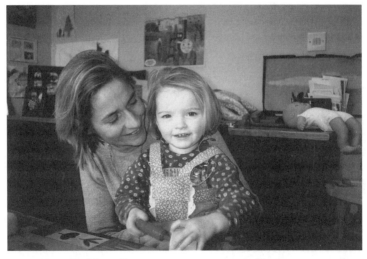

Figure 8.3. Developing parent/child interaction.

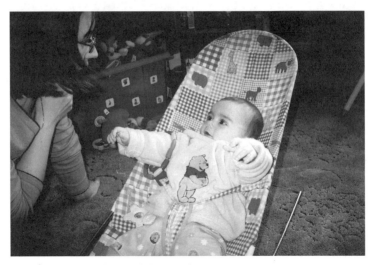

Figure 8.4. A young infant with her mother.

It is the parents who have the central role both in facilitating early language development and in helping the child make best use of the implant system. Successful rehabilitation of young deaf children largely depends upon the support and involvement of the parents who sometimes need help in avoiding a directive and controlling attitude towards communication and in establishing normal effective interaction. A parent training programme based on the Hanen Programme (Manolson, 1992) is used at Nottingham, combining group sessions with individual visits and using video to help parents analyse their communication style in a non-stressful way and to make positive changes in interaction (Figure 8.5).

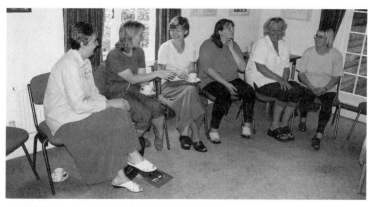

Figure 8.5. Parent interaction programme.

When we come to assess the progress of a child whose age is measured in months, rather than years, we need very careful observation, which will be facilitated by the use of video. A video recording of the infant on his mother's knee, looking at a pop-up card book, can be revealing. In this situation it is likely that the child's gaze will be directed toward the book, not his mother. Then, for example, if the book is about farm animals, one can look to see if the infant is responding in any way to sounds such as 'moo', 'baa', 'ee-ee' and so on. Does his face alter in expression, indicating that he has heard the adult's comments? Later on, does he begin to imitate the sounds? An infant cannot be asked to play co-operative listening games so skilled observation is a very important feature in monitoring progress and ensuring that activities are producing progress.

We now give some guidelines on helpful approaches with slightly older pre-verbal children, and also some practical suggestions, many of which can be adapted for use with young infants. They are described with reference to developing turn taking and auditory processing; additionally, suggestions for the development of meaningful vocalizations and the use of singing at the pre-verbal stage are included. For simplification, the adult is referred to throughout as 'she' and the child as 'he'.

Encouraging turn taking at the pre-verbal stage

A deaf child at the very earliest stage of language development, both before implantation and for some time afterwards, is likely often to be unaware of the adult's attempts to communicate with him. It can also happen that the adult is so keen to communicate that she misses what is in the child's mind. It is not possible to 'make' a young pre-verbal child understand us, any more than it is possible to 'make' him communicate. As with infant implantees, our initial approach needs to be on the lines of a mother with her hearing baby: to follow the child's line of gaze and comment on what he is looking at; to observe his activity and wait, giving him time to take the lead, to which her response will be meaningful. This is still the essential 'normal' baseline for pre-verbal three or four-year-olds; however, with these slightly older children there are additional strategies that may help to encourage turn taking, always bearing in mind the principles already mentioned.

The use of partner and parallel play

There are several ways of making the adult's presence interesting to a child at the pre-verbal stage. One answer is to become a partner – but the *less dominant* partner – in play; for example to be the patient to the child's doctor (Figure 8.6), the hungry person at the table waiting for the child to serve the dinner, the visitor knocking to be let in, and so on. It is at times such as these that the presence of another adult can be invaluable. One adult can be the naughty patient refusing medicine, while the other arouses interest in her and helps the doctor to administer suitable treatment.

Another way is to play 'in parallel' with an unresponsive child. Parallel play is a stage that normally comes between solitary and co-operative play. Children engage in the same activity, side by side, each of them modifying what he is doing because of the actions of the other child, though not actually playing

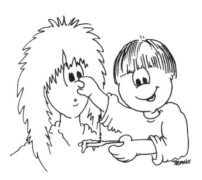

Figure 8.6. Promoting parallel play: who is the doctor?

with the other child. This form of play has been observed to occur much more rarely with hearing-impaired children (Gross, 1987) and that may well be because they have less auditory feedback to let them know what the child playing alongside is doing and planning to do. They therefore simply play alongside until they reach the stage of being able to join in co-operative play. For the adult to be the parallel (but again subordinate) partner in play can be a good way of promoting interaction in an unstressful, uncontrolling manner. One simply engages in the same activity that has been chosen by the child – for example playing with pastry – and does whatever the child does. Before long he becomes aware of this, and observes the adult's actions as well as his own, sometimes deliberately egging her on by unexpected behaviour (putting pastry on his nose, for example) thus giving lots of opportunities for one-to-one conversation and interaction dominated by the child (Figure 8.7).

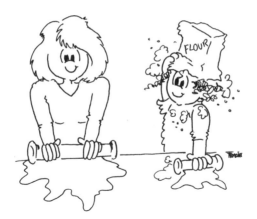

Figure 8.7. Developing adult/child interaction.

The use of familiar formats

The establishment of some 'format' (see Chapter 9) which catches the child's interest (and, if possible, causes amusement) is in our experience the most likely way of enabling appropriate turn taking to develop. An example follows from a one-to-one session with a profoundly deaf boy aged three, who has at this period very little receptive or expressive language. The adult's (A) and child's (C) 'turns' are presented in sequence. Notes on gestures and focus of visual attention are given in round brackets for the adult and square brackets for the child:

A: That's it! You're driving your car, and then we stop [sitting back], don't we, stop [policeman's 'stop' gesture], like that. [C looks at A throughout, until A gestures, then glances at gesture, and back at A.]

C: [Gestures 'stop', glancing at his gesturing hand, and back at A.]

A: 'Stop', the policeman says [glances at her hand] 'stop!' [with gesture], doesn't he. [C looks at A, then follows her glance at her hand by looking at both hands, and back at her.]

C: (St)o(p) [said without voice, with gesture, and a look at their gestures].

A: Stop. Yes, and then he says – [her arm is moving in preliminary to gesture] – 'go!' (gesture). [C has looked at her gesture preliminary, but looks back at her as she says 'go'.]

C: (G)o! [gesturing].

A: Go, that's right, and we'll drive our cars again.

Because this little routine is familiar to the child, it is very clear to him where his 'turn' comes. He is able to *take* his 'turn' first by gesture, then by gesture and a silent attempt at the appropriate word, and finally by a vocal attempt. This is very much the sort of process followed by the normally hearing infant in well known format-like routines.

The use of shared activities

Appropriate turn taking is a stage of the child's development. It cannot be imposed on him. What one *can* do is to provide situations where there will be some point taking his turn in the interaction. The shared activity (making a paper puppet) illustrated in Figure 8.8, is an example that shows how this might happen in practice.

The most important thing in all encounters is for the adult to be aware of any glances that come her way, to recognize the reason, and act contingently as previously described (Wood et

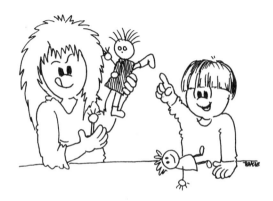

Figure 8.8. Developing turn taking: shared activities.

al., 1986). Any move a child makes toward the adult – and a glance in her direction is such a move – must be interpreted as communication and responded to as such. Similarly, one should treat any vocalization as intentional communication and respond to it, just as the mother of the normally hearing baby does, leaving pauses in the utterances that are long enough and frequent enough for the child to have a chance to take part. It is especially important to respond to any vocalization that the child makes during the adult's turn, and to relinquish one's own turn immediately. If a child takes a turn that has not been offered, it should be given to him. If many turns go by without his being able to take them, a brief return to a situation that he *can* recognize – a format – will help him get back into the conversation. This may take the form of a familiar 'joke'.

Turn taking is easier when the situation is predictable, which is why familiar formats and jokes play such an important part. Potentially fruitful activities are:

- playing with farm animals;
- playing with road and cars;
- cooking (real or pretend);
- model making;
- looking at pop-up books;
- cleaning shoes – or anything else;
- washing anything;
- setting the table;
- any games/activities that involve an element of surprise, such as items hidden in a bag.

Developing auditory processing: helping children to use their hearing at the pre-verbal stage

It is important not to give children the impression that 'listening' is something that only happens at special times, and thus losing the opportunity for incidental learning. There are advantages, however, in sound-making sessions whose main purpose is to make listening something that is exciting and fun. In the early days after initial tuning of the device the easiest activity for a child is to perceive the onset of sound because *he* is producing the sound himself and can observe its effects on others. For example, he plays percussion instruments and the adult reacts – perhaps marching while he plays a drum, and falling over (without looking at the child) when he hits the cymbal. The role of listener rather than producer of the sound need not be passive; for instance, the child hiding inside the playhouse and bursting forth when he has heard the sound (Figure 8.9). Similarly, it is great fun for him to listen for a sound and then send a skittle flying across the room.

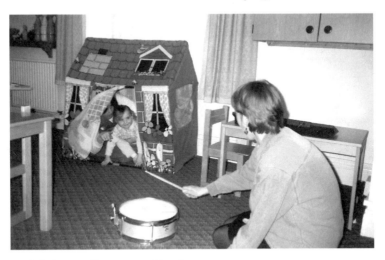

Figure 8.9. Responding to sound in play.

These are very simple examples, and there are many more adventurous things that can be done using more sophisticated instruments; but the basic idea *is* simple: the child makes a sound and observes its effect on other people. He sees these other people react to the sound he is making even when they are not looking at him. Also, he begins to be aware of sound, and of the person making it, when *he* is not looking at the sound source.

Although the child's auditory attention may be caught initially by the use of musical and environmental sounds, what one particularly wants him to be aware of is the human voice. Again, a child who is not a ready vocalizer may begin by simply using his voice to 'operate' the adult. For example, the adult may curl up in a comfortable chair, while the child attempts to 'wake' her or get her moving by vocalizing, illustrated in Figure 8.10. Then roles can be reversed so that the child is doing the listening.

As with the infant, we can assess the development of listening skills by using video recordings of the child in one-to-one interaction but we can also begin some listening activities to monitor responses. The Listening Progress Profile (LiP – see Appendix A) can be used to monitor the development of auditory processing

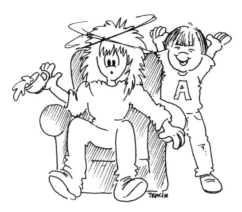

Figure 8.10. Using voice to great effect.

in children without spoken language skills and can be completed by skilled observation (Nikolopoulos, Wells and Archbold, 2000).

The role of singing with pre-verbal children

Singing is another activity that promotes listening and also goes a long way towards solving many of the early problems with eye contact, turn taking and vocalization. The idea of singing with a child who is not yet talking may seem a surprising one, but in fact it is in many ways easier for a young deaf child than conversation. This is because some of the 'rules' and conventions of spoken exchanges are waived in this activity. Eye contact, for example, is more straightforward in a simple action song, as the child does not need to look anywhere else for information in order to understand what is going on. Similarly, vocalizing comes more readily during singing because there is no need for turn taking. As eye contact and vocalization are pre-verbal skills, which one is trying to develop, an activity that encourages both in an enjoyable way is valuable. It has been found that young deaf children (wearing conventional hearing aids) at the pre-verbal stage maintain twice as much eye contact during the singing of simple action songs as they do during one-to-one conversational sessions with a known adult. With children at this stage there is seven times as much vocalization in singing compared with the talking situation. Additional benefits are that the children's voices are more varied in pitch and their utterances longer and more rhythmic (Tait, 1986). For all these reasons, singing is an activity to be recommended for all young children with implants, at any stage of their linguistic development, but particularly during the pre-verbal period.

The adult interacting with the child in singing needs to enjoy it and accept that being in tune is not important. What *is* important is to be near enough to be properly heard and seen, to sing at a reasonable volume and speed (not too slowly) and with rhythm. It is not necessary to try to make very young children watch the singer – they probably will watch if it is interesting enough, and most of all if the singer is enjoying it, as enjoyment is very contagious. On the other hand, a child who is not looking may very possibly be listening, particularly if he is showing signs of being involved in what is going on – vocalizing, for example, or doing the song actions. Similarly, it is better not to insist the child joins in; singing should be an enjoyable experience. In addition, children are most vocal under conditions of least control (Wood et al., 1986) and they will be more likely to join in positively, take the lead and suggest songs themselves if they are not pressured (Tait, 1986). Tapes of appropriate songs and suggestions for their use are available from the Nottingham programme.

To summarize: during the pre-verbal stage the development is taking place of:

- conversational turn taking;
- meaningful vocalization;
- auditory processing.

Once these skills become established the children will begin to understand speech and to use vocalizations and speech sounds in a meaningful way.

Working with older children who have developing communication skills

With young children the emphasis was on the development of early communication skills; with slightly older children, who have some communication abilities and are beginning to respond, or who have been implanted at an older age of four or five, more activities to facilitate listening and use of hearing are possible. The stages of response, followed by discrimination, identification and comprehension will follow, facilitated by the support programme. We next look at activities with environmental sounds, musical instruments and spoken language.

In planning appropriate activities for a child within these areas there may be great disparity between the child's linguistic age and chronological age. For a child deaf from birth or deafened at an early age, and implanted some years later, it may be taxing to find age-appropriate and interest-appropriate tasks. This is a common problem when working with deaf children, but with children who have not had any useful hearing for a number of years the problem may be even greater than usual. Listening activities must be meaningful and related to everyday activities in order that generalization can take place, rather than specific skills being learned in isolation, and this may necessitate some imaginative thinking on the part of the parent or therapist. The sudden acquisition of useful hearing after a number of years without audition will necessitate a number of adjustments for both the child and his or her carers. Those interacting with the child on a daily basis must change their expectations, while not subjecting the child to any pressure to 'perform'. This demands quite subtle changes of handling on the part of parents and educators if the best possible use is to be made of the implant system.

Listening to environmental sounds

For some, environmental sound discrimination is not an important part of the rehabilitation programme, but often the first observed responses are to environmental sounds, and it may be a major aim of implantation for safety reasons for parents (Eisenburg, 1985). At this stage the children enjoy 'listening' walks, indoor and out, responding to environmental sounds and drawing pictures of those that they can hear. The sounds within home or clinic can be used so that the child becomes aware of the diversity of sounds around and begins the early stages of discrimination. When a child has shown his first response to sound for many years, it is very easy to be too keen to test his listening skills, and he will soon not wish to co-operate. Opportunities for drawing attention to sounds in the environment must be made and taken casually without putting the child under any pressure. Saying 'there's the doorbell – let's go and see who's there', rather than questioning the child as to what made the sound, helps him to attach meaning to the sound in a relaxed way. Picture books that illustrate sounds in the environment and stories that refer to sound are all appropriate for this stage, helping the child to relate meaning to the new sensations being received. Picture cards showing sounds in the child's environment are readily available, and home-made picture books can be coloured and completed as responses to sounds are observed. This may be helpful in demonstrating new listening skills to parents at a time when apparent progress may be slow.

Listening to musical instruments

Whilst play with musical instruments will have formed a part of the rehabilitation work with children at the pre-verbal stage, with slightly older children it can be taken further (Figure 8.11). The term 'musical instruments' covers a wide range of sound makers. Fun may be had with toys that make a variety of sounds, with noisy toy animals, and with a whole range of sound-making equipment. The children develop the games played at the pre-verbal stage; for example, moving or responding to different musical instruments in a variety of ways, and playing musical statues or hide-and-seek in response to sound.

Once responses in play have been observed to a variety of musical instruments, then discrimination can begin. Naturally one begins discrimination games with musical instruments that are very dissimilar in sound, progressing to those that are more closely related. Children enjoy pretending to sleep and identifying the instrument that woke them up; different instruments can be played out of sight and the child can go to find them.

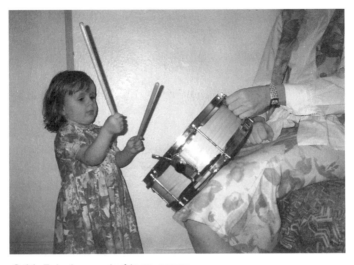

Figure 8.11. Enjoying musical instruments.

Children enjoy imitation games as rhythm and intensity are altered and pairs of instruments enable the adult and child to play alongside as imitative skills develop.

Children at this stage become more able to join in conventional songs and rhymes at school and teachers of the deaf often comment that a child is more able to participate in these activities following implantation, enjoying the repetitive songs that form part of the daily school routine. As with hearing-aided children, children with cochlear implants will often join in the repeated chorus of a well-known song, and many action rhymes enable children to respond with appropriate actions within a group (Figure 8.12), demonstrating developing listening skills, before they are able to join in the singing at all.

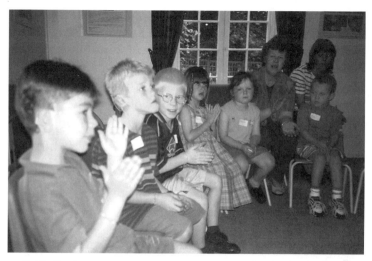

Figure 8.12. Singing in a group.

Listening to speech sounds: developing responses in play

Initially a variety of action toys will be useful in producing a reaction to speech sounds and an observable response from the child. Wind-up toys, which have to be told to 'go' and 'stop', are useful. The adult makes a sound to accompany their progress; for example the monkey goes 'oo oo'; the mouse goes 'ee ee'. These action toys interest a wide age range of children and provide an opportunity for repetitive sound making, encouraging recognition and imitation of speech sounds without stress.

Animals, vehicles, puppets and action toys give opportunity for hearing and making speech sounds in game formats. For example, jumping toy frogs into the pond on vocal command, or playing with farm animals, provide situations in which the child can hear and attempt to produce these sounds many times over in highly motivated situations. The animals can hide, pop out, go to market in turn in the lorry (accompanied by 'brmm brmm') and then settle down to sleep ('shh'). There are many books about animals that are appropriate for this stage and those that contain pictures for the child to open are most useful to encourage shared conversation and developing responses to speech sounds; these responses may initially be subtle and may only be observable on video.

Animal sounds have the advantage that with some ingenuity they can be used to cover the range of speech sounds, and children can be conditioned to associate a particular speech sound with a particular animal or toy. This proves useful in evaluating listening skills. Children at this stage may not be able to cope with formal imitation exercises or assessment of perception of Ling's five sounds (oo, ah, ee, sh, ss) (Ling, 1988) and, as clarified earlier, the early enforcement of repetition may not be productive. Perception of the five sounds can be assessed through play; observing the child's responses to 'sh' or 'ee' will enable even subtle changes in listening skills to be monitored.

Listening to speech sounds: developing discrimination

Once the child has developed responses to a range of speech sounds, the development of discrimination is encouraged. Once more this can be done through everyday, age-appropriate activities, but the aim is to increase, and monitor, discrimination in the following areas:

- a single sound versus a repeated sound; for example, a long train going 'choo, choo, choo' versus a short train going 'choo';
- a long sound versus a short sound; for example, a long snake going 'sssssss' versus a short snake going 'ss';
- a loud sound versus a quiet sound; for example, a large sheep making a loud 'baa' versus a lamb with a quiet 'baa';

- a high sound versus a low sound;
- one sound versus another; for example, 'moo' versus 'baa'.

Games to promote, and monitor, the discrimination of speech sounds include the following activities on hearing the appropriate speech sound:

- placing counters, or colouring on an appropriate picture;
- finding the appropriate hidden animal;
- throwing a ball or hoop at toy animals;
- racing animals (toy or puppet) along a track;
- racing vehicles along a track, making different noises for each vehicle;
- taking a pencil for a 'walk', varying the pattern in response to the sounds; for example, according to whether the stimulus was continuous or repeated;
- using a pencil or crayon to complete the path of a figure across a page, as in pre-writing left to right patterning activities; for example, moving the pram across the page in response to 'sh'.

Figure 8.13 shows some illustrations found useful for these activities.

Even young children can put counters on the long or short snakes according to whether the sound was long or short, or move a large or small animal along the track according to whether the sound was loud or quiet. Initially all these tasks are carried out with the child able to lipread if he or she wishes; gradually opportunity must be taken in play to perform these games when the child is not in eye contact, so that the extent of developing listening skills may be assessed and reliance on audition promoted. Face-watching opportunities should be withdrawn in a natural way, rather than by covering the mouth with one's hand. Children become very adept at speech reading even when one's mouth is 'hidden'; they look intently for other facial clues, and in reality may not be dependent on audition. It is possible to carry out listening activities side by side, with the child focused on the book, paper, toy or activity while one is talking, ensuring the child is not lipreading, but listening in a natural, unforced manner. The child may attempt the sounds himself and be in charge, so that the adult can move the appropriate animal or vehicle. If the adult prefers to act the fool and

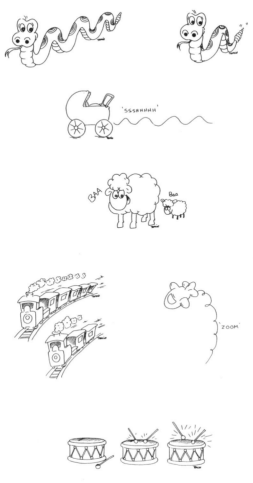

Figure 8.13. Examples of useful pictures for developing discrimination of speech sounds.

make silly mistakes the child will love to correct these (proving, of course, that he is able to perform the task himself).

We continue to emphasize that these activities should be used with imagination and care, as part of the whole child's programme; not as a series of daily exercises. With some thought, similar activities can be used as part of the child's everyday learning experiences; Robbins in Niparko et al. (2000) warns of the 'greenhousing' effect where children have learnt to perform such tasks but are not able to generalize the skill and utilize it. However, it is important that we are able to monitor the child's developing skills and these activities are one way of doing it. When the children are able to co-operate in the games described, and are able to demonstrate the ability to discriminate a range of speech sounds, they will usually be using some of these sounds in communication, will have developed an understanding of the rules of communication and be equal partners in conversation. Older children receiving implants because their hearing loss is a deteriorating one, or because of the relaxed audiological criteria, are likely to have developed functional spoken language and need a different approach.

Working with older children with functional spoken language

In the authors' programme, a small proportion of children have functional spoken language at implantation, but it is anticipated that the majority of implanted children will achieve functional spoken language within the first three years following implantation (see Chapter 10). At this stage, the children are able orally to:

- initiate conversation;
- comment;
- respond to questioning;
- question others;
- joke;
- contradict.

Children implanted at an older age, with functional spoken language, are likely to need some listening activities to help them to adjust to the new signal, and integrate their new hearing into a previously established communication system. However, communication and interaction at this stage become a great deal easier and some activities found useful in developing listening to environmental sounds, musical instruments and spoken language are described.

Listening to environmental sounds with older children

Although the emphasis is on providing access to spoken language via the *speech* processor, children at all stages may respond first to environmental sounds and those with functional language will be able to record their own listening progress in a variety of ways. They may be able to use written language, or drawings, to record their listening experiences completing their own checklists of sounds heard, and sorting into groups those they can and cannot hear, and those they can identify. Children who have had no significant auditory input for a number of years need opportunities to explore and comment on these sounds in their environment to enable them to begin to adjust to their new hearing. They also need to know that it is acceptable to indicate what they cannot yet hear or identify, and when there is no sound. Taped environmental sounds may give practice in learning to identify these new sounds, but care must be taken to introduce a few items at a time.

Listening to musical instruments with older children

The use of musical instruments can be developed further at this stage. They can be classified by the child into those he can or cannot hear, without the exercise being made at all stressful, or the child feeling under test. 'Sound' words may not have seemed very relevant previously and the use of musical instruments provides opportunity for discussion about the quality of sounds made and the introduction of appropriate vocabulary as words such as squeak, rattle, scrape begin to have an auditory meaning. An electric organ or music synthesizer is useful with older children who may enjoy experimenting with the different sounds it produces and children can learn to describe the sounds they can hear, as they become able to discriminate between loud/quiet, single/repeated sounds. The awareness of high/low discrimination seems a little more difficult for children, particularly those below the ages of seven or eight, but an electric organ provides many opportunities for experiment.

Older children enjoy using a personal stereo and listening to the usual 'pop' favourites; and for a child who has missed out on peer group interests in pop music, it can be an important social experience too.

Listening to spoken language with older children

Conversation

Once the child has developed some functional language the development of appropriate conversational skills is paramount.

The most practical approach will often be to use the one-to-one conversation session in a quiet situation to develop listening skills in a natural way. As always, the child's interests can be the basis of the conversation, and the child's own contributions encouraged with the adult creating the context of the conversation. Topics could include home, family, pets, hobbies, television or comic characters; the important thing to remember is that the adult must talk *with* the child, not *at* him or her (Webster and Wood, 1989), avoiding over-control by the adult. Prior to implantation, the child will have been unable to respond auditorily to spoken language; the child must now learn to use auditory clues and to take turns in conversation as we have described with children at an earlier stage. The adult can facilitate this change in focus from visual modality to auditory modality by gradually withdrawing physical prompts and limiting distractions, so that the child becomes reliant on auditory prompts such as his name or the command 'listen' (Webster and Wood, 1989). For children in total communication settings, the rehabilitation programme should gradually extend the emphasis from sign to audition, following the child's development of use of hearing.

The adult, as facilitator, bears some responsibility for ensuring that the listening environment for conversation is suitable for the child, particularly in the early stages following implantation, when listening in noise will be difficult. Background noise is difficult for cochlear implant users, as for hearing aid users. Classrooms should be acoustically treated to minimize reverberation, and parents should be aware that, at home, background noise from the television, washing machine, running water and so on will affect their child's ability to listen (Tye-Murray, 1992). Immediately after implantation, conflicting noise may well hinder children's developing confidence in their listening abilities.

Opportunities must also be provided in class for small group conversation, and child/child interaction encouraged. Group conversation requires an appreciation of turn taking at a higher level than on a one-to-one basis, and will provide the child with the experience of learning to follow the flow of conversation from one speaker to another with the conversation facilitated by an experienced adult.

Listening activities: spoken language

Discrimination of spoken language will be encouraged through the regular conversation sessions, but children at this stage still need some structured activities in order to develop reliance on audition and listening skills through the speech sound, word, phrase and sentence levels. Suggestions for activities to promote this development are now described; they must retain the element of fun and interaction that has already been emphasized and should be integrated into the child's everyday activities.

Figures with speech balloons into which the sound, word or phrase being given can be placed are adaptable for different children, and can be personalized. Speech balloons containing Ling's five sounds can be used for children to indicate with counters or by ticking which sounds they are hearing. The speech balloons may show family names (beginning with those of differing numbers of syllables) as the child learns to discriminate one family name from another; if the child is unable to read then photographs are used. Finger puppets, or card pictures of faces talking to each other provide opportunity to develop discrimination of words or phrases in an interactive setting.

Once the child has become able to discriminate single words, we need to develop the discrimination of two or three word phrases; for example, 'hello Mummy' versus 'bye bye Mummy'. Groups of pictures illustrating family members carrying out a variety of activities can be used to encourage discrimination of phrases; Mummy cooking, Mummy sleeping, for example.

Games previously used can easily be adapted to the child's interests using more complex language; favourite comic characters, vehicles, animals, puppets using oral instructions. In these games the teacher is able to provide opportunities for the child to develop listening further, and to observe the child's responses to spoken language as he plays the game appropriately. The child is engrossed in the game, and the adult is able to use familiar, repetitive language, while retaining a high degree of motivation. Older children and those with functional language are able to co-operate with an adult or other children and will enjoy turn-taking games, thereby also acquiring valuable communication skills that might not have been learnt prior to implantation.

Activities that are appropriate to develop the discrimination of speech for children with functional language include:

- races using oral instructions;
- following oral instructions: for example, drawing or colouring a picture, making a model, carrying out a physical activity;
- completing funny faces, figures or Mr Potato Head;

- Pelmanism (pick up pairs);
- bingo/lotto; particularly if the child is asked to guess the card the adult is describing;
- board games such as 'The House that Jack Built'; 'Quack Quack';
- memory games; for instance, lists can be given orally and each child repeats the list and adds another item of his choice;
- battleships, using oral clues;
- treasure hunts on a grid, given oral clues;
- map finding games, given oral clues;
- 'Guess Who?'
- 'Simon Says'
- 'Dot-to-Dot' pictures completed orally;
- Guess what I'm thinking of? The adult describes a picture or article and the child names it or draws it.

Teachers of the deaf commonly use communication games with children to promote effective communication between children and adult–child communication: that is, games in which children and teacher have to relay messages or instructions to each other effectively. Following implantation they are a useful way of giving the child a secure setting in which he can develop auditory skills. Conventional games such as Battleships, Guess Who?, following instructions to find the treasure or one's way about a map are all useful ways to motivate a child to wish to communicate. When trying to follow instructions on a map or grid, as shown in Figure 8.14, the difference between C1 and D1 is very difficult to ascertain without listening. Thus the child is placed in a non-threatening situation where he has to listen in order to be able to play the game. All these games can be useful means of involving other family members, including brothers and sisters, rather than only adults.

Developing listening through stories

Stories are an essential part of the child's learning to use sound in communication and have been found to play an important part in developing linguistic skills (Wells, 1981). Stories should have an amusing element; it helps both child and teacher to retain interest! Children enjoy personal contributions by their teachers, particularly if the teacher has done something they perceive as foolish; these personal stories can be illustrated and used as sequence

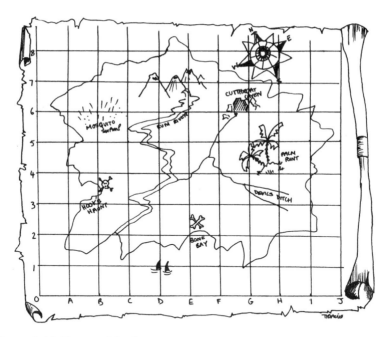

Figure 8.14. Treasure island game.

stories for repeated telling and enacting. Comics are a fruitful source of amusing stories and adapting the current favourite character can be profitable. Comic stories can be cut up into picture sequence so that they can be sorted and retold; the speech balloons can be blanked out so that the child can complete the story in his own words. Several goals can be achieved in this way: in retelling the story, the child can hear and experiment with different voices, learning to express a variety of feelings.

Children should have regular opportunity to hear a story and retell it, developing their own narrative skills with confidence. Speech and language therapists and teachers of the deaf at the Nottingham programme have developed a series of stories about a dragon family to promote the development of narrative skills and they have been used by the programme with a wide range of children (Nikolopoulos et al., 2000). Familiar and repetitive stories and rhymes give opportunity to develop confidence in listening, and children enjoy listening for deliberate mistakes made by teacher or parent in the retelling of a familiar story. Sequence stories in picture form are commonly used with deaf children and there are many sources of material. Once the pictures have been used to develop the storyline, with the child predicting events, then they can be used as a listening activity in which the child is asked to identify the appropriate picture by listening for the corresponding sentence, thus developing listening skills at a higher level than the phrase level.

There are many story books available today with no text, which are ideal for telling and retelling stories. Traditional fairy tales contain many repetitive elements, which again are ideal for children to retell or act out with their peers; those with finger puppets lend themselves to retelling by child and parent or teacher in a variety of ways.

Developing listening through written language

With school-aged children the reinforcement that comes with using the written word is very helpful; it can be introduced gradually, with a great deal of repetition in stories about themselves. As with a hearing child, the most useful way of introducing the written word is through the child's own story books about himself. For example, different members of the family may be illustrated involved in a variety of activities at home. Each picture may have a simple phrase or sentence written underneath at the child's own linguistic level. The more amusing the activities, the better the chance of gaining and sustaining interest. Older children tell us that seeing the written pattern while hearing it is helpful in learning to listen to spoken language. The consistent visual pattern appears to reinforce the new auditory pattern if simple stories about themselves with picture clues are written for the child to follow visually on paper while listening to the story being read by the adult. Stories containing four or five pictures are sufficient initially, and the use of speech balloons in the story encourages an interactive element. Shared reading reinforces our emphasis on meaningful interaction, and lack of adult control; sharing a book in this way provides an ideal means of assessing listening skills without putting the child in a 'test' situation (Figure 8.15). The focus of shared interest is naturally on the book and written word, and it is easy for the adult to assess the level of the child's understanding without lipreading.

Poems can also be useful, particularly amusing ones; they give the added clue of rhythm as the child attempts to follow the written script without lipreading. The adult may read and stop so that the child follows the written pattern and finds where the adult has paused. Amusing poems enable the teacher to use them several times for reinforcement, while retaining the child's interest and giving opportunity for shared enjoyment.

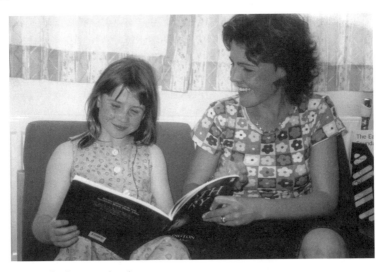

Figure 8.15. Sharing a book.

Connected discourse tracking (CDT) (De Filippo and Scott, 1978) is an accepted procedure for adults, which can usefully be adapted for children with functional spoken language. The adult reads the story in small phrases to the child, who then repeats each portion. If the child is unable to repeat there are several recognized strategies; repeating, rephrasing, breaking down further or using written or signed clues. The session is timed – it is usually about five minutes – and the number of words that the child has been able to repeat correctly per minute calculated. CDT is often used as a method of evaluation, with which there are many recognized difficulties (Tye-Murray and Tyler, 1988) but it can be a useful, meaningful rehabilitation task. We have adapted the Mr Men books (Hargreaves) for CDT: the child is at first able to see the picture but has to repeat the story, given initially with lipreading, then without. Later he repeats the story without pictures or preparation. A series such as the Mr Men books provides a wide variety of materials with the same format, and is of interest to children of a wide age range, making them very appropriate for use with the same child over time. The development of the ability to carry out CDT over time has been reported (O'Donoghue, Nikolopoulos and Archbold, 2000).

Along with the use of the written form as an aid to rehabilitation, we have found a phonic approach to reading very helpful. While recognizing the inherent problems in using a phonic approach with English and the fact that it emphasizes a weakness for deaf children (Webster and Wood, 1989), it does give a child learning to use audition confidence and word attack skills. Early play with letters and initial sounds gives opportunity for repetition of speech sounds with an additional helpful visual input. It may also enable the child to achieve age-appropriate success with his class peers. Games such as 'I-Spy' can be played at home and school alike.

Many teachers of the deaf and therapists use computer-based activities in their work, and children with cochlear implants find these helpful too. Language programmes and games with the child sitting side by side at the computer give opportunity for conversation while the focus of visual attention is on the screen; this provides a natural situation in which there is the need to be reliant on audition. The use of a language tape-card machine upon which material can be individualized involves the child in using relevant written words and sentences with opportunity for repeated listening and also for attempted repetition by the child. Similarly voice-activated software provides powerful opportunities for a child to use spoken language effectively to control a computer and produce a script.

Use of telephone

Many children find it very intimidating to use the telephone early in their use of the implant system and we have found that the best introduction is the way in which young hearing children first become accustomed to the telephone. That is, after a long period of confidence in spoken language, to be encouraged

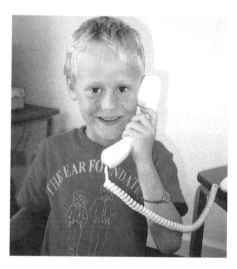

Figure 8.16. Developing telephone use.

to 'say hello to Daddy' (or any known adult), and to be allowed to do so over the telephone and to listen to the response and then say 'bye bye'. The child can then become accustomed to the sound of the voice over the telephone in a known format and develop confidence in its use. Children who are tested over the telephone at this stage by an overenthusiastic adult are often deterred by failure from further trials. Adult implant users report finding telephone training difficult, and children need sensitive handling in these early stages if they are to succeed.

A hearing child or an adult can be helpful in the beginning to encourage simple conversations, and children who can read find it very helpful to follow a simple script, which they have previously helped to write, over the telephone. The child and the adult on each end of the telephone each need a copy of the script, and read their part of the conversation. Once confidence has been built up in this way, children can then begin listening to simple 'tests' over the telephone: guessing who is being named (from a limited set at first); guessing what the weather is like at the other end; guessing what the other person is eating or doing. Children with implants enjoy games listening to the telephone, but, like all children, they can be intimidated by it and need to experience success in its use. The most powerful motivation will be when the child really needs to use the telephone to contact parents or friends to organize a social life!

Our telephone profile (Appendix B) was developed to monitor progress in these skills; it shows that these skills develop over a long time frame. Six and seven years after implantation, children are continuing to acquire the skill of telephone use (Tait, Nikolopoulos, Archbold and O'Donoghue, 2001).

Adolescents and cochlear implants

Although the emphasis in this book is on the implantation of young children, there are growing numbers of teenagers choosing to have a cochlear implant as the audiological criteria are relaxing, and a growing number of teenagers, implanted early, who are now facing new issues. These two groups deserve specific mention of their needs, and how they can be met. It is becoming clear that, teenagers, appropriately chosen, can become effective users of implant systems. They need to:

- be fully involved in the decision;
- be strongly motivated to using audition;

- be good hearing aid users, however little audition provided by conventional aids;
- use spoken language as the main means of communication, whether or not supported by sign;
- have strong oral/aural input at school and home;
- be counselled fully about the long-term outcomes from implantation;
- be counselled fully about the possible technical problems and long-term commitment required;
- have realistic expectations.

Teenagers who are using an implant for the first time need careful preparation. They need to be told directly (not via their parents) what implantation involves, and what the benefits are likely to be, and clearly need to have been fully involved in the decision. They need to know that speech is likely to sound strange at first, that they may not like it, that it may initially make lipreading more difficult, and that their own speech will not instantly improve. Parents of young children often get frustrated at the apparent lack of progress during the first year with the implant; teenagers too need to be prepared for the length of time it may take for benefit to be apparent.

Following cochlear implantation, these teenagers can learn to integrate the new signal into their own style, given time and appropriate activities for their age and interests. As suggested above, following scripts, using connected discourse tracking, reading texts from the school curriculum, are all appropriate. Support provided in helping them to learn to listen through the implant system must not disrupt their participation in the curriculum. In addition, however, they need:

- access to a peer group – deaf, but using cochlear implants rather than hearing aids;
- communication training – how to use appropriate strategies in difficult listening conditions;
- understanding of the technology they have received;
- understanding of the tuning process;
- understanding of the trouble-shooting process;
- knowledge of how to access the support needed should a problem arise with the equipment;

- ability to take on the long-term responsibility for the maintenance of the equipment.

All these will enable the teenager to take on ownership themselves of their implant system, and responsibility for its continued use and maintenance. In addition, those who are becoming
teenagers, having been implanted early, need similar opportunities, in order to come to terms with the decision made earlier for
them by parents. These teenagers need to understand, on their
own behalf, the technology within them, its possibilities and
limitations. The establishment of teenage support groups in the
UK is beginning to address these needs, and to help this growing
group of teenagers to take on responsibility for the care of their
cochlear implant systems themselves and to become adult users.
The advent of the widespread use of fax and email facilitates
contact for these teenagers, including those unable to use the
telephone. *Deaf@x* have begun a Web site for deaf children, and
this has tremendous potential for this group of teenagers too.

Comment

Helping children to learn to interpret auditory signals is not
new: many teachers have commented that, following implantation, children are able to participate in many activities that were
previously inappropriate as they required some useful hearing.
Children with cochlear implants may not require more rehabilitation or support than those with hearing aids; rather it may be
that the time spent with them after implantation will have a
different focus and different expectations from that prior to
implantation. Anecdotal evidence is that children may need
more support directly following implantation, but less later on,
as they come to use the system effectively.

For those implanted very young, it may be that the focus of the
rehabilitation programme is not with the child but with the family,
promoting the development of communication skills and hence
language, through the hearing provided by the implant system,
given appropriate interactions. It may also be that the child's
needs change as the use of hearing changes over time, and that
the appropriate management changes over time. This demands
flexibility on the part of implant teams to respond to changing
needs over time, and on the part of those working with the children and their families locally. The provision of this flexible

support, monitoring the changing use of audition over time, in close conjunction with the cochlear implant team, is a major challenge for local educational and speech and language services.

It is becoming increasingly apparent that the true benefits of cochlear implantation only accrue over several years, particularly with young children. Over time, there are tremendous possibilities: those of us involved in paediatric cochlear implantation have a responsibility to ensure that the children in our care have the time and opportunities needed to use their new auditory signals.

References

Allum D J (ed.) (1996) Cochlear Implant Rehabilitation in Children and Adults. London: Whurr.

Barker EJ, Dettman SJ, Dowell RC (1997) Habilitation: infants and young children. In Clark GM, Cowan RSC, Dowell RC (eds) (1997) Cochlear Implantation for Infants and Children Advances. San Diego, CA: Singular, pp. 171-90.

Bench J, Bamford J (1992) Speech Tests and the Spoken Language of Hearing Impaired Children. London: Academic Press.

Boothroyd A (1989) Hearing aids, cochlear implants and profoundly deaf children. In Owens E, Kessler DK (eds) Cochlear Implants in Young Deaf Children. Boston, MA: Little, Brown & Co.

Boothroyd A (1991) Assessment of speech perception capacity in profoundly deaf children. American Journal of Otology 12: 67-72.

Bruner JS (1983) Child's Talk: Learning to Use Language. Oxford: Oxford University Press.

Cooper H (1991) Training and rehabilitation for cochlear implant users. In Cooper H (ed.) Cochlear Implants: A Practical Guide. London: Whurr Publishers Ltd.

De Filippo CL, Scott BL (1978) A method for training and evaluating the reception of ongoing speech. Journal Acoustic Society America 63: 1186-92.

Dettman S, Barker E, Rance G, Dowell R, Galvin K, Sarant J, Cowan R, Skok M, Hollow R, Larratt M, Clark G (1996) Components of a rehabilitation programme for young children using the multichannel cochlear implant. In Allum DJ (ed.) Cochlear Implant Rehabilitation in Children and Adults. London: Whurr, pp. 144-65.

Eisenberg LS (1985) Perceptual capabilities with the cochlear implant: implications for aural rehabilitation. Ear and Hearing 6(3): 60S-69S.

Erber NP (1982) Auditory Training. Washington DC: Alexander Graham Bell Association for the Deaf.

Fryauf-Bertschy H (1992) Getting started at home. In Tye-Murray N (ed.) (1992) Cochlear Implants and Children: A Handbook for Parents and Teachers and Speech and Hearing Professionals. Washington DC: Alexander Graham Bell Association for the Deaf.

Gross H (1987) Social interaction and play in the deaf nursery school. Unpublished PhD Thesis, University of Nottingham.

Hargreaves R The Mr Men Series. London: Thurman Publishing Ltd.

Ling D (1988) Foundations of Spoken Language for Hearing Impaired Children. Washington DC, Alexander Graham Bell Association for the Deaf.

Manolson A (1992) It Takes Two to Talk. The Hanen Centre, Toronto, Canada.

Mellon NK (2000) Language acquisition. In Niparko JK, Iler Kirk K, Mellon NK, McConkey Robbins A, Tucci DL, Wilson BS (eds) (2000) Cochlear Implants: Principles and Practice. Philadelphia, PA: Lippincott, Williams & Wilkins.

Nevins ME, Chute P (1996) Children with Cochlear Implants. San Diego, CA: Singular.

Nikolopoulos T, Lloyd-Richmond H, Starczewski H, Gallaway C (in press) Using SNAP Dragons to monitor narrative abilities in deaf children following cochlear implantation.

Nikolopoulos TP, Wells P, Archbold SM (2000) Using Listening Progress Profile (LiP) to assess early functional auditory performance in young implanted children. Deafness and Educational International 2(3): 142-51.

Northcott W (1978) Curriculum Guide – Hearing Impaired Children 0-3 Years and their Parents. Washington, DC: AG Bell.

O'Donoghue GM, Nikolopoulos TP, Archbold SM (2000) Determinants of speech perception in children after cochlear implantation. The Lancet 356(9228): pp 466-8.

Osberger MJ (1990) Audiological rehabilitation with cochlear implants and tactile aids. Asha 32: 38-43.

Robbins AM (2000) Rehabilitation after cochlear implantation. In Niparko JK, Iler Kirk K, Mellon NK, McConkey Robbins A, Tucci DL, Wilson BS (eds) Cochlear Implants: Principles and Practice. Philadelphia, PA: Lippincott Williams & Wilkins.

Somers M (1991) Speech perception abilities in children with cochlear implants and hearing aids. American Journal of Otology 12: 174-8.

Tait M (1986) The role of singing in the social and linguistic development of nursery aged deaf children. Unpublished PhD Thesis, University of Nottingham.

Tait M (1987) Making and monitoring progress in the pre-school years. Journal British Association of Teachers of the Deaf 11(5): 143.

Tye-Murray N (1992) Cochlear Implants and Children: A Handbook for Parents, Teachers and Speech and Hearing Professionals. Washington, DC: Alexander Graham Bell Association for the Deaf.

Tye-Murray N (1993) Aural rehabilitation and patient management. In Tyler RS (ed.) Cochlear Implants: Audiological Foundations. San Diego, CA: Singular Publishing Group Inc.

Tye-Murray N, Tyler RA (1988) A critique of continuous discourse tracking as a text procedure. Journal of Speech and Hearing Disorders 53: 226-31.

Tyler RS (1993) Speech perception by children. In Tyler RS (ed.) Cochlear Implants: Audiological Foundations. San Diego, CA: Singular Publishing Group Inc.

Webster A (1992) Images of deaf children as learners. In Cline T (ed.) The Assessment of Special Educational Needs: International Perspectives. London: Routledge.

Webster A, Wood D (1989) Special Needs in Ordinary Schools: Children with Hearing Difficulties. London: Cassell.

Wells G (1981) Learning Through Interaction. Cambridge: Cambridge University Press.

Wood DJ, Wood HA, Griffith AJ, Howarth CI (1986) Teaching and Talking With Deaf Children. London & New York: John Wiley.

Appendix A: listening progress profile

LisProg2000

NOTTINGHAM PAEDIATRIC COCHLEAR IMPLANT PROGRAMME
LISTENING PROGRESS

Name:		CIN:	

| I/O | D/O | Key: I/O = Indirect Observation (left box); D/O = Direct Observation (Right box) (Both have equal scores) |

	Pre		6 mth		12 mth		24 mth		36 mth	
Behaviour										
Response to environmental sounds										
Response to drum (elicited)										
Response to musical instruments (elicited)										
Response to voice - elicited										
- spontaneous										
Discrimination between 2 different instruments										
Discrimination between: loud/quiet drum										
Discrimination between: single/repeated drum										
Identification of environmental sounds										
Response to: oo										
ah										
ee										
sh										
ss										
Discrimination between:										
Long/short speech sounds										
Single/repeated speech sounds										
Loud/quiet speech sounds										
2 of Ling's five sounds										
All of Ling's five sounds										
Discrimination between 2 family names of different syllabic length										
Identification of own name in quiet										

Scoring:		Scores:	
N (Never/Not known)	0	Pre ------------	24 ------------
S (Sometimes)	1	6 ------------	36 ------------
A (Always)	2	12 ------------	

Appendix B: telephone profile

Telephone1.2000

NOTTINGHAM PAEDIATRIC COCHLEAR IMPLANT PROGRAMME

TELEPHONE PROFILE

NAME: CIN:

	Pre	6 mth	12 mth	24 mth	36 mth
Response to ringing					
Identification of ringing					
Response to dialling tone					
Identification of dialling tone					
Response to voice					
Identifies known speaker					
Identifies: Hello					
Byebye					
Own name					
Follows structured conversation from prepared script					
Discriminates family names					
Discriminates four numbers					
Discriminates days of week					
Follows structured conversation without script					
Able to carry out open conversation with familiar speaker					
Able to carry out open conversation with unfamiliar speaker					

Scoring:		Scores:
N (Never)	0	Pre ------------
NK (Not known)	0	6 ------------
S (Sometimes)	1	12 ------------
A (Always)	2	24 ------------
		36 ------------

Chapter 9

Using video analysis to monitor progress in young cochlear implant users

Margaret Tait

Introduction

The majority of the children referred for cochlear implantation are under five years of age, with an increasing proportion under two to three years. Most are deaf from birth, with a sizeable number deafened very early in life, for example through meningitis. Most of these young children will have no spoken language and will therefore be considered to be pre-verbal, although they may understand and use some sign language, so would not in that case be considered to be 'pre-language'. They will need other methods to assess their progress than those that can be used with older children or with younger children who do have some understanding and use of spoken language (Osberger et al., 1991a; Miyamoto et al., 1992). In this chapter we look at a method of assessing the development of the pre-verbal skills which are an essential precursor to spoken language.

Research in recent years has identified several distinct, sequential stages that normally hearing infants pass through before the emergence of verbal communication. These stages start with attention seeking, use of crude gestures, and development of turn taking skills and vocalizations at appropriate junctures, and form the foundations of spoken language (Bruner, 1983). They include three important features of interaction: appropriate visual attention, turn taking by gesture and by vocalization and awareness of the appropriate time to take a turn from auditory monitoring. The ability to distribute visual attention between the parent or caregiver and the object of communication develops early in life (Bruner, 1983; Barnes et al., 1983;

302

Harris et al., 1986; Collis in Schaffer, 1977). At first it is the adult who follows the infant's line of gaze, but by four to six months the infant is beginning to follow the adult's line of gaze too. Such shared visual attention to objects in the environment promotes language development by establishing a context for associations between sounds and objects, and so helps infants to discover the significance of what is being said to them, provided that it is contingent upon what is occupying the child's attention (Baldwin and Markman, 1989; Harris, 2000; Crystal, 1997). Turn taking – the ability to take alternate 'turns' in dialogue, the normal practice in conversation – develops in the first months of life through the interactive behaviour of the parent or caregiver, and includes the use of intentional bodily gestures such as pointing (Zinober and Martlew in Barrett, 1985). Auditory monitoring is also evident early in life, as seen in the infant's response to the sound of the voice of the parent/caregiver by vocalizations and bodily movements (Brazelton in Tronick, 1982), and in the greater attentional response to the exaggerated pitch contours of infant-directed talk or 'motherese' (Cooper and Aslin, 1989; Werker and McLeod, 1989).

Comparable research into the pre-verbal development of deaf children indicates that the achievement of similar sequential stages predates the emergence of verbal communication (Wood et al., 1986; Tait and Wood in Crystal, 1987). Deaf children, too, need to develop the ability to distribute their visual attention and to take turns in dialogue. Good acoustic hearing aid amplification is known to promote the development of these early spoken language skills. One needs to know that the implant and speech processor are fulfilling a similar function for those children who have insufficient hearing to use acoustic hearing aids. Observation of the development of pre-verbal skills can show whether or not they are receiving appropriate auditory information from the speech processor, although of course there can be other causes of lack of progress in the development of these skills.

Assessment of pre-verbal skills as they develop is greatly assisted by video analysis. Video recordings of each child in interaction with a known adult, made at regular intervals, will enable us to monitor the development, over time, of eye contact and conversational turn taking. Auditory awareness and processing skills (the child's reaction to and interpretation of the sound of speech) can also be monitored through video analysis, by observing how a child reacts to speech when not looking at the speaker. A well-documented method of video analysis (Tait, 1993; Tait and Wood in Crystal, 1987; Tait and Lutman, 1997; Tait, Lutman and Robinson, 2000) has been developed to assess the pre-verbal and early verbal development of our young deaf children who receive cochlear implants while at a pre-verbal stage. This chapter describes the procedure, and through three illustrative cases discusses ways in which the analysis can provide indications of the effect of the implant on the child's communication. Finally, a resumé is given of current research into the possibility of using video analysis to predict future levels of performance in speech perception and intelligibility in children with cochlear implants.

Making a video recording: lighting, sound quality, frequency and length

Lighting

The room used for making the video needs to be light enough to make a clear recording. If the natural illumination is not sufficient, some form of extra lighting needs to be arranged and this should be placed discretely so that the child is not dazzled. However, making a video in daylight is usually possible. One should film away from the window with the child sideways on to it, so that the light falls on his face without his looking directly into it. This gives enough illumination to see the direction of the child's gaze when one is making the transcript. The camera needs to be pointing mainly at the child, but also taking in the adult in profile. One needs to see the child almost full face to be sure of the direction and focus of his gaze, whereas a profile view of the adult is sufficient to be able to tell where she is looking, her facial expression, and any signs, gestures or body language. (To avoid confusion, wherever possible 'she' is used to refer to the adult and 'he' to the child.) The child is usually filmed sitting side-by-side with the adult, or at right angles if he needs to see her face. This position makes it easy for him to look at the adult if he wishes, but does not 'require' it in the way that a face-to-face position can do.

Sound quality

The room in which the video is made should be reasonably quiet. This may seem obvious, but if one's hearing is normal it is easy to overlook background noise, which will make listening difficult for the child and also for the person doing the transcription afterwards. For the same reasons, a reverberant room is not ideal either. Very often the filming can take place in the child's home, where soft furnishings provide a good acoustic environment.

Frequency and length of video sessions

In Nottingham video films are made at the following intervals:

- pre-implant (two separate occasions);
- six months after initial tuning;
- 12 months after initial tuning, and thereafter only if necessary.

Filming lasts for between five and 10 minutes (longer only if there is difficulty in establishing interaction) with the aim of eventually transcribing no more than three minutes. This has been found to be long enough to get a good impression of the quality of interaction of which a child is capable, and it is also important to avoid unnecessarily prolonging the labour-intensive and time-consuming business of transcription. For this reason we now only analyse three of the four recordings: the second pre-implant, the six-month and the 12-month sessions.

Content of session

This depends on the age and communication ability of the child, but whatever stage he is at, the aim is to monitor what is emerging, not to enforce change. When filming, one needs to be guided by the child's role in the interaction, following his line of interest and trying to interpret what is in his mind rather than expecting him to interpret what is in the adult's mind – in other words, to be as normal and child centred as possible. This is particularly important with a very young child. When dealing with, say, a three- to four-year-old child who is in the early pre-verbal stages, without much (or any) receptive and expressive language, it is helpful to include a 'format' (Bruner, 1983) – a situation that has within it the possibility of enjoyable predictability. For example, toys such as a jack-in-the-box, toy train plus people, farm trailer plus sheep and cows, are all capable of being used in this way. These predictable shared activities solve, or at least make easier for the child, the problem of where to look and when to take a turn, and make the interaction relaxed and enjoyable. Similar situations can be used both before and after implantation, so that the videos can be compared.

An example of such a situation, using a farm vehicle and animals, is given below. The adult's and the child's 'turns' are presented in sequence.

Adult: Go, lorry, round, that's right. You'll have to tell it to –
Child: [gestures 'stop']

A:　– to stop, that's right. Can you –
C:　– [points at empty driver's cab]
A:　What's in there? No, there's no little man, is there, driving it, no. Stop, lorry. Get out, sheep. Now then, which of those shall we have?
C:　[picks up cow]
A:　A cow. The cow says 'moooo, mooooo, mooooo'
C:　Moooo, mooooo
A:　He wants a ride, mooooo.
C:　[gestures 'sleep']
A:　Go to sleep, that's right, go to sleep, cow.

Once the animal game has been initiated, the adult in this example is prepared to follow the child's lead at any point. From the way in which the child takes his 'turns' it is clear that he feels an equal partner in the interaction; he interrupts the adult twice, and by gestures ('stop' and 'sleep') suggests what is to happen next. It is also useful, particularly after the initial tuning sessions have taken place, to spend part of the time looking at a book. This is because it will be more natural for the child to look at the book than at the adult, and so the beginnings of auditory processing will become apparent – for example, in his repetition (without looking) of something that the adult has just said. It may be more difficult to get that information in a situation where adult and child are facing each other if the child has already established the habit of looking at the speaker's face.

Measures

Progress in pre-verbal development is monitored in the following areas:

Turn taking
- turn taking involving silent gesture/sign;
- turn taking involving voice and, eventually, words.

Autonomy/initiative
- vocal turn that cannot be predicted from adult's preceding turn (see below);
- gestural turn, which cannot be predicted from the adult's preceding turn.

Visual attention
- eye contact with the speaker;
- division of visual attention between speaker and object of reference.

Auditory awareness
Indications of auditory awareness in:
- repetitions (unsolicited) of words when not in eye contact with the adult;
- vocal turn taking after not having been in eye contact with the adult.

Making and analysing the transcript

Three transcripts, Figures 9.1, 9.2, and 9.3, show the scoring in detail.

Turn taking

This is marked on the transcript by an arrow every time it is clear that the adult has left a pause for the child to take part, or when the child has interrupted the adult's turn. It is useful, particularly when first using this approach, for two people to look separately at the video to see if there is reasonable agreement as to the points at which turns have been left. (The reliability of the analysis has already been established by a replicability study – Tait et al., 2001.) The total number of turns is then counted, the number of turns taken by gesture or by vocalization is counted, and the latter are then expressed as percentages of the total number of turns. Figure 9.1 shows how this works out in practice, but bear in mind that percentages are normally calculated from at least twenty turns.

The adult has left three turns – occasions when she has paused, still looking at the child, to give him the chance to take part if he wishes. (Of course, a child may decide to take a turn where he has not been left an opening, in which case the adult should give way to him.) How does the child in Figure 9.1 take the turns he is offered?

- on the first he does not respond;
- on the second he responds with a gesture;
- on the third he vocalizes.

Therefore, his responses have been as follows:

- gesture on one out of three occasions: 33%;
- voice on one out of three occasions: 33%;
- no response on one out of three occasions: 33%.

When monitoring a child's progress after implantation earlier sessions can be compared with later sessions, to see whether, for example, vocal turn taking is increasing.

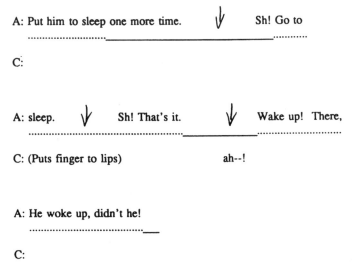

Figure 9.1. Transcript of conversational interaction, illustrating turn taking. Adult's and child's contributions are presented in parallel. Dotted and solid lines indicate eye contact (see text). Arrows mark the pauses left for the child's conversational turns.

Autonomy/initiative

We can also look at the amount of autonomy, or initiative, the child is showing in this situation. Is he simply repeating what the adult has said, and giving predictable responses to closed questions, or is he taking his turns in a manner that cannot be predicted from the adult's preceding turn, and showing progress towards more normal interaction? Examples of autonomy could include introducing new topics or information, contradicting the adult, joking, asking questions, and so on. The amount of autonomy he is able to exert will depend largely on the adult's conversational style; if she is very 'controlling', for example, asking a lot of closed questions, the child may not be able to show the autonomy of which he is capable.

The child's use of autonomy can be assessed by counting the number of turns in which he offers something that cannot be directly predicted from the adult's preceding remark, and then expressing that number as a percentage of the total number of turns. In this way we can see how much autonomy is being exercised vocally and how much gesturally. The child in Figure 9.1 does not show any autonomy. He takes part in the interaction that has been initiated by the adult but does not take control or change its course in any way. His percentage of autonomy is therefore 0%. Another child's use of autonomy is illustrated in Figure 9.2.

Here there are four turns, in three of which the child speaks, and in one of which she shakes her head. Therefore, calculating her turn-taking:

- she responds vocally on three out of four occasions: 75%;
- she responds gesturally on one out of four occasions: 25%.

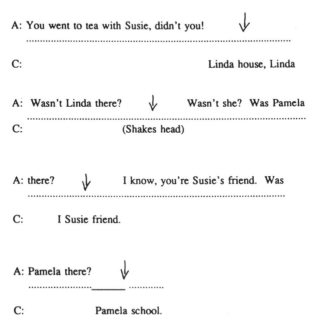

Figure 9.2. Transcript of conversational interaction, illustrating child autonomy (see text). Dotted and solid lines indicate eye contact (see text). Arrows mark the occasions when the child takes a conversational turn.

Her exercise of autonomy in the three vocal turns is as follows:

- in the first she introduces new information;
- in the second she insists on correcting what she sees as lack of understanding on the adult's part - she has gone to tea with Susie, not her sister;
- in the third she goes beyond the adult's closed question to give additional information.

Therefore, on each of these occasions she shows autonomy: 75%, expressed as a percentage of the total number of turns. Her gestural turn does not show autonomy, being a simple shake of the head. This child is exercising autonomy through the use of actual words, but autonomy can be observed in a child's vocal turns before he has reached the stage of being able to use words. He may, for example, vocalize forcefully (vocal autonomy), or touch the adult and point (gestural autonomy) to draw her attention to something.

Visual attention

The child's visual regard - the direction of his gaze and focus of his attention - can be shown on the transcript. This is a time-consuming activity, but very revealing. Instances that are very fleeting on the video film can be documented, affording more lengthy and detailed scrutiny. In our programme we do not now do this routinely for the whole transcript of every child. However, there may be children for whom it is desirable to document their visual attention in this way (for example, children with very complex needs) and the procedure is as follows:

The visual regard is added to the transcript as a dotted line just under the adult's words (or parts of words) for which the child is looking at her, and as a continuous line at a lower level under the words for which he is not looking (when he is looking at the object of discourse or elsewhere). At the latter points the focus of his attention is noted, in brackets. The total number of the adult's syllables is counted, then the number of syllables for which the child is looking at the adult. The latter ('looking' syllables) is expressed as a percentage of the former (total number of syllables).

This gives a broad measure, but the child's gaze can be examined in greater detail. For example, is he getting to be more likely to look away at the end of the adult's speaking turn instead of randomly during her turn? Are his glances towards the object of interest becoming more fleeting and his looks towards the adult becoming more sustained?

Answers to these questions are illustrated in Figure 9.1 (p. 308):

- A count of the adult's syllables gives a total of 23. The child is looking at her for 19 of these. Therefore his percentage of visual regard of the adult in this tiny excerpt is 83%.
- The focus of his attention is relevant. Each time he looks away from the adult he looks at the puppet, so that he is always either looking at the speaker or the object of interest.
- In this familiar situation he is becoming more likely to look away from the adult at the end of her speaking turn, rather than in the middle of it, and to return quickly after he has looked away. His looking at the adult is therefore well sustained.

Auditory processing

The occasions when it is necessary to show the visual regard on the transcript are to do with the observation of auditory processing. One of the clearest indications of auditory processing is that the child begins to take vocal turns when he has broken eye contact with the adult during her preceding turns. That is, he has looked away from her while she was speaking, and yet still comes in with a vocalization when she pauses to leave him a conversational turn. This suggests that he is beginning to register auditorily the points at which the adult stops speaking. Each vocal turn is therefore classified according to whether the child has, or has not, been in eye contact just before it – for the adult's last few words. These are the points where the child's visual regard needs to be plotted on the transcript. Then the percentage of 'non-looking' turns that have been filled vocally by the child is noted, and also the percentage of 'looking' turns that have been filled. If the child is not using auditory processing he is much more likely to fill the 'looking' than the 'non-looking' turns. As auditory processing develops he becomes progressively more likely to fill either sort of turn (Tait, 1986). Looking and non-looking turns are illustrated in Figure 9.3 (p. 312).

In the transcript shown in Figure 9.3 there are five turns taken vocally:

- The first is a non-looking turn. Although the child is looking at the adult when he actually says 'car', he has not been looking at her for her previous words.

- The second is also a non-looking turn, in the same way.
- The third is a looking turn, occurring simultaneously with the adult's.
- The fourth is another non-looking turn.
- The fifth is a looking turn, because he has been looking at the adult for the latter half of her preceding turn.

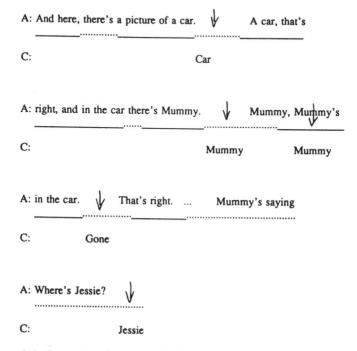

Figure 9.3. Transcript of conversational interaction, illustrating auditory processing, shown by the taking of non-looking vocal turns (see text).

Therefore his percentage of non-looking turns during this excerpt is 60%, and of looking turns 40%.

This child is beginning to use attempts at words, but the taking of non-looking vocal turns can be observed before actual words begin to emerge. Another noticeable indication of auditory processing is any repetition (unasked) of something the adult has said when the child was not looking at her. There are two examples of that in Figure 9.3 – the child attempts repetitions of 'car' and 'mummy', not having been in eye contact with the adult for either of these.

An early indication of the child's awareness of the sound of the adult's voice may be observed in his glancing up when the adult starts to speak or raises her voice, or uses an exaggerated intonation pattern, without any visual cue being given. An additional indication may be the development of intonation. In young deaf children who are acoustic hearing aid users, modulation of pitch in their voices is significantly related both to their hearing acuity and to their ability to identify words by listening alone (Tait, 1986). It is possible that in cochlear implantees, too, the development of varied and appropriate voice pitch may indicate efficient processing of sound.

Illustrative cases

The progress of three children, who by the time of implantation had very different communication skills, is outlined here to illustrate the method. The first, 'Brenda', already had good eye contact and some silent communication in signs. She might be described as being pre-verbal, but not 'pre-language'. The second, 'Martin', had very poor pre-verbal skills and little use of gesture. The third, 'Fiona', was congenitally deaf, with fairly good eye contact and some silent communication by gesture.

Brenda

Brenda was deafened at one year and two months, and thereafter 'total communication' was used with her by her parents and teacher (that is, spoken language supported by signing was used by the adults in contact with Brenda and she wore powerful hearing aids, which gave her awareness of sound at a vibrotactile level only). Brenda's understanding and use of signs was well established by the time of the implant operation, when she was aged two years and eight months. She used signs in one- or two- element combinations with considerable autonomy, and rarely vocalized. Figure 9.4 (p. 314) displays her vocal and gestural turn taking and autonomy over time.

Figure 9.4 shows how her use of vocalization (which six months after initial tuning consisted entirely of actual words) increased over time. Vocal autonomy started off more slowly but also increased materially over time. Conversely, turns taken by signing alone (without vocalization) decreased over the same period. By the second pre-implant session her visual regard was well established and structured, in that she was more likely to look away at the end of the adult's speaking turn than randomly during the turn. By the 12-month session (12 months after initial tuning), when conversing with her mother without any visual

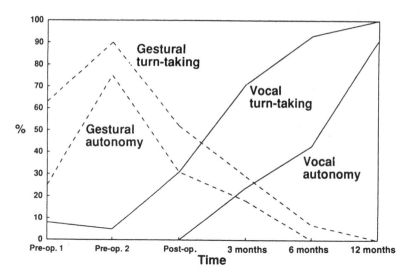

Figure 9.4. Measures of the first illustrative case: Brenda. Variations in percentages of vocal and signed turn taking and autonomy over the period from before implantation to 12 months after implantation.

aids to meaning, she maintained steady eye contact with her mother, and there were therefore few opportunities to observe auditory processing in non-looking turns. However, in a session filmed with her teacher on the same day, while looking at a book, her percentage of non-looking vocal turns was 76%. The two transcripts shown in Figures 9.5 and 9.6 demonstrate the changes in her communication. The first (Figure 9.5) is from the second pre-implant session. Brenda communicates by silent signing, shown in brackets, and the adult communicates in speech, signing the key words (signing not shown).

This extract from a longer transcript (five minutes) demonstrates Brenda's ability to communicate in signs, her willingness to take the lead in the interaction, and her facility in dividing her gaze between speaker and object of discourse. The percentages were as follows:

- Sign/gesture turn taking: 100% (percentage for complete session: 90%).
- Sign/gesture autonomy: 80% (percentage for complete session: 75%).
- Visual regard: 70% (percentage for complete session: 65%).

The second excerpt, shown in Figure 9.6, is from the session 12 months after initial tuning. The adult is now communicating

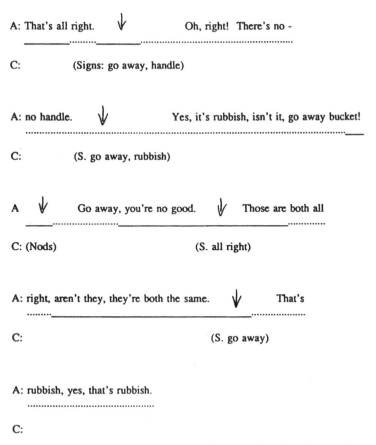

Figure 9.5. Transcript of excerpt from Brenda's second pre-implant session.

solely in speech. Brenda also signs most of the words she says
(signing not shown).

What is most noticeable here is the complete change-over, in
turn taking and autonomy, from silent signing to speech, with or
without the addition of signs. There was no great change in
visual regard, which was already well established, except that by
this 12-month stage she displayed the pattern of eye contact
normal to adult conversation – she looked at the person who
was talking to her, and looked away when she was speaking
herself. There was one indication of auditory processing: she
was not looking at her mother when the latter said 'Joan', but
repeated it. Percentages for turn taking, autonomy and visual
regard were as follows:

• Vocal turn taking: 100% (percentage for complete session:
100%).

- Vocal autonomy: 100% (percentage for complete session: 91%).
- Visual regard: 85% (percentage for complete session: 85%).

A: What about Joan and Kathy? ↓

C: Joan, Kathy. Long -- way--

A: It would be a long way, yes. ↓   Oh, too hard to walk.

C: Hard walk.

A: How would we get there? ↓   Long way to

C: Long way Kathy House.

A: Kathy's - oh, it's even further than that. ↓   Very

C: Hard (Signs: walk)

A: hard to walk, yes. How would we get on holidays? ↓

C: Better in

A: Better to go in the car, that's right, yes, I think so too.

C: car.

Figure 9.6. Transcript from Brenda's 12-month session. Arrows mark child's conversational turns, which are all taken by words, plus signing (not shown). Adult does not use sign.

During this 12-month period Brenda had received systematic tuning of the device and monthly rehabilitation sessions (fortnightly in the period immediately after the initial tuning sessions) where listening activities were pursued, leading to awareness and discrimination of speech features together with interactions fostering the development of vocal communication. There was at all times close liaison between the staff responsible for the tuning of the device and the implant centre teacher of the deaf and speech and language therapist, who also worked closely with the parents and local professionals.

Martin

Martin was deafened at two years eight months, and an oral approach was used by his parents and teachers, well supplemented by natural gestures and facial expression. He had lost all his understanding and use of spoken language, and seemed to have equal difficulty making sense of gesture. His visual regard and turn taking were at a very low level and there were only very moderate increases over a pre-operative period of six months. He was implanted at the age of three years five months.

Figure 9.7 displays his vocal and gestural turn taking and autonomy, over time. This shows his development of pre-verbal and early verbal skills over the 12-month period after initial tuning. His visual regard increased over the first six months, as pre-verbal skills became established, and then decreased as Martin gradually began to rely less on visual contact where his own turn taking was concerned. This was also shown by a rise over time in non-looking turns, the percentages for the post-switch-on, three-month, six-month and 12-month sessions being

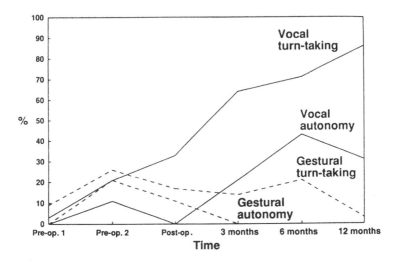

Figure 9.7. Measures of the second illustrative case: Martin. The variation in percentages of vocal and gestural turn taking and autonomy over the period from before implantation to 12 months after implantation.

33%, 56%, 50%, and 73% respectively. Vocal turn taking increased steadily over the whole period, while turn taking by gesture tailed off.

Two transcripts demonstrate the changes in his pre-verbal skills and early verbal communication. Both complete transcripts were five minutes in length. The first excerpt is from the second pre-implant session, and is shown in Figure 9.8.

A: Put them in. Like that. There, here's two more. ↓

C: (gestures:can't do it)

A: It won't go in, it won't go in, put it in that one. There

C:

A: now you can say bye-bye to them. Bye-bye. ↓ Bye-bye. ↓

C:

Figure 9.8. Transcript of excerpt from Martin's second pre-implant session.

Martin was engaged in the interaction to the extent that he was looking at the object of discourse, but his visual regard of the adult was at a low level. His turn taking was also at a low level, and entirely by gesture except on the two occasions (not shown) when reluctant voice was coaxed from him by offering the microphone. What autonomy there was also came via gesture. Percentages for turn taking, autonomy and visual regard were as follows:

- Gesture turn taking: 33% (percentage for complete session: 26%).
- Gesture autonomy: 33% (percentage for complete session: 21%).
- Visual regard: 17% (percentage for complete session: 18%).

The second excerpt is from the session 12 months after initial tuning, and is shown in Figure 9.9.

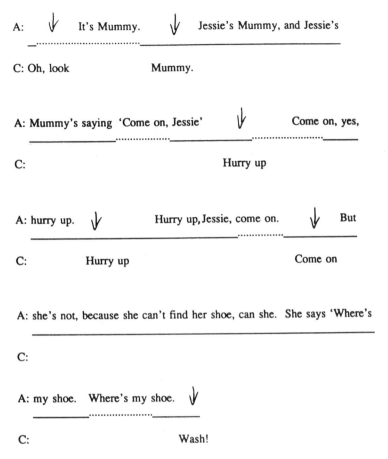

Figure 9.9. Transcript of excerpt from Martin's 12-month session. Arrows mark child's conversational turns, all of which are taken by words, without gesture.

Having acquired the pre-verbal visual regard skills, Martin showed at the 12-month stage that he was able to come in with his own vocal turn whether or not he had been looking at the adult for her turn, and to be capable of adding something new to the conversation. Percentages for turn taking, autonomy, visual regard and non-looking turns were as follows:

- Vocal turn taking: 100% (percentage for complete session: 86%).
- Vocal autonomy: 50% (percentage for complete session: 31%).
- Visual regard: 20% (percentage for complete session: 34%).
- Non-looking turns: 67% (percentage for complete session: 73%).

As was the case with Brenda (and with all the children implanted at Nottingham) Martin had received regular tuning of the device during this 12-month period. He had already been monitored by video analysis for six months prior to implantation, during which period development of pre-verbal skills was extremely slow. His progress after initial tuning was material, with steady increase in the pre-verbal skills which were necessary for his development of speech.

Fiona

Fiona was born profoundly deaf. Diagnosis and provision of hearing aids took place when she was eight months old, but she derived little benefit from amplified sound, her awareness being only at a vibro-tactile level. At the time of the implant operation she was aged four years and five months. An oral approach had been used by parents and teachers, but Fiona communicated mainly by silent gestures plus occasional vocalizations. Figure 9.10 displays her vocal and gestural turn taking and autonomy, over time.

Figure 9.10 shows how Fiona's use of vocalization, which by six months consisted almost entirely of actual words, increased over time. Her use of vocal autonomy shows a comparable increase. Conversely, gestural turn taking and autonomy

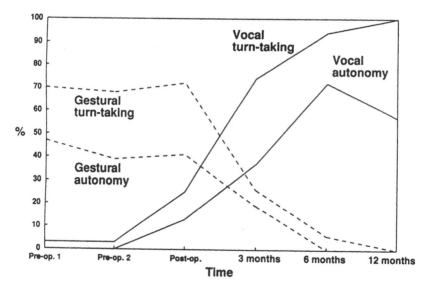

Figure 9.10. Measures of third illustrative case: Fiona. Variations in percentages of vocal and signed turn taking and autonomy over the period from before implantation to 12 months after implantation.

decrease over time. Her eye contact, 18% at the first pre-implant session, increases steadily over time, to 63% at 12 months. Non-looking turns go from 0% before implant to 50% after implant, and remain around that level. The two transcripts shown in Figures 9.11 and 9.12 demonstrate the changes in her communication. The first, from the second pre-implant session, shows Fiona communicating by silent gesture.

This excerpt from a longer session demonstrates Fiona's willingness to communicate by gesture and her readiness to take the lead in the interaction. The percentages were as follows:

- Gestural turn taking: 80% (percentage for complete session: 68%).
- Gestural autonomy: 60% (percentage for complete session: 39%).
- Visual regard: 27% (percentage for complete session: 31%).

The second excerpt, shown in Figure 9.12, is from the session 12 months after initial tuning.

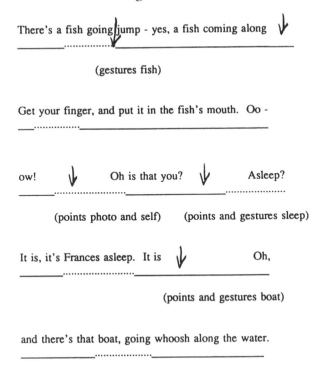

Figure 9.11. Transcript of excerpt from Fiona's second pre-implant session. Arrows mark the child's conversational turns, which are all taken by silent gesture, shown in brackets.

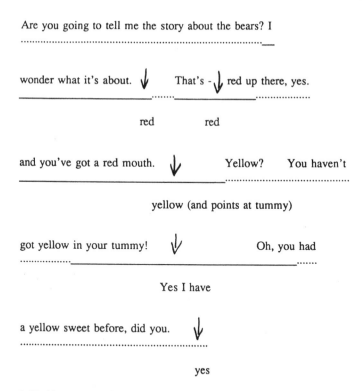

Figure 9.12. Transcript of excerpt from Fiona's 12 month session. Arrows mark child's conversational turns, which are all taken by words.

As with Brenda, what is most noticeable is the complete changeover from silent gesture to speech, both in turn taking and use of autonomy. Four of her five turns are non-looking, showing the development of auditory processing. Her percentages for vocal turn taking, vocal autonomy and visual regard are as follows:

- Vocal turn taking: 100% (percentage for complete session: 100%).
- Vocal autonomy: 80% (percentage for complete session: 57%).
- Visual regard: 62% (percentage for complete session: 63%).

Fiona was the first of the congenitally deaf children to be implanted at Nottingham. At four years and five months she was one of the older of the pre-verbal children, and, of course, had never had auditory stimulation. It is interesting that her progress is comparable with that of Brenda, who heard until she was one year and two months, and who was implanted at two years and eight months. Osberger and colleagues (1991b) reported that there was no obvious difference in speech perception abilities between children with implants who were born deaf and those who had hearing for one to three years before onset of deafness. Our results with born deaf children implanted in Nottingham have also shown the ability of cochlear implants to provide significant auditory receptive skills to young congenitally deaf children (O'Donoghue et al., 1998).

Research findings

Our work with video analysis in the Nottingham programme has given rise to research in several areas: comparison of early communicative behaviour in young children with cochlear implants and with hearing aids; the predictive value of post-implant and pre-implant video analysis measures of pre-verbal behaviours on later outcomes from cochlear implantees; and a repeatability study of the analysis methods. The findings are summarized below:

- Comparison of early communication behaviour in young children with cochlear implants and with hearing aids (Tait and Lutman, 1994). In a repeated measures design video analysis techniques were used to follow the development of emerging communication skills in nine children with multi-channel cochlear implants, and also in two groups of nine severely or profoundly deaf children who wore hearing aids, one group having better hearing and making more efficient use of their aids. The implanted children were found to develop an auditory/vocal style similar to but in advance of that of the efficient hearing aid users, during their first year with an implant. The video method was able to distinguish clearly between the three groups and was shown to be sensitive to differences within children over time, and between children.
- The predictive value of measures of pre-verbal communicative behaviours in young children with cochlear implants (Tait and Lutman, 1997). A longitudinal study of young children with cochlear implants showed that the extent of auditory/vocal pre-linguistic behaviour, measured 12 months after implantation, predicted their ability to perform accurately on speech perception tasks, measured three years after

implantation. Auditory/vocal behaviour at 12 months was assessed by constructing a composite measure, adding together vocal turn-taking, vocal autonomy and non-looking vocal turns, and subtracting gestural (silent) turn taking and gestural autonomy. This composite measure correlated highly with three-year outcome speech perception measures.

- Pre-implant measures of pre-verbal communicative behaviour as predictors of outcomes in children with cochlear implants (Tait, Lutman and Robinson, 2000). This work set out to examine whether post-implant measures of speech perception in young children with cochlear implants could be predicted from pre-verbal communication measures obtained before implantation. The results showed that up to a fourth of the variance in speech identification performance three years after cochlear implantation could be predicted from characteristics that were inherent to the child before implantation; in particular by the demonstration of autonomy in pre-verbal communicative interactions, whether by vocalization or by gesture.

- Pre-implant predictors of benefit in young children (Tait and Nikolopoulos, 1999). A study up-dating the results of the previous paper provided strong evidence that pre-verbal children whose pre-implant communication showed autonomy were likely to have better speech perception and speech intelligibility outcomes three, four and five years following implantation.

- Assessment of pre-verbal communication behaviours from video analysis: consistency amongst observers (Tait et al., 2001). Three observers analysed twelve video samples independently, according to the established protocol. There was a very high level of accord amongst observers, all correlations between scores being statistically significant.

Conclusions

Progress towards understanding and use of spoken language, through audition, cannot be predicted before implantation, and it is vital to monitor indications of development as they occur. It is, therefore, important to transcribe the videos within a short time of making the recordings. The measures used – vocal turn taking, vocal autonomy and non-looking vocal turns in particular – are sensitive indicators of use of the processor. We have found that percentages in these measures have fallen sharply if for any reason there has not been consistent use of the processor.

Even with consistent use, progress measured in understanding and use of actual words can be very slow where young pre-verbal children are concerned. The techniques of video analysis make it possible to observe minute changes over time in turn taking and auditory processing. The analysis provides objective evidence, before children are able to undertake formal speech and language evaluations, whether there is progress in the pre-verbal skills, which are the prerequisite of spoken language.

References

Baldwin DA, Markman EM (1989) Establishing word-object relations; a first step. Child Development 60: 381–98.

Barnes S, Gutfreund M, Satterly D, Wells G (1983) Characteristics of adult speech which predict children's language development. Journal of Child Language 10: 65–84.

Brazelton TB (1982) Joint regulation of neonate-parent behaviour. In Tronick EZ (ed.) Social Interchange in Infancy. Affect, Cognition and Communication. Baltimore, MD: University Park Press.

Bruner JS (1983) Child's Talk: Learning to Use Language. Oxford: Oxford University Press.

Collis GM (1977) Visual co-orientation in maternal speech. In Schaffer HR (ed.) Studies in Mother-Infant Interaction. London: Academic Press.

Cooper R, Aslin R (1989) The language environment of the young infant: implications for early perceptual development. Canadian Journal of Pyschology 43: 247–65.

Crystal D (1997) The Cambridge Encyclopaedia of the English Language. 2 edn. Cambridge: Cambridge University Press.

Harris M (2000) Social interaction and early language development in deaf children. Deafness and Education International 2(1): 1–11.

Harris M, Jones D, Brookes S, Grant J (1986) Relations between the non-verbal context of maternal speech and rate of language development. British Journal of Developmental Psychology 4: 261–8.

Miyamoto RT, Osberger MJ, Robbins MS, Myers WA, Kessler K, Pope ML (1992) Longitudinal evaluation of communication skills of children with single- or multi-channel cochlear implants. American Journal of Otology 13(3): 215–22.

O'Donoghue GM, Nikolopoulos T, Archbold SM, Tait M (1998) Congenitally deaf children following cochlear implantation. Acta Oto-rhino-laryngologica Belgica 52: 111–14.

Osberger MJ, Miyamoto RT, Zimmerman-Phillips MS, Kemink JL, Stroer BS, Firszt JB, Novak MA (1991a) Independent evaluation of the speech perception abilities of children with the Nucleus 22-channel cochlear implant system. Ear and Hearing 12(4), supplement.

Osberger MJ, Todd SL, Berry SW, Robbins AM, Miyamoto, RT (1991b) Effect of age at onset of deafness on children's speech perception abilities with a cochlear implant. Annals of Otology, Rhinology and Laryngology 100: 883–8.

Tait DM (1986) Using singing to facilitate linguistic development in hearing impaired pre-schoolers. Journal of the British Association of Teachers of the Deaf 10(4): 103–8.

Tait DM (1987) Making and monitoring progress in the pre-school years. Journal of British Association of Teachers of the Deaf 11(5): 143–53.

Tait DM (1993) Video analysis: a method of assessing changes in preverbal and early linguistic communication after cochlear implantation. Ear and Hearing 14(6): 378–89.

Tait DM, Lutman ME (1994) Comparison of early communicative behavior in young children with cochlear implants and with hearing aids. Ear and Hearing 15(5): 352–61.

Tait DM, Lutman ME (1997) The predictive value of measures of preverbal communicative behaviours in young deaf children with cochlear implants. Ear and Hearing 18(6): 472–8.

Tait DM, Lutman ME, Robinson K (2000) Pre-implant measures of preverbal communicative behavior as predictors of cochlear implant outcomes in children. Ear and Hearing 21(1): 18–24.

Tait DM, Nikolopoulos TP (1999) Pre-implant predictors of benefit in young children. Paper presented at British Cochlear Implant Group meeting, York, April.

Tait DM, Nikolopoulos TP, Lutman ME, Wilson D, Wells P (2001) Video analysis of preverbal communication behaviours: use and reliability. Deafness and Education International 3(1): 38–43.

Tait DM, Wood DJ (1987) From communication to speech in deaf children. In Crystal D (ed.) Child Language Teaching and Therapy 3(1): 1–16.

Werker J, McLeod P (1989) Infant preference for both male and female infant-directed talk: a developmental study of attentional and affective responsiveness. Canadian Journal of Psychology 43: 230–46.

Wood DJ, Wood H, Griffiths AJ, Howarth I (1986) Teaching and Talking with Deaf Children. Chichester: John Wiley & Sons.

Zinober B, Martlew M (1985) The development of communicative gestures. In Barrett MD (ed.) Children's Single Word Speech. Chichester: John Wiley & Sons, pp. 183–215.

Chapter 10

Monitoring progress: the role and remit of a speech and language therapist

Dee Dyar, Thomas P Nikolopoulos

This chapter will consider the following aspects involved in monitoring progress:

- the principles of effective casework and liaison with a range of professionals;
- measurement issues relating to the establishment of baseline linguistic assessment outcomes; and
- the classification of deaf children's linguistic competence before and after implantation.

It will also provide an overview of a computer-based speech and language therapy assessment and outcomes protocol that has been devised as part of an interdisciplinary clinical database. Examples of current global measures of communication benefit after cochlear implantation will be given. Finally, we will consider some identified gaps in current practice and how implant programme based speech and language therapists are considering innovative and more time-effective ways of working collaboratively with implanted children's families and local support professionals.

As authors, our considerations are based on findings reported in the literature and international paediatric cochlear implantation conference proceedings as well as insights gained in actual practice as members of the Nottingham Paediatric Cochlear Implant Programme. The philosophy of this implant programme is to provide a seamless management regime. This implies a flexible and stress-free programme of care for the child, family and local support professionals.

In the case of young implanted deaf children the purposes of monitoring progress by the implant team speech and language therapist (SLT) are the following:

- To *assess* and *describe* the individual child's current communication skills and ongoing needs before cochlear implantation.
- To *document* an individual child's progress in communication skills over several years after implantation and to provide progress updates on all children within the implant programme at specified assessment intervals.
- To *investigate* the possibility of unforeseen non-sensory difficulties in the case of deaf children who present as 'under functioning' cochlear implant users.
- To *observe* the child in a range of everyday settings as well as in performance-based tasks, to guarantee the representative nature of assessment findings.
- To *share* information and appropriate advice on strategies to develop the child's communication skills, with his or her family and a range of local professionals, and by doing so, to complement the work of the implant team teachers of the deaf in particular.
- To *contribute* to interdisciplinary team audit and monitoring procedures by providing information to the implant programme co-ordinator on SLT assessment and intervention outcomes.

In addition to these identified priorities an SLT may be requested to contribute to implant-programme initiated research studies on focused groups of cochlear implant users, for example, extremely young candidates or pre-verbal or low-verbal deaf children. This may require the use of descriptive techniques such as video time sampling and criterion-referenced approaches as a precursor to norm-referenced or standardized linguistic performance measures.

Along with the audiological scientist and the teacher of the deaf, a team SLT may be called upon to identify factors that appear to have a high correlation with successful use and the linguistic benefits gained by deaf children fitted with cochlear implants. For this reason it is important that systematic and, ideally, validated measurements of language, voice and speech production skills are used even in the case of extremely young deaf children.

Most implant-programme based SLTs share a commitment to more uniform data collection across different spoken languages and cultures and are willing to learn more about computer-based data collection and analysis techniques in order to facilitate the exchange of information at an international level.

Ways of working

The development of a paediatric cochlear implant programme has already been described (Chapter 3). The recommended frequency of contact, and the nature of a speech and language therapy support programme provided for families and the deaf child's support professionals should be explicit and convey a sense of good interdisciplinary collaboration between all members of the paediatric cochlear implant programme.

In Nottingham the outreach service involves both an implant programme teacher of the deaf and an assigned SLT for each deaf child accepted for cochlear implantation. The outreach role includes sharing information, advice, reassurance and support with parents and a range of local professionals as well as working directly with a deaf child before and after cochlear implantation.

The purposes of monitoring the progress of the deaf child after cochlear implantation will vary depending on the professional background and perspective of individual team members – medical, scientist, educator or therapist. For this reason it is important that a paediatric cochlear implant programme adopts a genuinely 'interdisciplinary' rather than a multidisciplinary management approach. An interdisciplinary management approach implies a child-sensitive way of working with planned opportunities to share insights and concerns with implant programme colleagues as well as with the child's family and the professionals involved. A multidisciplinary approach, on the other hand, may simply mean a large number of professionals working in parallel. It frequently results from split-site locations of work as this affects the opportunity to liaise routinely on a daily or weekly basis in a cross-disciplinary manner. Working in parallel may seem to be an effective way of working within a discipline – but it can be stressful for the deaf child's family for two reasons. Firstly, the parent has to act as a go between, sharing assessment outcomes with a number of different professionals. Secondly, parents may choose to use the implant team advice selectively in the absence of team collaboration. For these reasons, it seems important to stress the rewards of peer support and enhanced perspective that result from regular cross-disciplinary team meetings and established feedback systems. As part of demonstrating effectiveness, an implant programme co-ordinator relies increasingly on the ability of all team members to maintain a sense of professional autonomy while also working flexibly within the context of an interdisciplinary team.

Deafness affects everyone in the family. An outreach professional must always keep in mind the notion of a family as a system in which all parts are intimately and inextricably linked (Luterman, 1987). It is important that the implant programme SLT establishes a confident rapport and also an 'active' working relationship with the deaf child's family and local professionals from the start. Implant programme outreach professionals must guard against situations that force them to work in a highly didactic manner or to be perceived as an 'expert' rather than a 'specialist resource person'.

During the 1980s and 1990s traditional SLT practice in the UK usually meant that deaf children received speech and language therapy in a clinic or a school setting. The emphasis in traditional therapy tended to be placed on high levels of direct contact with the child and an SLT driven programme of rehabilitation or intervention. In a traditional SLT approach opportunities for feedback among professionals, joint planning and rehabilitation sessions were affected by the constraints of the clinic schedule or school timetable and dependent on the goodwill or flexibility of the professionals involved with the child.

An outreach programme such as that provided by a number of paediatric cochlear programmes throughout the UK may be considered a non-traditional way of working. To be effective it requires flexible time management, comprehensive record keeping and an aptitude for forward planning by the outreach professional. In an outreach model, SLT direct contact sessions with the implanted child may be two to three months apart, rather than on a traditional weekly or monthly basis. The SLT, however, may choose to work with the child at home, school or in another context as appropriate. There is generally more opportunity for siblings and grandparents as well as parents to observe sessions or participate in rehabilitation activities.

Implant programme SLTs build upon a personal style of

working. Ideally they should perceive parents and local professionals as 'active' partners and co-workers, so that requisite assessments can be completed and communication skills objectives planned and implemented jointly. To paraphrase Luterman (1987), an outreach professional must be empathetic to the time lag involved before families adjust to the new reality of a deaf child with a cochlear implant. Outreach professionals, both therapists and teachers, need to acknowledge and build on a range of diverse coping strategies used by different families. This extract from a recorded interview with the mother of a profoundly deaf child provides a thought-provoking perspective on home-based speech and language therapy provision for her child:

> *Live discussion* at the time problems and difficulties arise is by far the best.
>
> *Joint sessions* because they give me a great deal of hope, because you can see the improvement. You've always stressed the things he *can* do rather than the things he can't . . . It's nice to see them at a time when you say 'Right, that is not happening yet, but we can do this and this to make it happen.' So it almost doesn't matter that I am seeing things he can't do because at the same time I am getting ideas and hope that they will happen. I like to have the *written report* but given that I have the other two opportunities, I could do without them.

As professionals, perhaps it is time to consider the amount of time spent on report writing rather than live discussions, joint sessions and the provision of more skills-based training opportunities for parents.

Assessment phase

In response to changes in the international selection criteria in the mid-1990s and subsequently significant agreed changes to the audiology criteria, described in Chapter 4, the Nottingham programme established a joint disciplinary assessment as part of the selection phase process. A joint session with a teacher of the deaf (usually the programme co-ordinator) and a speech and language therapist is now scheduled routinely after the initial audiological appointment. The purpose of this assessment session is to identify and describe the prospective cochlear implant candidate's current interaction and communication skills and ongoing linguistic needs. A written summary is made after this assessment with the aim of assisting the implant programme co-ordinator to identify casework issues and priorities that need to be addressed further – before a decision to proceed with cochlear implantation can be confirmed. It also provides written documentation for other members of the team, for example, surgeon or psychologist, when they see the child. In the case of some complex cochlear implant candidates an SLT who has been involved in the initial communication assessment may also be present at the hospital appointment with the surgeon and programme co-ordinator, when parents give consent to proceed with cochlear implantation for their child. Experience in Nottingham suggests that a joint clinic model of service delivery confirms the interdisciplinary nature of support that will be offered during the surgery phase and after implantation and it therefore provides reassurance for prospective families in the earliest stages of making a decision on behalf of their child. If a decision is reached not to proceed with surgery, the programme co-ordinator may involve an SLT along with other professionals in the provision of support for the family. At this time parents and families need time to discuss the contraindications and reasons why cochlear implantation may not be a feasible option for their deaf child on more than one occasion. Ideally, they should also have an opportunity to discuss alternative ways of enhancing their child's communication skills in the future.

Candidature for implantation in young children depends on a number of factors in addition to degree of hearing loss; these include medical and developmental conditions, the deaf child's linguistic background and educational environment. Other factors include parental attitudes and styles of communication and the amount and nature of locally available support. In order to investigate these factors from an interdisciplinary perspective, the Children's Implant Profile (ChIP) (Nevins and Chute, 1996) is used, routinely, as part of the Nottingham programme clinical database, as described in Chapter 3.

The ChIP profile consists of 12 factors that are likely to affect a deaf child's ability to use a cochlear implant (Table 10.1). These include demographic details of the children:

- chronological age;
- duration of deafness;
- medical and radiological conditions;
- audiological assessment outcomes;
- language and speech abilities;
- multiple handicaps or disabilities;

- family structure and support;
- educational environment;
- the availability of support services;
- expectations of the family and deaf child;
- cognitive abilities;
- learning style.

Table 10.1. Children's Implant Profile (ChIP) factors

FACTS LEVEL	F1	Chronological age
	F2	Duration of deafness
INVESTIGATIONS LEVEL	F3	Medical/radiological issues
	F4	Audiological assessment outcome
	F5	Language and speech abilities
	F6	Multiple handicap/disabilities
EXTRINSIC LEVEL	F7	Family structure and support
	F8	Educational environment
	F9	Availability of support services
	F10	Expectations of family/child
INTRINSIC LEVEL	F11	Cognitive ability
	F12	Learning style

In a clinical audit of the first 200 children selected for cochlear implantation by the Nottingham Programme (Nikolopoulos, Dyar and Gibbin, accepted) the ChIP profile was used with the results shown in Figure 10.1.

Chronological age at the time of assessment (before implantation) was the most common factor of great concern (9% of the children studied) and the pre-implant language and speech abilities of the children was the most common factor of mild to moderate

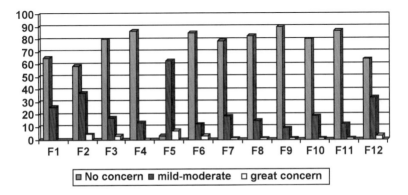

Figure 10.1. Children's Implant Profile: Distribution of the first 200 implanted children according to the ChIP factors. Percentage scores for each factor by no concern, mild/moderate concern, great concern.

concern, affecting 63% of the children. The second most common factor of mild to moderate concern was duration of deafness (37%) and the third was the learning style of the children (33%). Availability of support services was the least factor of concern as 179 children (90%) did not have any problems in this area.

Current candidature trends suggest that two increasing groups of appropriate referrals – extremely young profoundly deaf children and school-aged deaf children with some useful pre-operative hearing, will reduce the incidence of major concern under ChIP factor 1 (chronological age) and concerns under ChIP factor 5 (language and speech abilities) in the future. Further studies are needed into the effects of cognitive ability (Pisoni, 2000).

Once a deaf child has been selected for a cochlear implant, the implant programme SLT may receive a live, telephone or written enquiry for help from the child's local SLT. Not all of the deaf children selected for cochlear implantation receive speech and language therapy at the local level. At the time of writing approximately 70% of the implanted children in the Nottingham programme have access to a local SLT. The percentage of children under the care of a local SLT may change yet again in the future as more school-aged deaf children with some pre-operative hearing are considered to be suitable candidates for cochlear implantation. An implant programme SLT is assigned to all children during the selection phase in Nottingham in order to provide support and guidance to the deaf child's family and local professionals as appropriate, in conjunction with an implant programme teacher of the deaf.

An informal review of the most commonly occurring local SLT enquiries received since 1989, suggests that concerns and queries can be broadly centred in three areas:

- How much and what form of training should a child have before s/he receives a cochlear implant?
- What is the philosophy of the Nottingham Programme in relation to families and local educational services who use a sign bilingual approach?
- How will the assigned implant programme SLT interface with the deaf child's local SLT and other support professionals?

Guidance and information should be given on the frequency and purposes of an SLT outreach visit and the opportunities to work collaboratively before and after the child has a cochlear implant.

Cochlear implantation has now become a comparatively routine option for profoundly deaf children. Such local SLT enquiries therefore appear to reflect commitment and initiative rather than the high anxiety associated with enquiries handled by outreach professionals during the early 1990s when paediatric cochlear implantation was considered a radical alternative to acoustic hearing aids. As more SLTs become interested in working with deaf children with cochlear implants, it is gratifying to report improvements in speech and language therapy undergraduate training as well as continuing professional development opportunities at the post-qualification level.

The purposes of an SLT when working at in local contexts at home or at a deaf child's school can be summarized as follows:

- To document current progress and to identify the child's ongoing communication needs in everyday settings.
- To ensure that appropriate and realistic rehabilitation aims and objectives are being set for recently implanted deaf children.
- To promote a collaborative or joint management approach between implant programme and local support professionals in the baseline assessment of a deaf child's communication skills and subsequent linguistic changes observed during the first few years after cochlear implantation.
- To influence the attitudes of local agencies towards the potential benefits of a cochlear implant by sharing up-to-date information on evidence-based outcomes and candidacy trends reported in the international research literature.
- To provide reassurance and share rehabilitation techniques and strategies with a child's family and primary caregivers.

An SLT outreach visit may include a request for an in-service training presentation. The primary purposes of an implant programme therapist or teacher of the deaf when responding to such requests are to demystify the mythology of cochlear implants and deaf children as described by Laurenzi (1993), and to promote robust expectations and effective classroom management of the implanted child. Experience suggests that, with direction, deaf or hearing classmates, like siblings, can be wonderful allies in effecting changes in an implanted deaf child's everyday communication style and linguistic attainments if they are encouraged to be so.

At all times, an outreach SLT should encourage contributions from the child's local speech and language therapist or teacher of the deaf, for example, sharing representative video samples of the child's spontaneous communication, planning or co-writing progress reports. As part of establishing an effective local and long-term support regime, an implant programme SLT may need to challenge or modify the short-term rehabilitation goals of the child's local support professionals. This usually occurs when the expectations of the child's family or local professionals are too ambitious as a result of understandable enthusiasm in the early months after implantation. Perhaps more surprisingly, therefore, it has also been found necessary to increase expectations in some cases of school-aged profoundly deaf children who have been fitted with cochlear implants when support professionals appear excessively cautious, pessimistic or over-reliant on their know-ledge of the child's capabilities before implantation. An implant programme SLT has a unique opportunity to work with deaf chil-dren across a wide chronological age group and also a wide range of linguistic and learning abilities. That said, however, it is import-ant to view each implanted child through the eyes of the family's local support professionals, as these professionals may have been supporting the child's family and working regularly with the deaf child from the time a diagnosis of deafness is made.

Deskilling of local professionals can occur unintentionally if an implant programme SLT projects an image of unattainable expertise when working with the child at the implant centre or on an outreach visit to the child's home or school. Once an initial casework rapport and working relationship has been established, it is important that the outreach SLT facilitates improvement in the child's overall language and speech skills, by demonstrating what the child can do, for example, when speech reading without sign support in closed-set tasks, and later using an implant without lipreading – as well as describing the child's ongoing communication needs.

An *active* local management regime results from a collabora-tive perspective and the sharing of information communication objectives and outcomes in an *accessible* way. For example:

- Using the child's parent or local teacher/therapist as the adult interactor in video samples.
- Enhancing the perspective of a local SLT by sharing video extracts of implanted children at the same or a 'soon-to-be achieved-stage' of linguistic competence of the child under discussion. Composite video extracts of the same deaf child

at different stages of spoken language attainment have been found to provide a great deal of reassurance and aspiration for parents and less experienced support professionals.

- Providing a written summary of SLT visit/session outcomes immediately. Ideally this summary includes some positive feedback on the local management of the child's communication needs as well as information on ideas and strategies for implementing further appropriate rehabilitation goals.
- Organizing timetabled discussion time to share insights and feelings as well as formal assessment findings with the child's local support professionals – to ascertain whether the SLT session outcomes are typical of the implanted child's current spontaneous communication skills or to talk through difficult or amorphous one-to-one sessions outcomes – especially in the case of implanted children with complex linguistic or learning difficulties.
- Written recommendations must be concise and both developmentally and linguistically appropriate for the child. They must also be measurable and time effective.
- Deaf children's local teachers and SLTs are frequently encouraged to try out the recommended activities and strategies with non-implanted children.

The amount and nature of support required by the deaf child's family and local support professionals may vary, in several ways, from the support required by a adult who has chosen to have a cochlear implant. Informal evaluation of SLT practice in Nottingham reveals a 60:40 weighting of direct and indirect contact with each child's family during the first year after implantation. By the third year, however, this weighting has been reversed to 40:60 direct and indirect contact with a gradual reduction in reliance on the visiting SLT as children demonstrate their ability to learn spoken language more 'independently'. This usually coincides with the establishment of a collaborative and effective management regime between the implant programme outreach professionals and the child's local support professionals. In the future, it seems likely that the nature of outreach support programmes will continue to change as more deaf children are fitted with cochlear implants in the pre-school years and an increasing number of support professionals request training opportunities and workshops that enable them to share information and ideas on their own ways of working with implanted children.

Measurement issues

The Nottingham Programme SLT assessment and outcomes protocol is a component of a specifically designed multi-professional clinical database (IMPEVAL, 1993; BCS Clinical Database, 1999). The following factors have been identified as most likely to influence the implant team professional's choice of assessment when investigating a deaf child's communication skills before and after cochlear implantation:

- The *appropriateness* of a language or speech assessment measure in relation to the child's age and interest level.
- The *language level* required to attempt or complete an assessment with reliability.
- The *time effectiveness* of the selected assessment, not only in terms of test administration and concentration required by the child, but also the time required to analyse, interpret the data and to complete clinical database entries for ongoing implant programme audit and research initiatives.
- Selected assessment procedures should be *repeatable* and allow *comparisons* to be made – within a particular child and across children over time and with other standardized linguistic measures.
- A high level of *inter-user reliability* is desirable and this should be monitored when newly appointed professionals start to use an established language and speech assessment protocol. Any adaptations made to an assessment measure should be explicit and used consistently by all users of the implant programme assessment protocol.
- Ideally the assessment and outcome measures used by different professionals in a paediatric cochlear implant programme should complement rather than duplicate findings at *auditory, cognitive,* and *neurolinguistic* levels.

Making an initial communication skills assessment

Ruben (1992) points out that measures of language need to take into account the syntax, prosody and age appropriateness of the child's language and also reflect the communication style or 'child-directed speech' used by his or her primary caregivers. Tyler and Fryauf-Bertschy in Tye-Murray (1992) outline three useful categories for describing a deaf child's communication style: *passive, interesting* and *demanding*. These authors state that many variations of each style exist and the same child may exhibit different styles at various times.

Wanner and Gleitman (1989) refer to the writings of Bloomfield (1933) and Chomsky (1965) and describe two crucial facts about the human use of language – it is both rule governed and creative. Increasingly, parents are requesting information on deaf children's performance on standardized or age-equivalent language and speech measures. During the first 12 months or so after implantation the use of language assessment techniques designed for children or adults with established language skills before the onset of deafness may be inappropriate for a profoundly deaf child who is functioning at a 'pre-verbal' stage of spoken language acquisition. It is no longer a widely held view that language development is completed between the ages of 18 months and five years. In hearing infants the production of recognizable words is expected around 12 months of age. However, developmental phonology studies on hearing infants (Vihman, 1996) suggest that although the foundations for learning an ambient language are laid down during the first year of life the process goes on much longer than the pre-school years. In the case of hearing children, for example, speech development is not always completed between five and seven years of age. Referring to the persistent theme in the language development literature of a critical period, Robinson in Gregory et al. (1998) defines the biological considerations and parameters of such a critical period as occurring between two years and the onset of puberty. He continues by stating that physiologists today write about 'sensitive' rather than critical periods as there is recent evidence to suggest that the adult brain continues to adapt and reorganize. Likewise Haynes in Mogford and Sadler (1989) argues that overall language acquisition continues until at least adolescence. Haynes stresses the need to acknowledge that language develops in different children at different rates and this is linked to a child's rate of development in non-linguistic areas. She cites five interrelated areas of development: *cognitive, perceptual, motor, social* and *linguistic*. Any deficiencies in one or more of these domains may impact on the child's development of linguistic competence.

Lund and Duchan (1993) outline the purposes of language and speech assessment. The professional needs to establish:

- Whether a language problem exists.
- What is causing the problem?
- What are the areas of deficit?
- What are the regularities in the child's language performance?
- What is recommended after assessment for the individual child?

A comprehensive baseline assessment of communication before cochlear implantation should include a video-recorded sample of the child's spontaneous communication and interaction skills and not just 'performance-based' measures of language and speech. According to Dowell in Clark, Cowan and Dowell (1997), video-taped samples of conversation can be useful in the evaluation of speech production, language and pragmatics as they allow repeated viewing of the interaction for analysis purposes and provide a more representative picture of communication than formal testing. McConkey Robbins in Niparko et al. (2000) states that the potential for incidental language learning is perhaps the most compelling hypothesis to explain language enhancement from cochlear implants (see also Chapter 8).

In the case of some school-aged cochlear implant candidates, criterion or norm-referenced linguistic measures may continue to be required as not all school-aged cochlear implant candidates can complete standardized or norm-referenced tests with reliability. Implant programme SLTs need to be aware that some school-aged deaf children may be functioning at the pre-verbal or 'low verbal' stage of spoken language development, and the appropriateness of relative ranking scores such as percentile scores, age-equivalent or standard scores, may appear to provide limited information before implantation. However age-appropriate language and speech protocol measures must be administered routinely on all selected candidates in order to ensure that changes in both implant candidacy trends and technological advances in device and programming strategies can be monitored effectively.

An SLT may need to consider *who* needs the test or particular assessment procedure? In Nottingham we have found it useful to make an informal evaluation of new assessment procedures from the deaf child's perspective in terms of the amount of time required to complete the task the linguistic complexity and even the cultural appropriateness of test items, toys and pictures.

Dyson in Booth and Swann (1987) cautions professionals against the use of an assessment simply as a means of demonstrating their own competence, to justify or estimate the merits of a particular developmental test, or to reinforce the justifications for professional decisions that have already been made, such as a school placement. He states that the traditional view of the need to assess a child's special needs is self-evident: you have to identify needs in order to be able to meet them. Implant team professionals should consider whether similar test results reflect the limitations or strengths of test measures or the actual outcome in terms of linguistic benefit to the implanted child (Haggard, 1992). Haggard recommends that implant programme professionals need to look at outcomes in terms of language, cognition and communication as a whole. By implication, in the case of young deaf children, measures that can show 'soft' or subtle changes in the implanted child's interaction and everyday communication skills may be as important as the results obtained using standardized procedures during the first year after initial device programming. Assessments must only test what is assessable. A good assessment should allow a range of responses as children of different linguistic abilities may give answers of different complexity. In conclusion, an implant programme communication assessment and outcomes protocol should reflect the continuum of language and speech abilities ascribed to deaf children.

Recent international changes in selection criteria indicate that there are now three increasingly significant groups of referrals for cochlear implantation that warrant careful assessment of their rate of progress in the acquisition of spoken language. The first group consists of deaf children who present with hearing loss with a progressive rather than sudden onset. Such children frequently function in a similar manner to partially hearing children. The second group includes a small but increasing number of cochlear implant candidates who present with some useful pre-operative hearing. Both of these groups contain deaf children with a comparatively small cognitive-linguistic gap and to some extent, an established persona as 'auditory' learners. In a majority of cases these children appear to be acquiring spoken language following a recognized sequence of development and in some cases may be at or near age-level in comparison to hearing peers. The third and inevitably increasingly large group of referrals consists of deaf children in the first 18 months of life. In the UK, these infants will have had an adequate trial with acoustic hearing aids before a referral to be considered for a cochlear implant is made.

The development of the Nottingham SLT protocol has been influenced by the language acquisition perspectives and research findings reported in the cross-linguistic research literature (Vihman, 1996; Ferguson et al., 1992). For example, the feasibility of looking at two or more languages in a 'language specific' way (with the assistance of fluent co-workers when necessary) or considering the effects of different interaction and language input styles in a bilingual learning environment. Many born profoundly deaf children and their families, however, rely on some form of sign language system as their primary means of everyday communication, before implantation. At the time of writing, the Nottingham programme is supporting approximately 30 children (circa 10%) from a bilingual home background – that is, where there are two spoken languages. A majority of these selected candidates were classified as profoundly deaf and therefore they also needed to learn British Sign Language (BSL) to convey their needs and views effectively before they received their cochlear implants. In Nottingham, the agreed 'monolingual' SLT assessment and outcomes protocol is applied routinely on all candidates selected for cochlear implantation. In the future perhaps there are parallels to be explored further in the developmental linguistics research findings on hearing infants from bilingual backgrounds as we endeavour to compare the progress of deaf children from sign bilingual or multi-lingual home environments with deaf children from monolingual backgrounds after cochlear implantation. Because of the diverse linguistic backgrounds and the wide chronological age range of paediatric cochlear implant candidates, assessment and outcomes protocols should include measures that enable deaf children to respond using a variety of language forms when it is appropriate to do so – especially in the baseline assessment phase (ICSLT, 1998). The effects of sensory impairment on language and cognitive development are complex and implant programme professionals may need to consider the interrelationships between the development of symbolic play (Brown 1999) and the 'child directed speech' used by parents and caregivers on implanted children's rate of progress in communication and language development (Kretschmer and Kreschmer, 1999).

During the selection phase the role of an implant programme SLT is to contribute an initial opinion on the child's overall development, interaction and communicative style and to identify issues to be addressed further in collaboration with the child's family and support professionals, as well as the implant programme coordinator.

Classification of linguistic status

Unlike the widely accepted audiological criteria on the severity and likely consequences of severe or profound sensorineural hearing loss in the pre-school years (Boothroyd in Tyler, 1992), the literature remains divided on the most effective way of describing the effects of deafness on a deaf child's linguistic competence. The lack of agreed criteria for looking at language and speech skills acquisition makes sharing linguistic outcomes after cochlear implantation a challenge for researchers and practitioners even across English-speaking populations. The following international classification for describing the onset of deafness has been used in some but not all of the Nottingham language and speech production studies after cochlear implantation: congenital (from birth); pre-lingual (onset before two years of age); peri-lingual (onset between two and four years of age); and post-lingual (onset after four years of age).

The terms 'oral-aural' and 'total communication' when used to describe a deaf child's primary mode of communication, may disguise a continuum of language modalities. This may range from *ideal* for one child's current communicative competence and linguistic needs at home and at school to *well-meaning but inappropriate* for a variety of reasons, not least the impact of the child's profound deafness on parents and professionals as interlocutors (Wood et al., 1986). In Nottingham we are looking at ways of defining deaf children's reliance on sign language before and after implantation less ambiguously. One aim of the Stories/Narrative Assessment Procedure (SNAP) research was to develop 'evidence-based' categories and definitions of the stages of development of narrative skills (Starczewski and Lloyd, 1999). It was hoped that this would enable both SLTs and teachers of the deaf to describe the rate at which individual children make (or do not make) a modality 'shift' from sign to spoken language as the preferred means of everyday communication after cochlear implantation in a more effective way.

In 1993 an informal audit of candidates presenting for cochlear implantation suggested no less than six sub-categories of speech production at the time of implantation:

- profoundly deaf children who presented with a full phonological repertoire (FPR) or system of spoken language;
- children who presented with a deterioration in speech
  production abilities, after acquisition of a full phonological
  repertoire;
- pre-school profoundly deaf children who presented with
  mild or moderately delayed acquisition in spoken language
  abilities including connected speech intelligibility;
- deaf children who presented with severely delayed or atypical acquisition of spoken language and/or speech production
  abilities;
- deaf children who were described as functioning at the 'pre-
  lexical' stage of spoken language development irrespective of
  their competence in sign language.

A comprehensive evaluation of the deaf child's linguistic competence should include an investigation of the child's use of
language, its content and form (Lahey, 1988). *Use* refers to the
child's ability to use language in context, *content* represents the
way the child conveys meaning, and *form* includes the surface
aspects of language such as syntax, morphology and phonology.
This principle suggests that a systematic assessment of deaf children's spoken language skills after cochlear implantation
involves more than performance-based tests of speech perception, listening and speaking. Crystal (1992) advocates looking at
the whole person and seeing his or her language system as a
whole, including all the interactions among different levels of
language structure. He states that phenomena at one linguistic
level can influence those at another level. In the case of deaf
children who use total communication (sign language +
speech), this should therefore include monitoring modality
dominance and any changes in the child's reliance on sign
language after cochlear implantation.

Outline of a recommended speech and language therapy assessment and outcomes protocol

Research findings still suggest that pre-verbal or low-verbal deaf
children continue to make steady progress and may even accel-
erate their rate of progress in communication skills as late as
three or even five years after implantation. The following SLT

assessment intervals – before implantation and at one, three, five, seven, and 10 years after implantation have been designated as essential or priority intervals for outcomes data collection. An additional SLT assessment is recommended at 15 years after implantation if the child has not already transferred to an adult implant programme for long term maintenance.

Profile of Actual Linguistic Skills (PALS)

In 1993, the Profile of Actual Linguistic Skills (PALS) (Allen and Dyar, 1997; Dyar et al., 2000) was developed to facilitate the exchange of information on the children's progress in communication skills in a systematic way and to promote the need for a developmental perspective. The PALS profile is a criterion-referenced procedure that was developed specifically to monitor a deaf child's ability to use oral language, effectively, in everyday linguistic and learning environments.

The aims of the PALS profile are:

- To provide a systematic means of assessing and monitoring a deaf child's progress at five interrelated linguistic levels: (a) everyday communication skills, (b) receptive skills, (c) expressive skills, (d) voice skills, and (e) speech skills.
- To complement and extend the traditional classification of deaf children – congenital, pre-lingual, peri-lingual and post-lingual, which is based exclusively on a child's chronological age (rather than language age).
- To substantiate the potential usefulness of a criterion-referenced 'descriptive' approach as a precursor to standardized or norm-referenced linguistic assessment measures.
- To identify deaf children who appear to be making (a) an average rate of progress, (b) an accelerated rate of progress, or (c) a less than expected rate of progress in the acquisition of language or speech skills after cochlear implantation.
- To indicate the possibility of unforeseen non-sensory disabilities that may require further investigation.
- To provide a linguistically principled approach to remediation by profiling 'actual' as well as predicted linguistic outcomes after cochlear implantation.

This developmental framework approach of PALS makes it an appropriate precursor to norm-referenced language performance measures. It can be applied in a language-specific way in the case of deaf children from a two-spoken-language background as well as children from a sign bilingual background.

As a criterion-referenced profile, PALS can be applied to infants from the age of nine months and it has no upper age limit. It has been designed to complement rather than to replace norm-referenced language assessments. There are a number of appropriate standardized measures that can be used with children from around nine months of age, for example, the Pre-school Language Scale – PLS 3 UK (Boucher and Lewis, 1997; Brinton in RCSLT, 2001) or the Reynell Developmental Language Scales 111 (Edwards et al., 1997). The PALS profile has been designed to complement rather than replace such measures hence its emphasis on the less visible but nonetheless important 'precursors' to rule-based spoken language. The PALS profile has been found to be a relatively stress-free way of documenting changes in deaf infants' and toddlers' spontaneous communication skills once acoustic or digital hearing aids have been fitted and prior to confirming a decision to proceed with cochlear implantation. During the selection phase for a cochlear implant it has been used to monitor the rate of linguistic progress made by

- deaf infants during the first 18 months of life;
- deaf children with childhood degenerative hearing losses; and
- deaf children who present with asymetric hearing losses.

The PALS profile is applied as a baseline measure before implantation on all selected candidates in Nottingham. The recommended follow-up intervals after cochlear implantation are (six months), one year, three years, and five years after the baseline assessment. Therefore it can be used as a middle- and long-term measure of linguistic benefit as well as monitoring individual children's progress in the first 12 months after implantation. It has been found to be a sensitive and time effective means of 'profiling' changes in the spontaneous communication/linguistic skills of profoundly deaf children who are functioning at the pre-lexical stage of language acquisition – when other more formal language and speech assessments are inappropriate.

PALS is equally useful when providing reassurance to the parents and support professionals of pre-school or school-aged deaf children who are functioning at the pre-lexical stage in spoken language development or deaf children with complex linguistic or learning needs. Identified 'gaps' in the PALS profile, enable the SLT to identify immediate communication goals for the deaf child in collaboration with the child's local support professionals. As an outcome measure rather than a test, PALS can provide global data on the linguistic capabilities and achievements of both large and focused groups of cochlear implant users over time. It has also been found to be clinically useful when profiling the 'mismatched' linguistic abilities of children with acquired deafness of sudden onset in middle or late childhood.

The PALS Individual Profile considers the effectiveness (success) of the deaf child's communication at five non-hierarchical but interrelated linguistic levels.

Using comprehensive written criteria, the user of a PALS profile makes a decision about the child's current communicative competence five times, at each of five interrelated linguistic levels (Table 10.2). The child's current competence at each of the 25 features on the PALS Individual Profile (Appendix 1, p. 380) is described using the following categories:

- *Pre-verbal:* the child is functioning at the pre-lexical stage of spoken language acquisition. As PALS has been designed as a language specific procedure the user must specify which language is being profiled for example, English, Welsh, Urdu, or British Sign Language.
- *Transitional:* the ability to use recognizable words and simple formulaic expressions is reported by the child's parents or other well-known adults. It is possible to elicit some single words or social phrase patterns in a familiar closed-set context on a minimum of two occasions.
- *Functional language:* the deaf child demonstrates the ability to use language(s) spontaneously and in a systematic or rule-based way. A knowledge of meaning and awareness of the syntactic rules of the ambient spoken language is apparent. It has been both reported and observed by the child's parents and support professionals. Linguistically equivalent features are emerging in the spontaneous communication used by deaf children who use sign language (or a spoken language other than English) as their primary means of everyday communication.

Table 10.2. PALS performance profile: five interrelated linguistic levels

Linguistic Level	Area of Investigation
1 Everyday Communication Skills	Use of language, pragmatics, discourse skills, social skills
2 Receptive Skills	Perception: auditory, visual and tactile considerations Comprehension: semantics, syntax and lexis
3 Expressive Skills	Expressive language (production): semantics, syntax, morphology and lexis Mode considerations
4 Voice [Skills]	Prosodic features: non-segmental aspects of speech [production]
5 Speech [Skills]	Speech [production features]: articulation, phonology and connected speech intelligibility

At the *everyday communication skills* level PALS profiles a deaf child's use of non-linguistic and linguistic communication strategies to convey needs and views. At the *receptive skills* level the child's functional understanding at home or at school is profiled rather than the outcomes obtained on formal tests of language comprehension. The less commonly investigated areas of speech perception and language modality shifts – from 'vision' to 'vision plus audition' to 'audition alone' is also described. As Boothroyd in Tyler (1992) states, it is important to recognize the distinction between auditory capacity and auditory performance.

Profoundly deaf people need two things if auditory capacity is to be revealed in auditory performance – hearing aids and listening experiences. During the first year after implantation it is important to monitor the child's development of sound awareness at the non-linguistic level also, for example, the ability to detect and localize environmental sounds. A strong relationship between speech perception and speech production is reported in the literature.

At the *expressive skills* level PALS profiles changes in the quantity of spoken language used by the deaf child in different everyday contexts as well as any changes in language modality dominance after implantation. When used with very young or older low verbal deaf children it aims to complement the traditional emphasis on assessments of vocabulary and syntax and morphology. At the *voice skills* level PALS looks at the non-segmental or prosodic features of speech production. For example, changes in the phonetic-level features of pitch and loudness and, at a later stage of spoken language development, the phonological features of prosody such as the rhythm of connected speech and the use of appropriate intonation contrasts.

At the *speech skills* level PALS profiles the status of a deaf child's spontaneous speech production patterns in terms of speech sound repertoire and the articulation and phonological precursors of intelligible connected speech patterns.

The results obtained using the PALS procedure on a large group of children before and after cochlear implantation are illustrated in Figure 10.2. All of the subjects in this study were profoundly deaf and at a pre-lexical stage of spoken language acquisition at the time of implantation. The global outcomes illustrated in Figure 10.2 supports the research findings that it takes at least 12 to 18 months after cochlear implantation for 'pre-verbal' deaf children to reach the 'rule-based' stage of spoken language in their everyday environments.

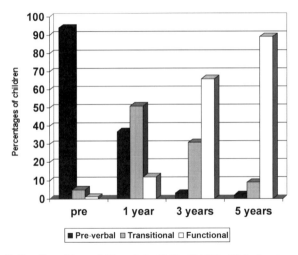

Figure 10.2. Profile of Actual Linguistic Skills (PALS): Global outcomes on 100 children before and one, three and five years following implantation; reaching the pre-verbal, transitional and functional language stages.

Figure 10.3 illustrates how the emphasis on current skills and ongoing needs rationale of the PALS can be used to reassure the parents and support professionals of deaf children with additional non-sensory needs. The 16 subjects in this group included children with significant learning difficulties, cerebral palsy or autistic spectrum disabilities. Finally, Figure 10.4 shows the percentage of the 100 children who had progressed through the pre-verbal and transitional stages of PALS to reach the functional language stage in each area of spoken language acquisition – within one, three or five years following implantation.

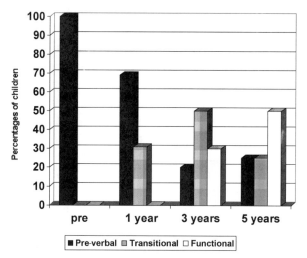

Figure 10.3. PALS: Global outcomes obtained on 16 children with complex linguistic or learning disabilities before and one, three and five years following implantation; reaching the pre-verbal, transitional and functional language stages.

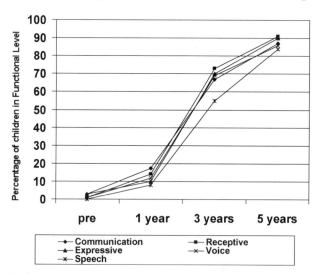

Figure 10.4. PALS: Percentage of 100 children classified as at the functional language level of spoken language ability in the five areas of spoken language acquisition, before and one, three and five years following cochlear implantation.

The Pragmatics Profile of Everyday Communication Skills (PPECS)

The Pragmatics Profile of Everyday Communication Skills (PPECS) (Dewart and Summers, 1988, 1995 and 1996) is a series of informal interview schedules (pre-school, school-age and adolescent/adult). The PPECS profiles are used by SLTs to investigate the social, interaction and conversation abilities of children who present with a wide range of spoken language impairments. The PPECS enables an implant programme SLT to ascertain and document the views of parents about their child's ability to communicate in everyday situations 'in their own words'. The information obtained provides a useful if qualitative outcome. The PPECS findings can be used to promote a dialogue between the family, the child's local therapist and teacher of the deaf and implant programme outreach professionals (Inscoe, 1999).

An adapted version of the PPECS pre-school summary form is illustrated in Appendix 2 (p. 381). For the purposes of collecting data that provides both a scientific and a clinically relevant outcome we have added an extra dimension to the PPECS summary form in order to record the pragmatic skills of deaf children from a sign bilingual background or a two-spoken-language background. The left column on the PPECS summary form is used to record the child's current status in spoken English. The right column is optional but it can be used to record the bilingual child's competence in another language. This column must be completed in collaboration with a fluent user of the non-English language.

The pre-school PPECS results obtained on 100 children are illustrated in Figure 10.5. A three-point progressive scoring system has also been introduced to demonstrate the children's rate of progress over time:

- absent (not observed or reported);
- developing (used inconsistently); and
- established skill.

Smith and Leinonen (1992) describe the cognitive, motor and perceptual developmental precursors that infants and pre-school children must acquire – as part of the transition from pre-intentional to intentional communication. When used with profoundly deaf children, we have found that the PPECS profile helps an SLT to confirm or out rule the presence of additional interaction or non-sensory difficulties that may be affecting a child's rate of linguistic progress especially in the pre-school years.

Test for Auditory Perception of Speech (TAPS)

The assessment battery known as TAPS (Reid and Lennhardt, 1993) was designed by Cochlear AG to look at the perceptual

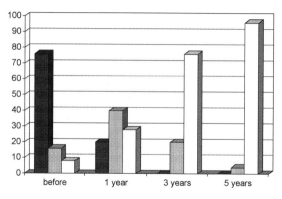

■ absent or not observed ▨ developing skill □ established skills

Figure 10.5. Pragmatics Profile of Early Communication Skills: pre-school outcomes PPECS: Median percentage of spoken language skills before implantation and one, three and five years following implantation in pre-lingually deaf children implanted younger than six years.

skills of children between the ages of two and 15 years. The TAPS consists of a common set of research-based measures that have been adapted for use with English, French and German speaking children as follows:

- Category 1: this category assesses the child's awareness of speech sounds (presence or absence) using auditory cues alone.
- Category 2: this category assesses the child's ability to differentiate between segmental speech features, using durational and intensity cues via auditory cues alone.
- Category 3: this category assesses the child's ability to identify spoken words and simple picture–related sentences by differentiating spectral information via auditory cues alone.
- Category 4: this category assesses the child's ability to identify the word stimulus from a group of three words, two of which are visually homophonous, using auditory and visual cues.
- Category 5: this category assesses the child's ability to recognize speech related to a particular topic in a modified open-set format using auditory cues alone. A production-level response is required in Category 5 (Reid and Lennhardt, 1993).

In 1993, approximately 75% of the profoundly deaf candidates selected for implantation in the Nottingham programme were functioning at the pre-verbal stage of spoken language acquisition. In such cases it was not always possible to administer TAPS for the first time until the 12 months or sometimes the 24 months assessment interval after implantation. Since 1998, however, the relaxation in the audiological criteria and subsequent increase in appropriate referrals of suitable school aged candidates with some pre-operative hearing has made TAPS a more useful component of the baseline SLT assessment battery. Our recent clinical experience in Nottingham suggests that a majority of children with cochlear implants can complete part or all of the TAPS battery between the 12- and 24-months interval. Candidates who are functioning at the two-word-level or above stage of spoken language ability at the time of implantation may achieve reliable results on TAPS categories 1,2 and 3 within the first 12 months after implantation – using listening without the support of lipreading.

Reynell Developmental Language Scales (RDLS)

The Reynell Developmental Language Scales 111 (Edwards et al., 1997) are considered to be a clinically practical assessment in that even very young children readily co-operate with test procedures (Edwards et al., 1999). The RDLS 111 is based on the original test (Reynell, 1977) but the new scales have been constructed to reflect current knowledge and to incorporate findings from up-to-date research on structural and lexical development in children. In Nottingham the RDLS 111 is administered to all cochlear implant candidates up to a chronological age of nine years before implantation, and again at one, three, five and seven years as appropriate after implantation. The RDLS 111 Comprehension Scale has been standardized on children from 1;6 years. The RDLS Expressive Scale has not been standardized on children younger than 1;9 years. For this reason use of the RDLS with infants and toddlers may need to be complemented by more developmentally appropriate measures such as PPECS (Dewart and Summers, 1995; Edwards et al., 1999).

Test for Reception of Grammar (TROG)

The Test for Reception of Grammar (TROG) (Bishop, 1989) is a multiple-choice test of language comprehension which consists of 80 four-choice test items. It is appropriate for a wide range of children from 4 years to 12 years of age and has been standardized on a UK population, including some normative data on adults. No expressive speech is required from the subject in this test. Picture and vocabulary test stimuli have been selected to ensure low ambiguity and the control of non-linguistic factors such as plausibility. The TROG test results may be interpreted both quantitatively and also qualitatively. For example, an SLT may wish to investigate whether the child's errors (grammatical confusions) are predominantly lexical or grammatical. As a standardized assessment, the TROG results may be correlated with the findings obtained on other standardized comprehension tests, notably, the British Picture Vocabulary Tests (Dunn et al., 1982) and the Reynell Developmental Language Scales (Edwards et al., 1997).

As a language comprehension test, TROG has proved of value in the assessment of children presenting with specific language disorders, deafness, mental delay and cerebral palsy. It is appropriate for children aged four to 13 years and it has been standardized on over 2,000 British children who did not have any known learning difficulty, hearing loss, or any other disability.

The TROG can be presented to a subject using spoken, written, or signed modality. A block is passed only if all four items in that block are responded to correctly. The probability of a subject getting all four items correct and passing a block by chance is 0.004. Depending on the number of complete blocks passed, the TROG results can be converted into a centile score, a standard score or an age-equivalent score (when this is appropriate). Detailed description of the test and the methods of scoring can be found elsewhere and the test has been found to be suitable for American as well as British subjects (Bishop, 1989; Abbeduto, Furman and Davis, 1989).

In a large group study the TROG was used to assess the comprehension of spoken language grammatical features of 153 profoundly deaf children implanted under the age of 11.5 years and to compare findings with the comprehension of grammar abilities of hearing peers (Nikolopoulos et al., in press).

The strength of a centile score is that it allows a direct statistical comparison of a deaf child's performance with hearing children of the same age. In other words, it is an index of the percentage of hearing children expected to obtain a score equivalent to or below that obtained by the subject. For example, if a subject scored at the tenth centile, this would mean that only 10% of hearing children would be expected to obtain a score equivalent to or below the one obtained by the subject, and conversely, 90% of hearing children would do better. The TROG centile scores can be used to report changes in the spoken language comprehension abilities of implanted children from four to 13 years of age. This is a constraint of the TROG test (and some other standardized tests) as long-term longitudinal studies are difficult to carry out and different children may fall within the required age limits at each interval. Moreover, if children under four years of age at the time of implantation were excluded, the rate of progress of younger implanted children in their understanding of the grammatical features of spoken language would not be taken into account. On the other hand TROG enables comparisons to be made between deaf children with cochlear implants and hearing children of the same age, making the previously mentioned constraint less important.

The results from a preliminary large group TROG research study revealed that before implantation, 91% (N = 112) of profoundly deaf children in the study were below the first centile of age-matched normally hearing children, 5% were between the first and 25th centiles, 2% between 25th and 75th centiles, and 2% between 75–100th centiles (Nikolopoulos et al., in press). By the three-year interval after implantation the respective percentages (N = 97) were 63%, 31%, 3% and 3%. The children continued to show increased understanding of the grammatical features of spoken language between three and five years after implantation, and by the five years' assessment interval, the respective percentages (N = 36) were 39%, 42%, 14% and 5%. In a future study it will be interesting to look at the potential outcomes obtained using TROG on a more homogeneous population of deaf children fitted with cochlear implants in the pre-school years.

Functional Lipreading and Listening Skills (FLLS)

The FLLS profile (Nottingham Paediatric Cochlear Implant Programme, 1993) has been designed to monitor a deaf child's emerging lipreading and listening skills at the one word level and later at a sentence level after cochlear implantation.

The single case study over time (Table 10.3) was chosen to demonstrate how many months or years a profoundly deaf child

Table 10.3. Functional Lipreading and Listening Skills (FLLS): a case study record over three years following implantation

Date & Audio information	WLR (A)	WLR X2	LR (AV)	LR X2	Written	TC	NR	Initials of Rater
BKB PR Sentence Lists ——— Pre-implant	CNT	CNT	CNT					
12 months post	CNT	CNT	CNT					
24 months post	CNT	–	44%	37&	–	6.5%	12.5%	
30 months	–	–	87.5%	12.5%				
36 months post	81%		12.5%	6.5%				

Functional Lipreading & Listening Skills: Scoring Codes:
WLR	= without lipreading (auditory alone)
WLRX2	= without lipreading + single repetition
LR	= lipreading and listening (AV)
LR X2	= lipreading and listening + single repetition
Wr	= written cue
TC	= Total Communication
NR	= No response
CNT	= Could not test

may take before being able to complete a sentence level task by listening alone. The child in this example was classified as pre-verbal at the time of implantation. The onset of deafness was two years, eight months and he received a multi-channel cochlear implant in 1989 at the age of three years and eight months. The graphic style of the FLLS profile demonstrates clearly how the child progressed from a 'could not test' phase during the first 18 months after cochlear implantation. This was followed by a relatively long phase of reliance on lipreading as well as listening before he was able to complete the Bamford, Kowal and Bench Picture-related Sentence Lists using listening alone (Bench and Bamford, 1979). By 30 months after implantation good progress is noted at the combined 'lipreading and listening' level. This phase is followed by an even more rapid rate of development between 30 and 36 months, when this child begins to achieve high-level scores in closed-set tasks using listening alone. It may be of historical interest to record that these results were achieved by the first child fitted with a multi-channel cochlear implant in the UK. Recent research findings suggest that young profoundly deaf children with a shorter dura-tion of deafness who are fitted with up-to-date implant electrode arrays and device programming strategies are likely to achieve faster (if not better) results at the listening alone level.

Story/ Narrative Assessment Procedure (SNAP)

Narratives play an important role in a child's language develop-ment and later academic achievement (Starczewski, Lloyd and Robinson in Waltzman and Cohen, 2000; Starczewski and Lloyd, 1999; Lloyd and Starczewski, 1998). The Stories/Narratives Assessment Procedure (SNAP) is a child-centred assessment that has been specifically developed for deaf children following cochlear implantation:

- SNAP materials/stimulus stories. The SNAP Dragon assess-ment battery consists of a set of 14 picture based stories. The set includes an introductory book, five assessment stories, and eight practice stories, written and illustrated specifically for pre-school deaf children. The books feature a family of dragons involved in everyday events throughout the year, which is appealing to this age group.
- SNAP sample collection: children are introduced to the key characters in the stories via hand puppets or the introductory book. A selected story is then told by an adult using a picture book with a separate text. Using the picture book as a prop, the child is then encouraged to retell the story. The adult is allowed to use phatic or supportive comments but other types of prompts, for example, questions are discouraged and are monitored carefully on the video-recorded samples.
- SNAP data transcription and analysis: a video recording is made of the child both listening to and retelling the story in their own way. A broad-based phonetic transcription (incor-porating an additional coding system adapted from Parker 1999) is made to document the range of communication modes used by the child. This may include one or more of the

following modality categories: gesture, sign, mixed, speech and sign, or speech (Starczewski, Lloyd and Robinson in Waltzman and Cohen, 2000).

Following this phonetic transcription the child's preferred mode of communication is identified and his or her storytelling abilities are assigned to one of eight categories as illustrated in Table 10.4.

Table 10.4. Story Narrative Assessment Procedure (SNAP): stages of narrative skills development

Narrative Stage	Story grammar	Narrative behaviour
1	Pre-analysis	Child is not ready to respond to the task
2	Pre-analysis	Child is happy to look at the book while the adult tells the story, but is not ready to retell the story.
3	Child labels or comments on pictures	Child needs prompting / scaffolding to retell the story (>3 prompts)
4	1 or 2 story categories used. Not a complete episode.	Some prompting needed (<3)
5	1 complete episode.	Spontaneous retelling. No prompting needed. Can include a "verbatim" stage
6	1 episode complete and second nearly complete (2/3 categories)	Verbatim stage may persist
7	2 complete episodes	Confident storytelling
8	> 2 episodes. Internal responses used increasingly to show reasoning of characters.	Confident and creative story-telling

Stages of narrative skills development

In a preliminary study using the SNAP procedure on 18 children between three and nine years of age, the conclusion reached was that SNAP can be used to document progress in language and communication skills in deaf children with very limited language as well as competent storytellers whose preferred communication mode is speech (Starczewski, Lloyd and Robinson in Waltzman and Cohen, 2000). Current narratives research in Nottingham suggests that it is possible to show a statistically significant increase in deaf children's narrative abilities over time. Prior to implantation, a majority of the young profoundly deaf children are functioning at the 'pre-structural' level and can at most label or make simple comments about the story pictures. By two years after implantation, however, many of the children have surpassed one or two categories (see Table 10.4) and are capable of completing at least one episode in their spontaneous retelling of a story. Individual case studies have also demonstrated that the children do not reach their maximum potential in narrative abilities until several years after implantation. As children are not under pressure to use any particular communication mode during the SNAP assessment procedure, the shift towards a preference for retelling the stories using speech may very well be attributed to the role of a cochlear implant in developing auditory and speech skills.

South Tyneside Assessment of Syntactic Skills (STASS)

The STASS provides information on changes in the clause, phrase and morphological patterns of spoken English. As a picture-based syntax screening procedure STASS (Armstrong and Ainley, 1986) has been adapted from the Language Assessment Remediation Assessment Procedure (LARSP) developed by Crystal, Fletcher and Garman (1989). An additional code of modifications is used when transcribing the spontaneous language production of deaf children.

The STASS has been found to provide a clinically useful baseline measure of the spoken English syntax of most young cochlear implant candidates including deaf children from a sign bilingual background. It has also been used with school-aged deaf children of low verbal level during the first few years after implantation.

Voice Skills Assessment (VSA)

Voice Skills Assessment (VSA) is a criterion-referenced rating scale that was devised as part of a computer-based clinical database (IMPEVAL, 1993; Bawtry Computer Services, 2001). The aim of the VSA is to describe the absence or presence of non-segmental features of speech production (prosody) that may contribute to a deaf child's overall speech intelligibility.

In Nottingham the VSA (Table 10.5) is completed as part of the initial communication assessment, before implantation, and at one, three, five, seven and 10 years after implantation. As a criterion-referenced rating scale, the VSA has no lower or upper age limit. It can therefore be used to provide preliminary information on the voice skills of all paediatric cochlear implant candidates – children and adolescents. The VSA takes an experienced rater approximately 15 minutes to complete. Users of the VSA rating scale should have an in-depth knowledge of commonly occurring voice features associated with deafness. Ideally, the SLT will have observed and worked with the child in more than one context either in a clinic, home or school context before completing the VSA rating scale. During the first year after implantation it has been found useful to check the VSA findings at the same time as completing video-based assessments.

The VSA rating scale is a measure of the deaf child's voice skills in spontaneous communication. For this reason an SLT or teacher may like to complete the VSA jointly with a deaf child's parents or local support professionals.

Table 10.5. Voice Skills Assessment (VSA): record form

	Phonetic level voice features	Outcome
1.1	Air stream type	
1.2	Air stream control	
1.3	Voice quality	
1.4	Pitch range	
1.5	Pitch control	
1.6	Loudness control in quiet or one-to-one context	
1.7	Loudness control in noisy or group context	
1.8	Resonance	

	Phonological level voice features	Outcome
2.1	Rhythm in words	
2.2	Rhythm in connected speech	
2.3	Use of spoken English intonation contrasts	
2.4	Rate of connected speech	

VSA scoring system for computer-based clinical database:
Absent = not observed or reported = 0; Developing skill: used inconsistently = 1;
Established skill = 2 based on detailed written criteria at each VSA level.

CID Phonetic Inventory: suprasegmentals

The CID Phonetic Inventory suprasegmental aspects, allows the examiner to assign up to 21 points based on the child's imitation of syllables or strings of syllables with different duration (5 points), intensity (2 points), pitch (5 points), and breath control (3 points). In addition, a possible six points are assigned for overall voice quality in different vowel contexts (Tobey in Tyler, 1993; Moog, 1988).

In Nottingham the suprasegmentals component of the CID Phonetic Inventory has been used to provide time effective and clinically relevant information on the voice features of deaf children during the first few years after cochlear implantation.

The Fundamental Speech Skills Test (FSST) is a comprehensive assessment that can be used with deaf children who have sufficient established spoken language to complete a performance-level test with reliability.

The FSST investigates the following fundamental or basic aspects of speech production: breath stream capacity, elementary articulation, pitch control, syllabification, stress and intonation contours.

Speech Intelligibility Rating (SIR)

Speech intelligibility is a function of the skills of listener and speaker and so intelligibility ratings or summaries are relative not absolute (Parker and Irlam in Wirz, 1994). The reason for the development of the Speech Intelligibility Rating (SIR) rating scale (Table 10.6) was to document deaf children's rate of progress and the stages involved in reaching connected speech intelligibility. SIR was designed primarily as an outcome measure rather than test of speech production.

A series of research studies have now been published using the SIR rating scale (Allen, Nikolopoulos and O'Donoghue, 1998; Allen et al., 2001). The first of these published studies, was a prospective study following 118 consecutively implanted deaf children with up to five years of implant use. Using the Mann Whitney U-test, the results of this study showed that the differences between the SIR categories increased signifi-cantly each year for four years. For the first two years the median rating remained 'pre-recognizable words' or 'unintelligible speech'. It was not until the three-year interval that the median intelligibility rating became Category 3 (intelligible speech if someone

Table 10.6. Speech Intelligibility Rating (SIR): five categories

Speech Intelligibility Rating (SIR) Criteria	SIR Category
Connected speech is intelligible to all listeners. The child is understood easily in everyday contexts	SIR Category 5
Connected speech is intelligible to a listener who has little experience of a deaf person's speech. The listener does not need to concentrate unduly	SIR Category 4
Connected speech is intelligible to a listener who concentrates and lipreads – within a known context/topic	SIR Category 3
Connected speech is unintelligible. Intelligible speech is developing in single words (or social phrases) when context and lipreading cues are also available	SIR Category 2
Pre-recognizable words in spoken language. The child's primary mode of everyday communication may be manual	SIR Category 1

concentrates and lipreads). At the four-year interval 85% of children had some intelligible connected speech. This improvement continued and at the five-year interval the median speech intelligibility was Category 4 (intelligible speech to a listener with little experience of deaf speech) and the mode was Category 5 (intelligible speech to all listeners) (Allen, Nikolopoulos and O'Donoghue, 1998). The overall conclusion of this study (see Figure 10.6) was that congenital and pre-lingually deafened children gradually develop intelligible speech that does not plateau over five years after implantation.

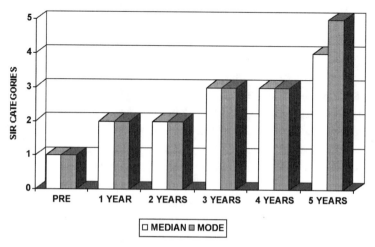

Figure 10.6. Speech Intelligibility Rating (SIR): Outcomes from the first 118 consecutively implanted deaf children over the first five years of implant use.

The importance of chronological age at implantation and the acquisition of connected speech intelligibility

The results of a second SIR study on 141 children, suggests that there is a correlation between the rate of development of speech intelligibility after cochlear implantation and a deaf child's age at implantation, duration of deafness and primary mode of communication. In this study 90% of the children were rated as 'pre-recognizable words' (SIR Category 1) before cochlear implantation. Three years after implantation, 58% of the children had achieved some connected speech intelligibility and were rated as SIR Category 3 or above (SIR Category 3-45%; SIR Category 4-10%; SIR Category 5-3%). Four years after implantation a total of 85% of the children had reached the upper categories of the rating scale: SIR Category 3-55%, SIR Category 4-20%, SIR Category 5-10%. The conclusion of this study was that 'connected speech intelligibility' is an achievable goal for a majority of deaf children after cochlear implantation.

The inter-observer reliability of SIR has now been formally assessed and a high rate of agreement between observers has been found (Allen et al., 2001). A third research investigation is being conducted using the SIR procedure to look at the effect of chronological age at the time of cochlear implantation on a deaf child's rate of development of connected speech intelligibility (see Figure 10.7).

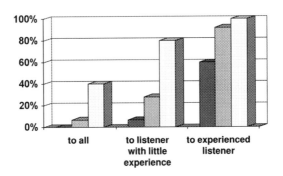

Age at implantation
■ 5-7 years old ▨ 3-5 years old □ < 3 years old

Figure 10.7. Speech Intelligibility Rating: a comparison of age at implantation with the development of speech intelligible to all, to a listener with little experience, and to an experienced listener four years after implantation.

Profile of Actual Speech Skills (PASS)

The Profile of Actual Speech Skills (PASS) is a video-recorded sampling technique looking at the spontaneous vocalizations and speech patterns of profoundly deaf children before they are linguistically ready to complete standardized tests of speech production. Its design was strongly influenced by the findings reported by Osberger in Owens and Kessler (1989) and Osberger et al. (1991).The PASS enables an SLT to establish a baseline of speech production in young cochlear implant candidates (age range nine months to two years and six months) and to continue to monitor spontaneous speech production over time. It also provides clinically relevant information on any pre-school or school-aged child with limited spoken language abilities. Approximately 65% of the children selected for implantation in Nottingham have required a PASS analysis before implantation. The procedure is repeated during the first year after implantation at the six-month and 12-month assessment intervals. By the two year assessment interval most of the implanted children have progressed sufficiently to attempt more formal or standardized tests of articulation or phonology.

A PASS profile consists of:

- A detailed phonetic transcription of a video-recorded sample of the deaf child interacting with a well-known adult. The emphasis must be on the child's spontaneous rather than elicited or 'modelled' speech production patterns
- A six-minute representative sample is selected by the PASS rater for analysis purposes. This may be a consecutive or composite sample.

The PASS initial comprehensive profile looks at the low-verbal deaf child's utterances, in terms of speech, speech-like, non-speech and other patterns. There is a choice of three additional analytical procedures: a consonant and vowel summary, a summary for place of articulation and a voice, place, manner error pattern analysis that can be made once the initial comprehensive profile has been completed.

The PASS data can then be interpreted with reference to recent research findings in developmental phonology on hearing infants.

Experience in Nottingham suggests that the PASS profile provides information on the changing status of implanted children's spontaneous speech production patterns during the first year after cochlear implantation that has both scientific and clinical relevance. The outcomes obtained in a large group pilot study demonstrated a fourfold increase in the quantity of vocalizations/utterances produced by deaf children fitted with cochlear implants – between the baseline and 12-months post-implant assessment intervals. It must be said that not all these speech production patterns were either meaningful or intelligible. For this reason, we are looking in more depth at the range of developmental dynamic or 'infra-phonological' (Vihman, 1996) processes that occur most frequently during the first year after implantation.

PASS is usually not suitable for prospective implant candidates who already have established spoken language skills. As well as investigating the deaf child's speech at the spontaneous utterance and single word levels, it is strongly recommended that deaf children with cochlear implants complete a comprehensive phonological assessment of their speech production – when they are linguistically ready to do so. It is acknowledged that some profoundly deaf children make a rapid and smooth transition from 'no speech' to intelligible connected speech patterns, but a majority of 'average' cochlear implant users may benefit from further systematic assessment of their speech production systems. In the UK, the most widely used phonological procedure with deaf or hearing-impaired children and adults is the Phonological Evaluation and Transcription of Audio-Visual Language (PETAL) (Parker, 1999). The PETAL investigates a child's vowel and diphthong system (monophthongs and diphthongs): it looks at whether consonant sounds are used contrastively; at the range of intonation patterns with reference to a child's ambient spoken language, and finally, it looks at a child's overall intelligibility in more than one context. A phonological analysis usually involves a video or audio-based recorded sample of target words and phrases. The Phonological Assessment of Child Speech – Toys (PACS) (Grunwell, 1985) is also used with pre-school children who present with high levels of established spoken language.

Edinburgh Articulation Test (EAT)

The Edinburgh Articulation Test (Anthony et al., 1971) is a standardized articulation test used by SLTs in the UK. It has been included in the Nottingham assessment and outcomes protocol so that a comparison of speech articulation findings can be made between a deaf child with a cochlear implant and a hearing peer. According to its authors, the aim of the EAT assessment is to provide a sensitive and economical instrument for looking at the spoken language of very young children. As a measure of speech production, however, the EAT is concerned only with consonant articulations. No attention is given to vowels, rhythm, intonation or voice quality (Abercrombie in Anthony et al., 1971). Prior to the availability of cochlear implants in the early 1990s, the limitations of both the quantitative analysis and to a lesser extent the qualitative analysis level of the EAT were self-evident. The measure was avoided, actively disliked or considered to be inappropriate for profoundly deaf children, by specialist SLTs who worked primarily with a deaf or hearing-impaired client group. Recent improvements in implant devices and programming options, however, and the trend towards mainstream educational placements by parents of pre-school profoundly deaf children have increased the need for SLTs to investigate and describe the articulation patterns of pre-school cochlear implant users in comparison with hearing peers as well as with deaf peers who use hearing aids. The EAT quantitative level analysis, enables clinicians or researchers to convert raw scores into a standardized outcome that has been norm-referenced on British children. During the first few years after implantation, the EAT qualitative level analysis may provide a useful indicator of a deaf child's resolving articulation difficulties over time or identify specific articulatory (rather than phonological level) difficulties that may require remediation. The EAT has been found to provide information on the articulation aspects of an implanted deaf child's speech production in an accessible format. It has also been used successfully to make a stress-free baseline assessment of children's established speech-production skills – in the case of deaf children with progressive hearing losses, those with established spoken language and those children who have become deaf after language was established.

Overview of assessments

Table 10.7 provides an overview of the rationale and areas of emphasis of all the selected assessment measures that have been described here.

Table 10.7. Speech and language therapy assessment and outcomes protocol

Linguistic level* (PALS)	Title of measure	Origin	Type of test	Area of emphasis	Implemented using Speech	Gesture/sign
Level 1 Everyday communication	Pragmatics Profile of Everyday Communication Skills (PS) (S) or (A) version	UK	Interview Schedules: Pre-school/ School/ Adolescent Versions	Communicative functions, pragmatics, social, interaction & conversation skills: Pre-school version (9 months to 4 yrs11mo); School version (5yrs to 11yrs) Adolescent/Adult version (from 11 years onwards – if appropriate)	+ + +	+ + +
Level 2 Receptive	Test for Auditory Perception of Speech (TAPS)	Europe	Test for area of deficit	Speech perception	+	+
	Reynell Developmental Language Scales 111 (Receptive Language Scale)	UK	Standardized/ Norm-referenced UK population	Language comprehension	+	
	Test for Reception of Grammar (TROG)	UK	Standardized/ Norm-referenced UK population	Language comprehension	+	
	BKB Picture-related Sentence Lists	UK	Test for area of deficit	Listening alone: sentence level task	+	+
Level 3 Expressive	Reynell Developmental Language Scales 111 (Expressive Language Scale)	UK	Standardized/ Norm-referenced UK population	Expressive language	+	

(contd)

Table 10.7. (contd)

Linguistic level* (PAIS)	Title of measure	Origin	Type of test	Area of emphasis	Implemented using	
					Speech	Gesture/sign
	Story/Narrative Assessment Procedure (SNAP)		Test for area of deficit	Narrative skills	+	+
	South Tyneside Assessment of Syntactic Skills (STASS)		Test for area of deficit	Spoken language syntax	+	+
Level 4 Voice	Voice Skills Assessment rating scale	UK	Criterion-referenced Rating scale	Non-segmental features of speech production (prosody)	+	
	CID Phonetic Inventory: suprasegmental aspects	USA	Rating scale	Suprasegmental aspects of speech production	+	
Level 5 Speech	Speech Intelligibility Rating (SIR)	UK	Criterion-referenced	Speech intelligibility	+	
	Profile of Actual Speech Skills (PASS)	UK/ USA	Recorded time sampling	Spontaneous speech patterns	+	
	Edinburgh Articulation Test (EAT)	UK	Test for area of deficit	Articulation	+	

Factors influencing rate of progress

As with tactile and acoustic hearing aid users the form or level of training provided to implanted children may be an important variable in determining the type of communication skills they ultimately acquire (Alcántara et al., 1990). Along with scientists and teachers of the deaf, an implant programme SLT is likely to be involved in enabling the child to develop a set of basic perceptual skills and also to establish basic motor skills at the speech-production level after implantation.

A realistic framework of short-term monitoring or (re)habilitation goals has been described by Dyar (1996). The recommended short-term goals for young deaf children during the first year after cochlear implantation were:

- to detect different noises and tones;
- to learn how to control and improve their voices;
- to perceive the sounds of speech and speech rhythm;
- to obtain improved understanding when implant and lip-reading are used;
- to achieve some understanding of speech without lip-reading;
- to improve speech production;
- to document changes in emerging linguistic skills using skilled observation or video-recorded sampling and analysis techniques.

Between one and three years after implantation the mid-term (re)habilitation goals for extremely young or older low verbal implanted children were:

- to monitor the views and training needs of the child's parents and primary caregivers using questionnaires or rating scales;
- to involve parents and support professionals in planning and implementing communication goals for the child that can be carried out easily at home or at school;
- to identify the child's current skills and ongoing linguistic needs using language- and age-appropriate performance measures.

Between three and five years after implantation, the long-term (re)habilitation goals for young children fitted with cochlear implants were:

- to monitor the child's 'self generating' linguistic skills in everyday home and school contexts;
- to monitor the child's linguistic effectiveness and ability to cope as an independent learner.

An SLT aims to develop and consolidate the child's capacity for speech memory and recall of speech patterns after direct training has been removed. This includes an ability to transfer trained speech skills to new contexts. When monitoring an implanted child's speech-production abilities, implant programme SLTs have a responsibility to maintain an up-to-date knowledge of the implications of technology advancements and device-programming strategies. When working with deaf children in the first few years of life SLTs need to learn how to identify what is being attempted by the child, what is being accomplished and what conditions promote or impede success. It has been suggested that normal hearing children need to be exposed to language before the age of three years for them to develop a language system effortlessly (Tyler and Fryauf-Bertschy in Tye-Murray, 1992). In the Deafness Management Quotient (DMQ), Northern and Downs (1978) outlined five factors that may contribute to a deaf child's ultimate progress:

- residual hearing;
- central intactness;
- intellectual factors;
- family constellation; and
- socioeconomic status.

Geers and Moog (1987) in the Social Language Predictor Index (SLPI), investigated the effects of five similar but not identical factors that are likely to impact on the eventual speech prognosis of a profoundly deaf child:

- residual hearing capacity;
- language competence;
- non-verbal intelligence;
- family support; and
- the deaf child's speech communication attitude.

Finally, 12 potential areas of further investigation were identified as part of a detailed study of the development of spoken language skills after cochlear implantation (Dyar, 1992):

- Communication: uses of language, social skills and conversation abilities. An investigation of both deaf child and adult attitudes to communication, styles of interaction and also appropriateness of expectation levels after cochlear implantation.
- Receptive (input): the actual rate of development of listening skills rather than the predicted rate based on auditory acuity or implant device settings; the rate of transition from 'vision' to 'vision plus audition' and finally to 'audition alone' as the 'dominant' modality for language learning; reasons why some children continue to use a bi-modal approach to language learning; the rate of development of the child's spoken language comprehension skills after cochlear implantation – at vocabulary, meaning and syntax levels.
- Expressive: the child's expressive (production) abilities at speech, sign and written levels; the rate of expressive language development – at vocabulary, meaning and syntax levels.
- Speech production: oro-motor capacity and skills development, phonetic and phonological encoding skills.
- IQ and academic attainments: Non-verbal IQ; academic attainments; child's attitude to (re)habilitation.
- Social needs and opportunities: an investigation of age appropriate opportunities for independent communication outside school and home.
- Emotional development: ability to share affect in age appropriate ways.
- Personality: an investigation of the child's self-image, coping and compensatory strategies and learning style.
- Friendships: ability to mix and make friends with other deaf and hearing children; ability to sustain friendship with school peers.

An implant programme SLT may also need to investigate communication and language difficulties associated with non-deafness-related conditions. For this reason it has been found useful to maintain or develop links with SLTs who have specialized with other communication impaired populations – for example, cleft palate, specific language impairment or autistic spectrum disorders.

The decision about selecting the most appropriate educational setting for a young deaf child with a cochlear implant remains difficult for many families. McCracken and Sutherland (1991) give the following guidelines:

- parents/families should consider both the current and predicted development of their children's language and speech;
- they should consider the child's potential capacity to convey his or her needs and views independently;
- the personality of their child;
- the child's general mental (cognitive) ability – insofar as it can be ascertained, and whether the child has additional special educational needs apart from deafness.

Ultimately, these authors conclude it is the child who must decide the pace of progress.

Future trends, issues and concerns

Initial and subsequent changes to a deaf child's implant device settings may result in subtle changes in the deaf child's typical behaviour and communication skills. It is recommended, therefore, that implant programme professionals discuss, at an inter-disciplinary level, when and why changes to device settings are made. Such collaboration also assists implant programme professionals to conduct well-planned interdisciplinary research studies that meet peer review standard. Parents and deaf children's local support professionals continue to request clear guidance on the length of a hearing aid trial required before cochlear implantation. It will be interesting to observe the impact on referrals for cochlear implantation as digital hearing aids become more widely available in the UK. The feedback from participants at a series of weekend workshops asked for more support and ideas on how to evaluate the benefit of cochlear implants for deaf children with additional cognitive, linguistic or oro-facial/oro-motor disabilities. As more cochlear implant users transfer to post-primary educational settings, local SLTs and teachers of the deaf are requesting help with monitoring the changing needs of these children.

The adaptation of TAPS (Reid and Lehnhardt, 1993) was a pioneer attempt at developing a speech perception measure based on linguistically 'equivalent' vocabulary and sentence patterns across more than one spoken language. More recent findings in developmental linguistics research suggests that there are still many inherent difficulties in the construction of 'cross-linguistic' assessment measures, even when the goal of multi-centre and even multi-cultural shared data is an admirable one.

Techniques for the assessment of deaf infants' pragmatics skills, such as the use(s) of language, social interaction and conversation strategies in everyday situations appear to be back in favour as implant programme professionals endeavour to monitor the initial progress of extremely young children who have been fitted with cochlear implants.

Clinical sociolinguistics is perhaps a less developed area (Ball, 1992), but professionals with an interest in sociolinguistics may wish to look further at the implanted child's linguistic competence in relation to class membership, sex, regional background, ethnic background, age and the use of language varieties. Sociolinguistics may also encompass studies of language from a bilingual or multilingual perspective. Most SLTs who have chosen to specialize in hearing impairment have a particular interest in sign bilingualism. The role and linguistic effects of sign language on deaf children's linguistic and academic attainments after cochlear implantation require further scrutiny.

The literature on the linguistic outcomes obtained by implanted children who were in the linguistically developing stage at the time of implantation remains sparse (Ruben, 1992). While this statement is no longer true, Ruben's reminder that the essential purpose of the intervention in the case of a linguistically developing child is to enable the child to develop optimal language (not speech perception or speech intelligibility) remains valid. At times the research literature seems to concentrate on 'star' performers but as implant programme professionals we also need to reflect on the reasons for outcome variability if we are to improve future practice. The importance of reporting individual scores is emphasized by Tyler in Tyler (1993). He states that reporting average scores across individuals does not specify the most critical information. It can also be misleading to report the percentage of children scoring above chance before and after surgery as this fails to indicate the magnitude of the pre- and post-operative differences. What is important is the absolute level of performance for each child. For this reason a solution may be to show individual data in scattergrams or bar graphs.

As well as reporting reasons for device failure, implant programme professionals need to investigate and share findings on other potential intrinsic or extrinsic reasons for poor performance in those children who appear to be making a less than average rate of progress in linguistic skills development.

The traditional view of the role of an SLT as 'correcting' children's speech production on weekly visits to an outpatients clinic has become an outmoded one (Webster and Wood, 1989). Speech and language therapists can make significant contributions to the overall management of deaf children's communication skills development before and after cochlear implantation. Increasingly SLTs are demonstrating a willingness to

- work collaboratively with parents and professionals;
- to implement clinical audit procedures;
- to participate or provide specialist induction training; and
- to plan and deliver skills-based training on aspects of communication, language and speech development for a range of professional groups associated with paediatric cochlear implantation.

The authors of this chapter support the view that the assessment of very young children necessitates the development of specific measures rather than adapting those designed for an adult programme (Archbold, 1992). The overall philosophy of the Nottingham programme is that changes in young implanted children's social adjustment, early communication, linguistic and educational attainments should be monitored by professionals with experience of this age group.

Haggard in Cooper (1991) argued for robust exportable rehabilitation methods so that local rehabilitation support professionals may contribute to and continue the (re)habilitation goals initiated by the implant programme with continuity of methods. It is hoped that this view has been mirrored in the rationale of the SLT assessment and outcomes protocol described in this chapter. As professionals associated with one of the largest paediatric cochlear implant programmes in the world, the authors have found it necessary to constantly revise their expectations about the long-term linguistic capabilities of deaf children who use cochlear implants. Association with a dedicated paediatric cochlear implant programme has afforded opportunities to improve interdisciplinary team work; to consider deafness-related communication difficulties from a range of different perspectives; and to accept and attempt to overcome the challenges associated with 'evidence-based' research outcomes. It has also taught us to appreciate the phenomenal role of audition in the acquisition of effective and 'self generating' spoken language skills.

References

Abbeduto I, Furman L, Davis B (1989) Relation between the receptive language and mental age of persons with mental retardation. American Journal of Mental Retardation 93: 535-43.

Abercrombie J (1971) Introduction to the Edinburgh Articulation Test. In Anthony A, Bogle D, Ingram T, McIsaac M (eds) The Edinburgh Articulation Test. Edinburgh: Churchill Livingstone.

Alcántara JI, Whitford LA, Blamey PJ, Cowan RSC, Clark GM (1990) Tactile features recognition by deaf children. Journal of the Acoustical Society of America 88(3): 1260-74.

Allen MC, Nikolopoulos TP, Dyar D, O'Donoghue GM (2001) The reliability of a rating scale for measuring speech intelligibility following pediatric cochlear implantation. American Journal of Neuro-otology 22(5): 631-3.

Allen MC, Nikolopoulos TP, O'Donoghue GM (1998) Speech intelligibility in children following cochlear implantation. American Journal of Otology 19(6): 742-6.

Allen S, Dyar D (1997) Profiling linguistic outcomes in young children after cochlear implantation. American Journal of Otology 18: S127-S128.

Allum DJ (ed.) (1996) Cochlear implant rehabilitation. In Allum DJ (ed.) Children and Adults. London: Whurr.

Anthony A, Bogle D, Ingram T, McIsaac M (eds) (1971) The Edinburgh Articulation Test. Edinburgh: Churchill Livingstone.

Archbold SM (1992) The development of a paediatric cochlear implant programme: a case study. Journal of the British Association of Teachers of the Deaf 16(1): 17-26.

Armstrong S, Ainley M (1986) STASS: South Tyneside Assessment of Syntactic Skills. Northumberland: STASS Publications.

Ball M (1992) Clinician's Guide to Linguistic Profiling of Language Impairment. Kibworth: Far Communication.

Bawtry Computer Services (2001) BCS System for Cochlear Implant Centres. Info@bawtry.net.

Bench J (1992) Communication Skills in Hearing Impaired Children. London: Whurr.

Bench J, Bamford J (1979) Speech-Hearing Tests and the Spoken Language of Hearing Impaired Children. London: Academic Press.

Bishop DVM (1989) Test for Reception of Grammar (TROG). 2 edn. Available from the author, MRC Applied Psychology Unit, 15 Chaucer Road, Cambridge.

Bloom L, Lahey J (1978) Language Development and Language Disorders. New York: John Wiley.

Bloomfield L (1933) Language. New York: Henry Holt.

Boothroyd A (1992) Profound deafness. In Tyler RS (ed.) Cochlear Implants: Audiological Foundations. London: Whurr.

Boucher J, Lewis V (1997) The Pre-School Language Scale PLS-3 (UK). The Pyschological Corporation Ltd. Harcourt Brace.

Brinton J (2001) Measuring language development in deaf children with cochlear implants. In Royal College of Speech and Language Therapists (2001) Conference Proceedings: Sharing Communication.

Brown PM (1999) Early development in deaf and hard of hearing children: the state of play. Australian Journal Education of the Deaf. Vol. 5.

Chomsky N (1965) Aspects of the Theory of Syntax.

Clark GM, Cowan RSC, Dowell RC (eds) (1997) Cochlear Implantation for Infants and Children. San Diego, CA: Singular.

Crystal D (1992) Profiling Linguistic Disability. 2 edn. London: Whurr.

Crystal D, Fletcher P, Garman M (1989) Language Assessment and Remediation and Screening Procedure (LARSP). London: Whurr.

Dewart H, Summers S (1988) Pragmatics Profile of Early Communication Skills. Windsor: NFER-Nelson Publishing Company.

Dewart H, Summers S (1995) The Pragmatics Profile of Everyday Communication Skills (Pre-school, School Age). Windsor: NFER-Nelson Publishing Company.

Dewart H, Summers S (1996) The Pragmatics Profile of Everyday Communication Skills in Adults (Adolescents). Windsor: NFER-Nelson Publishing Company.

Dowell RC (1997) Pre-operative audiological speech and language evaluation. In Clark GM, Cowan RSC, Dowell RC (eds) Cochlear Implantation for Infants and Children. San Diego, CA: Singular Publishing Group Inc, pp. 83-111.

Dunn LM, Dunn CM, Whetton C, Pintilie D (1982) British Picture Vocabulary Scale. Windsor: NFER-Nelson.

Dyar D (1992) The development of spoken language skills after cochlear implantation: results obtained from one child during the 0-3 years interval after cochlear implantation. Presentation at the First European Symposium on Paediatric Cochlear Implantation: Nottingham, September 1992.

Dyar D (1996) Assessing Auditory and Linguistic Performances in Low Verbal Implanted Children. Basel: Karger pp 139-46.

Dyar D, Allen S, Nikolopoulos TP, Inscoe J, Harrigan S, Allen MC, England R (2000) Profiling the range of oral language abilities after cochlear implantation. Presentation: Fifth European Symposium on Paediatric Cochlear Implantation, Antwerp, June 2000.

Dyson S (1987) Reasons for assessment: rhetoric and reality in the assessment of children with disabilities. In Booth T, Swann W (eds) Including Pupils with Disabilities. Milton Keynes: Open University Press.

Edwards S, Fletcher P, Garman M, Hughes A, Letts C, Sinka I (1997) The Reynell Developmental Language Scales 111 (The University of Reading Edition). Windsor: NFER-Nelson.

Edwards S, Garman M, Hughes A, Letts C, Sinka I (1999) Assessing comprehension and production of language in young children: an account of the Reynell Developmental Language Scales 111. International Journal of Language and Communication Disorders 34: 2; 151-91.

Ferguson CA, Menn L, Stoel-Gammon C (eds) (1992) Phonological Development Models Research Implications. Maryland: York Press Inc.

Geers A, Moog J (1987) Predicting spoken language acquisition of profoundly hearing impaired children. Journal of Speech and Hearing Disorders 2: 84-94

Geers AE, Moog JS (eds) (1994) Effectiveness of cochlear implants and tactile aids for deaf children. The Volta Review 96: 5.

Grunwell P (1985) Phonological Assessment of Child Speech (PACS). Windsor: NFER-Nelson Publishing Company.

Haggard MP (1991) Introduction: cochlear implants in perspective. In Cooper H (ed.) Cochlear Implants: A Practical Guide. London: Whurr.

Haggard MP (1992) Health economics aspects of paediatric cochlear implantation. Keynote address: First European Symposium on Paediatric Cochlear Implantation. Nottingham, September 1992.

Harrigan S, Nikolopoulos TP, Inscoe J, Allen MC, England R, Dyar D (2000) Effect of parent interaction training programmes on the communication skills of the parents of implanted children. Poster presentation: The Fifth European Symposium on Paediatric Cochlear Implantation. Antwerp, June 2000.

Hasenstab S (1993) Cognitive and linguistic changes in children using Nucleus multichannel cochlear implants. Proceedings of the Third International Cochlear Implant Conference. Innsbruck, Austria, April 1993.

Haynes C (1989) Language development in the school years – what can go wrong? In Mogford K, Sadler J (eds) Child Language Disability: Implications in an Educational Setting. Clevedon: Multilingual Matters.

Hellman SA, Chute PM, Kretschmer RE, Nevins ME, Parisier SC, Thurston LC (1991) The development of a children's implant profile. American Annals of the Deaf 136(2): 77–81.

ICSLT Guidelines for Good Practice working with Clients with Cochlear Implants (1998) Implant Centre Speech and Language Therapists (ICSLT) National Policy Document sponsored by British Cochlear Implant Group.

IMPEVAL (1993) Nottingham Paediatric Cochlear Important Programme Protocol. Nottingham, UK

Inscoe J (1999) Communication outcomes after paediatric cochlear implantation. International Journal of Pediatric Otorhinolaryngology 47: 195–200.

Kretschmer R, Kretschmer L (1999) Communication and language development. Australian Journal Education of the Deaf. Vol. 5.

Lahey M (1988) Language Disorders and Language Development. New York: Macmillan.

Laurenzi C (1993) The bionic ear and the mythology of cochlear implants. British Journal of Audiology 27: 1–5.

Lloyd H, Starczewski H (1998) Using narrative to measure benefit from paediatric cochlear implantation. Presentation: The Fourth European Symposium on Paediatric Cochlear Implantation. 's Hertogenbosch, Holland.

Lund N, Duchan J (1993) Assessing Children's Language in Naturalistic Contexts. 3 edn. Englewood Cliffs, NJ: Prentice-Hall.

Luterman D (1987) Deafness in the Family. San Diego,CA: College Hill Press.

McConkey Robbins (2000) A Rehabilitation after cochlear implantation. In Niparko JK, Iler Kirk K, Mellon NK, McConkey Robbins A, Tucci DL, Wilson BS (eds) Cochlear Implants: Principles and Practices. Philadelphia, PA: Lippincott Williams & Wilkins, pp. 323–67.

McCracken W, Sutherland H (1991) Deaf Ability not Disability: A Guide for Parents of Hearing Impaired Children. Clevedon: Multilingual Matters.

Moog J (1988) CID Phonetic Inventory. St Louis, MO: Central Institute for the Deaf.

Nevins ME, Chute MP (1996) Cochlear Implants in Educational Settings. San Diego, CA: Singular.

Nikolopoulos TP, Dyar D, Archbold SM, O'Donoghue GM (in press) Proceedings of Third Congress of Asia Pacific Symposium on Cochlear Implant and Related Sciences, Osaka 5–7 April 2001.

Nikolopoulos TP, Dyar D, Gibbin KP (accepted) Assessing candidate children for cochlear implantation with the Children's Implant Profile (ChIP): the first 200 children.

Niparko JK, Iler Kirk K, Mellon NK, McConkey Robbins A, Tucci DL, Wilson BS (2000) Cochlear Implants: Principles and Practices. Philadelphia, PA: Lippincott Williams & Wilkins.

Northern J, Downs M (1978) Deafness Management Quotient (DMQ). In Northern J, Downs M (eds) Hearing in Children. Baltimore, MD: Williams & Wilkins.

Nottingham Paediatric Cochlear Implant Programme (1993) Cochlear Implant Evaluation Database (IMPEVAL) - Speech and Language Therapy Protocols. Nottingham UK.

Osberger MJ (1989) Speech production in profoundly hearing impaired children with reference to cochlear implants. In Owens E, Kessler D (eds) Cochlear Implants in Young Deaf Children. Boston, MA: College-Hill Press.

Osberger MJ, Robbins AM, Berry SW, Todd SL, Hesketh LJ, Sedey A (1991) Analysis of spontaneous speech samples of children with a cochlear implant or tactile aid. American Journal of Otology 12 (supplement): 151–64.

Parker A (1999) PETAL: Phonological Evaluation and Transcription of Audio-Visual Language (PETAL). Oxon: Winslow.

Parker A, Irlam S (1994) Intelligibility and deafness: the skills of listener and speaker. In Wirz SL (ed.) Perceptual Approaches to Speech and Language Disorders. London: Whurr.

Pisoni DB (2000) Cognitive factors and cochlear implants: some thoughts on perception, learning and memory in speech perception.

Reid J, Lennhardt M (1993) Speech perception test results for European children using the Nucleus cochlear implant. Proceedings of the 3rd International Cochlear Implant Conference. Innsbruck, Austria, April 1993.

Reynell J (1977) Reynell Developmental Language Scales. 2 edn.

Robinson K (1998) Cochlear implants: some challenges. In Gregory S, Knight P, McCracken W, Powers S, Watson L (eds) (1998) Issues in Deaf Education. London: David Fulton Publishers.

Ruben RJ (1992) The paediatric cochlear implant. Keynote address: First European Symposium on Paediatric Cochlear Implantation. Nottingham, September.

Smith BR, Leinonen E (1992) Clinical Pragmatics. London: Chapman & Hall.

Snow CE (1972) Mother's speech to children learning language. Child Development 43: 549–65.

Starczewski H, Lloyd H, Robinson K (2000) Stories/Narratives Assessment Procedure (SNAP) for children with cochlear implants. In Waltzman SB, Cohen N (eds) Cochlear Implants. New York: Thieme Medical Publishers.

Starczewski H, Lloyd H (1999) Using the Stories/Narrative Assessment Procedure (SNAP) to monitor language and communication changes after a cochlear implant; a case study. Deafness and Education International 1(3): 137–54.

Tobey EA (1993) Speech production. In Tyler RS (ed.) Cochlear Implants: Audiological Foundations. London: Whurr.

Tyler RS (1993) Speech perception in children. In RS Tyler (ed.) Cochlear Implants: Audiological Foundations. London: Whurr.

Tyler RS, Fryauf-Bertschy H (1992) Hearing abilities of children with cochlear implants. In Tye-Murray N (ed.) Cochlear Implants for Children: A Handbook for Parents, Teachers, Speech and Hearing Professionals. Washington, DC: Alexander Graham Bell Association for the Deaf.

Tyler RS, Gantz BJ, Woodworth GG, Fryauf-Bertschy H, Kelsay DMR (1997) Performance of 2- and 3- year old children and prediction of 4 year from 1- year performance. The American Journal of Otology 18: S157–S159.

Vihman MM (1996) Phonological Development. The Origins of Language in the Child. Cambridge, MA: Blackwell.

Wanner E, Gleitman L (1989) Language Acquisition: The State of the Art. Cambridge: Cambridge University Press.

Webster A, Elwood R (1986) The Hearing Impaired Child in the Ordinary School. London: Croom-Helm.

Webster A, Wood D (1989) Special Needs in Ordinary Schools: Children with Hearing Difficulties. London: Croom Helm.

Wood D, Wood H, Griffith A, Haworth I (1986) Teaching and Talking with Deaf Children. Chichester: Wiley.

Yoshinaga Itano C, Sedey AL, Coulter DK, Mehl AL (1998) Language of early- and later-identified children with hearing loss. Pediatrics 102: 5.

Zimmerman I, Steiner V, Pond R (1969) Pre-School Language Scale (PLS). The Psychological Corporation Limited. Harcourt Brace. UK Adaptation: Boucher J, Lewis V (1997) The Psychological Corporation Limited. London: Harcourt Brace & Company Publishers.

Appendix 1

Profile of Actual Linguistic Skills (PALS): individual profile

Name Assessment Interval	Date
1. Everyday Communication Skills 1.1 Use of spoken language pattern for communication 1.2 Range of communicative intentions 1.3 Response to verbal communication from others 1.4 Effectiveness of communication 1.5 Sociolinguistic variation	P T FL
2. Receptive Skills 2.1 Use of hearing 2.2 Use of situation cues 2.3 Listening and lipreading 2.4 Listening without lipreading 2.5 Ability to carry out performance measures	P T FL
3. Expressive Skills 3.1 Use of non-verbal strategies 3.2 Use of spoken language to communicate 3.3 Level of spontaneous spoken language 3.4 Level of syntax and morphology 3.5 Ability to carry out performance measures	P T FL
4. Voice Skills 4.1 Use of voice 4.2 Phonetic level voice features 4.3 Elicited voice features 4.4 Phonological level voice features 4.5 Ability to carry out performance measures	P T FL
5. Speech Skills 5.1 Use of spontaneous speech 5.2 Speech sound repertoire 5.3 Phonogical system 5.4 Speech intelligibility 5.5 Ability to carry out performance measures	P T FL
Overall PALS Classification: Pre-verbal ☐ Transitional ☐ Functional Language ☐	

Appendix 2

Pragmatics Profile of Early Communication Skills: Pre-school Summary

A	COMMUNICATIVE INTENTIONS	Spoken English	Other language [specify]
A1	Attention Directing		
A2	Requesting		
A3	Rejecting		
A4	Greeting		
A5	Self-expression & Self-assertion		
A6	Naming		
A7	Commenting		
A8	Giving Information		
B	RESPONSE TO COMMUNICATION	Spoken English	Other language [specify]
B1	Gaining Child's Attention		
B2	Interest in Interaction		
B3	Understanding of Gesture		
B4	Acknowledgement of Previous Utterance		
B5	Understanding of Speaker's Intentions		
B6	Anticipation		
B7	Responding with Amusement		
B8	Response to 'No' and Negotiation		

Pre-school Summary (cont.)

C.	INTERACTION AND CONVERSATION	Spoken English	Other language [specify]
C1	Participating in Interaction		
C2	Initiating Interaction		
C3	Maintaining an Interaction or Conversation		
C4	Conversational Breakdown		
C5	Conversational Repair		
C6	Request for Clarification		
C7	Terminating an Interaction		
C8	Overhearing a Conversation* (* 'overlooking' a "signed" conversation)		
C9	Joining a Conversation		

Adapted scoring system
Absent: not observed or reported 0 Developing skill: used inconsistently 1
Established skill 2
Sources: IMPEVAL 1993 and BCS Clinical Database 1999.

Chapter 11
Family perspectives

HAZEL LLOYD-RICHMOND

The role of the child's family has been stressed throughout this book. This chapter considers the family's perspective of the implantation process from initial decision making, through to living with an implanted child on a day-to-day basis. Some contributions to this chapter are taken from diaries kept by parents and by older children themselves, some from articles written for our newsletters and others from responses to questionnaires. All names have been changed to protect the children and their families. Outcome measures of performance from cochlear implantation are becoming increasingly important and the role played by the family can directly affect the optimal outcomes that we seek.

The close involvement of parents, as partners, in all aspects of the care of implanted children is vitally important, especially as some of the outcomes take several years to accrue. Services that are shaped to accommodate parental needs are the most likely to obtain optimal outcomes from the intervention (Nikolopoulos et al., 2001).

We have always recognized the importance of the role played by the parents, siblings and the wider family circle, and in this chapter we acknowledge this role, giving the parents an opportunity to speak for themselves.

The decision-making process

The decision to have, or not to have, a cochlear implant for their child, is now often taken earlier and earlier in a young child's life, and an implant may well be discussed with parents very soon after diagnosis of deafness has been made. The speed at which this happens should be taken into account by professionals dealing with the situation, for as Tait (1998) says: 'The impact that the diagnosis of deafness has on a family should never be underestimated.' Parents need time to come to terms with the child's deafness before being faced with the decision of implantation. For parents of children who have acquired deafness after meningitis there may be a short time limit if ossification is a consideration, but otherwise there should be a reasonable time to allow families to recover from the shock of the diagnosis of deafness and have time to grieve. It is also important to remember that parents can sometimes be treated like 'forgotten experts' (Tait, 1998). Parents have special and intimate knowledge of their children, which is sometimes not used by 'the experts' and when the diagnosis of deafness is confirmed they sometimes experience a feeling of relief at getting their suspicions taken seriously (Gregory et al., 1995). Getting to know the family and their emotional needs should be an important consideration before broaching the subject of implantation.

Families who have older children who are being considered for implantation will have to make various decisions. How much they should say to their child about cochlear implantation and how to discuss it might be an issue. If they are too positive and implantation is not appropriate for their child, will this create problems for the family? On the other hand, if they are not positive enough, the child may not see the implant as a reasonable option. Giving and discussing balanced information creates dilemmas for the family.

In the early years of cochlear implantation there was little written about implantation in young children and it was difficult to find suitable material for parents to access information either in written form or video format. Now there is a wealth of information on television and in newspapers, to which parents and families have easy access. Some families may also access information through the Internet. However, this information is not always useful or helpful and some families feel bombarded with too much information. Additionally, it is almost impossible to ensure that the information is up-to-date and accurate. It is important to recognize the varied needs of the families. Some families have a great thirst for knowledge, want to see and hear everything and can pick out what is relevant for them, helping them to reach a decision. Other families need simple facts presented at a basic level taking into consideration only what is appropriate for them and their children at that particular time.

Professionals working with families need to listen to their needs and provide information appropriately. Information also should be presented at different levels according to the members of the family. Young siblings might require simple format of pictures with no print. Older siblings may want more information using print and pictures (cartoon format is often enjoyed at this stage). Grandparents may require information and parents may require any amount of information at whatever level they feel is appropriate for them. A range of information should be available at every implant centre. Information should also be available in other languages as necessary, and with subtitling and signing options on videos.

Parents and families should also be encouraged to talk to as many people as possible, including families who already have an implanted child. In the UK, this information can be obtained independently from the Cochlear Implant Children's Support Group (CICS) (Figure 11.1), who have a directory of implanted children throughout the country. The group will try to match families with similar circumstances, including other difficulties apart from deafness, for example, syndromes. In other countries there are similar groups providing this level of support, and in Europe, the European Cochlear Implant Users' Group provides useful meetings.

The time of diagnosis has always been considered stressful (Gregory and Knight, 1998). It is important to consider that parents of a newly diagnosed deaf child will find themselves the recipients of a great deal of advice from many different professionals, and this advice may be conflicting. The consideration of a cochlear implant at this stage will introduce more professionals into their lives and could add more tension to what is an already difficult period. Professionals working with families need to take this into consideration when organizing visits to the family home.

Two families describe their very different approaches to making the decision:

> We wanted to have all the information that was available. I spent hours trawling the Internet, whilst my wife searched the local libraries. Then we put everything together, sorted out what was relevant for us and finally came to a decision.

> We don't read a lot and didn't want to be flooded with complicated explanations that we couldn't really understand. What we wanted were the basic facts which were relevant to us. Talking to other families like us helped a lot and talking to each other of course.

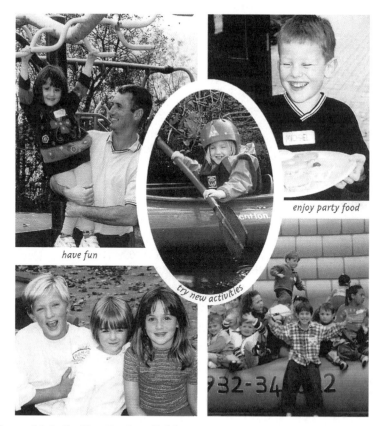

Figure 11.1. Cochlear Implant Children's Support Group, CICS.

At no point during the entire assessment period, which may take many months, should parents or children be pressured regarding their final decision. They may well find it helpful to talk to families who feel that implantation is not the way forward for their child. It is most important that each family is satisfied that they have explored all avenues open to them, before making an informed decision on behalf of their deaf child.

Making the decision on behalf of a young child, without the child's real knowledge or understanding of what is to happen to him or her, is perhaps what contributes to the difficulty of the decision. For Tom's parents, making the decision to allow their four-year-old son to have a cochlear implant was to give their son a choice in later life. They wrote:

> Our son is a healthy, robust, happy, deaf young man. He uses Sign Supported English to make his needs known to us, and we talk and sign to him. He was born hearing and suffered with meningitis at the age of two years, when he lost his hearing almost completely. After wearing

high-powered hearing aids for two years, with no apparent benefit, we decided to find out if he was a suitable candidate for a cochlear implant. Why did we feel a cochlear implant would be appropriate for our son? Because we wanted to give him a choice in later life. As our son is using sign language, and attends a unit for hearing-impaired children, where he is taught using Sign Supported English, we know that he will always have this facility of communication available to him. However, we also want to give him the opportunity to be part of the hearing community, hence a cochlear implant, to help him to hear and to learn to speak. If in later life, after using the implant consistently throughout his learning years, he chooses only to be part of the deaf community, all he has to do is not wear his speech processor. What we hope is that he will choose to belong to both worlds, the deaf and the hearing.

Six years after receiving his cochlear implant Tom has just completed his first term at his local secondary school. He talks to his peers and hopes to be chosen for the school football team, he is also a keen drama student. He also continues to visit the local Deaf Club to keep up his signing skills and is happy in either world and a great source of pride to his family.

Discussing the decision with the child's school can be important. Carol's father reported discussing implantation with his daughter's headteacher, who was an avid supporter of British Sign Language and of deaf culture. The headteacher asked him numerous questions about the decision he and his wife were about to make, to allow their young daughter to have a cochlear implant. After several hours of deep discussion, many disagreements and some agreement, the headteacher finally commented that, although she personally did not agree with cochlear implants for young children, she felt that she had given the father a thorough interrogation into his reasons for making the decision and that he was justified in saying that his decision was well informed. She then confirmed that the child's school would do whatever was necessary to help make sure the implant was successful.

For Tania's parents, making the decision to allow their daughter to have a cochlear implant after losing her hearing through meningitis was an attempt to restore a sensation of hearing of some kind:

Watching our young daughter suffer this dreadful debilitating illness, leaving the hospital unable to walk, sit up, hold a cup and most devastating unable to hear, and eventually after a few weeks unable to talk, made us determined to do anything and everything within our power to help make some kind of amends to her. When we first heard of cochlear implants at an open information evening we were determined that putting our daughter back into hospital for a major operation was not the answer for us. At first we were told that she was only partially deaf and that with the help of good hearing aids and lots of patience she would learn to talk again. However, it soon became clear not only to us, but also to local professionals, that this was not to be the case. It was then that we decided to try sign language. This too was hard work and although we slowly made some progress we still wanted to hear our little girl talk again. Once more we considered a cochlear implant, only to be told, wrongly, that we must raise the money ourselves. Amazingly, through the support of our family and friends and the local community we raised enough money and took the major step to find out if our daughter was a suitable candidate.

After the first assessments, we were still not totally convinced that we were doing the right thing, so we made contact with an adult who had an implant and it was through talking to her that finally made up our minds that this was the right way forward for our daughter.

It took Tania some time to adjust to her implant but now, eight years later, she attends an oral school for the deaf and says that her implant is so much a part of her that she often forgets to take it off when she has a bath or shower! She both talks and uses some sign language.

For Colin's parents, going back to hospital for the medical assessments, after the trauma of meningitis, proved too thought provoking and they decided that they could not go ahead with the operation. Twelve months later they felt better prepared emotionally and decided to go ahead with the operation for their young son. All parents need to be sure in themselves that they are ready to cope with the operation and ensuing period of tuning and rehabilitation.

Rowena's parents referred to the time of initial diagnosis of deafness as 'living through a nightmare'; when their daughter's deafness was first diagnosed, they were told that a cochlear implant was not suitable for congenitally deaf children. With the realization that she was gaining no benefit from hearing aids, although she wore them constantly, they decided that she should attend a school for the deaf. She settled there very quickly and made enormous progress, all through sign-based communication in a total communication environment.

Conceptually she was certainly always on a par with her hearing peers, but her spoken language was non-existent. Naturally, as hearing parents our worries for the future were many and constant.

Some time later we attended Cochlear Implant Information Day. What we heard made us think again and offered new hope. We persuaded our local ENT Consultant to refer Rowena and there the story of her path to hearing began.

Rowena has now had her cochlear implant for five years. She attends her local primary school and is maintaining the standards set by her peers of the same chronological age. Her favourite activity is listening to tapes, preferably in her tent outside in the garden!

For some of the families with older children, what to say to the child can be a major dilemma. Obviously the child is well aware that something is happening. Why all the visits to the hospital? How much should parents say and what should they say? Parents want neither to frighten their child in any way, nor to raise expectations too high, in case an implant is not possible, for whatever reason.

Christine's parents agonized for weeks over how to discuss with their nine-year-old daughter that all the tests she had undergone at the hospital may be leading to an operation for a cochlear implant. Eventually it was decided that her father should bring the topic up, whilst mum and Christine's older sister were out. With the help of a booklet produced by the implant programme, Christine's father was able to explain that they were thinking about a very special hearing aid. It would be different to the ones she was wearing now, and would help her to hear environmental sounds and people talking; however, she would need to have an operation. Her father waited with trepidation for what his daughter was going to say. He wasn't the least bit prepared. 'OK', she said! When her mum and sister arrived home she greeted them with: 'I'm going to have an operation to have a new hearing aid. Did you know?' 'Yes', said mum, who was rather taken aback that her daughter was so matter-of-fact. 'Right' said Christine, 'I'm going to watch *Neighbours* [a television programme] now, actually I read all about it in the book you kept under the settee!' And this ended the conversation.

Christine had her operation seven years ago. She has always been an oral child and she continues to use spoken language appropriate for her age. She now attends a local secondary school that has a unit for hearing-impaired pupils. Christine is in mainstream classes for 95% of her school week. She receives support in some subjects and will take five GCSE examinations next summer. She is expected to gain passes in all subjects. She enjoys shopping for clothes with her friends, going abroad with school and attending local discos.

Kirsty's mother recalls telling her daughter about the imminent operation only to find that the operation posed no apparent problems for her eight-year-old daughter, probably because mum herself had undergone mastoid surgery at some point and had a scar in the same place as that of an implant operation. Kirsty was very positive thinking about an operation that would possibly help her to hear and talk. However, she was adamant that no one was going to cut off any of her long hair, and this was the major problem for her. Loss of hair can be extremely traumatic, especially for the older children, and this issue was always discussed and addressed very carefully by all concerned. The headshave at the time of operation is now minimal, if any, and the incision is very small, behind the ear, and therefore less traumatic for the children.

For Anthony's parents the route to obtaining a cochlear implant for their son was very complex. Anthony was born congenitally deaf and at the time when his parents were contemplating an implant for their child, there were no teams in the UK who would consider implanting a congenitally deaf child.

We spent lots of time and effort looking at every possibility available for our young son. We started the John Tracy correspondence course and everyday I sat opposite Anthony doing set activities and giving him all the language to go with them. I sat my son in his rocker on the draining board and talked about dirty cups, the soap bubbles and the clean plates. A fly on the wall would have thought I was completely mad!

Although Anthony enjoyed these experiences we still felt that it just did not seem to be enough. We then decided to go to signing classes to help give our son a language for communication purposes. A peripatetic teacher visited Anthony at home, but was not in favour of signing and we began to realize what a contentious issue this was: to sign or not to sign! It was at this point that an auditory/verbal therapist began working with Anthony. We decided to contact a paediatric cochlear implant team to discover (at that stage) that they were only implanting children with acquired deafness. However, we were given the address of the New York, Iowa, Hannover and Melbourne programmes and we wrote to them all. After numerous tests at a London hospital to find out if Anthony was suitable for an implant at all, I contacted the original programme again to find out if their policy had changed and enquired whether they would be willing to carry out the rehabilitation, if Anthony had an implant abroad.

In June, we had a reply that they were not yet in a position to implant a congenitally deaf child and neither could they fragment their programme. It is one of the very few occasions that a letter has reduced me to tears!

Eventually, however, it made us more determined to achieve what we felt was necessary for our son. A visit to the Manhattan Eye, Ear and Throat Hospital and a day spent with the family of an implanted child made us feel more optimistic, but the prospect of moving to the US for several years seemed rather daunting. The next to try was the programme in Hannover, which at the time had the most experience of implanting young children. After more tests Anthony was offered an operation in Hannover and we decided to take up this option. The final decision to implant our deaf son was not easy. The issue of a congenitally deaf child being born to the deaf community is a huge one that had weighed heavily on our minds for months. We know that Anthony will always be a deaf person and we accept that. We are not trying to change him into a 'hearing' person, but he was born into a hearing family and a hearing world. If he can comprehend even the smallest amount of sound, surely it will make life easier for him as an adult, in the world at large. He is our child and, like all parents, we can only do what we feel is best for him.

This was perhaps one of the most traumatic routes for any family to have to contemplate to enable their son to have an implant. It reflects the difficulties encountered by families and professionals in the UK when introducing implant programmes for children amidst considerable opposition from parents, professionals and the deaf community.

Surgery period

Once the assessments and testing are completed and the decision to go ahead has finally been made, the next hurdle for the family is to overcome the operation itself. Making the decision and signing the consent form on behalf of children who are happy and healthy, to put them through a four-hour elective operation, is stressful enough. However, living with that decision over the next few weeks until the operation day arrives can be even more stressful. At this time the support of the local professional services is crucial. As parents are obviously more familiar with local professionals, it is natural that they should be the ones that parents turn to for support at this time.

It is important that parents attempt to prepare their children for surgery in a way that is appropriate to their needs and abilities. Young children need to be made aware that they are going to hospital again and that they will go to sleep and wake up with a big bandage on their head, and also a drip in their hand. It is most important for parents to stress that they will be there when the child wakes up and for the whole time the child is in hospital, in the same way as children are prepared for any operation. To help young children understand what is going to happen to them simple colouring books are available to parents to use with their children to help to explain what is going to happen to them (Figure 11.2).

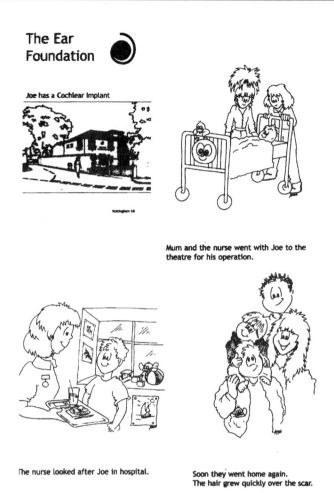

The Ear Foundation

Joe has a Cochlear Implant

Mum and the nurse went with Joe to the theatre for his operation.

The nurse looked after Joe in hospital.

Soon they went home again.
The hair grew quickly over the scar.

Figure 11.2. Joe has a cochlear implant.

Older children require more detailed explanation and in the case of one bright seven-year-old, he wanted to know everything that was going to happen to him, right down to what the 'knife' looked like that the surgeon would use. Paul's parents write:

Our son was seven years old when we decided to go ahead with a cochlear implant. Paul had good communication through sign language and he wanted to know exactly what was going to happen to him whilst he was in hospital. We told him honestly and sensitively everything we knew, but to ensure that Paul had fully understood everything we asked his local teacher of the deaf for her help. She decided that together with Paul she would 'act out' what would happen to him. Paul would be surgeon, the teacher would be the nurse and teddy bear would be the patient. Together they acted out what would happen. Teddy would come into hospital with mum and dad. Paul, the surgeon, would begin by listening to his chest to make sure he didn't have a cough or cold. Paul used the toy stethoscope to listen to his chest. 'Are you well?' he asked. 'Have you got a cough?' 'No, I'm fine', signed teddy bear (with help from the nurse)! 'First you must have some medicine to make you sleep, then some magic cream on your hand. You won't feel the needle in your hand. Then you will go to sleep.' Paul signed to teddy. 'Now where will we go?' asked the nurse. 'To theatre on the "train" trolly', signed Paul.

With the help of a dummy implant, a toy scalpel (plastic knife from the wendy house), a razor (with no blade) and a big bandage, Paul performed his cochlear implant operation on his teddy bear, taking great care to put the electrodes into the cochlea, 'Just like a snail', signed Paul. Then teddy was wheeled back to the ward to see his mummy and daddy.

This exercise not only helped Paul to understand what was going to happen to him, it also enabled his teacher of the deaf to check that Paul had no misconceptions about the operation and to allay any fears he might express.

As parents we felt happy in the knowledge that we had given our son all the information he needed to help prepare him for the operation.

Paul was implanted eight years ago. He enjoys wearing his speech processor and says that it is now part of him. He attends an oral school for the deaf and is about to take nine GCSE examinations; he hopes to get good passes in all subjects. He is a keen footballer and plays in goal for his school team.

At the time of operation, naturally, parents are extremely concerned and worried that everything should go well for their child. It is often while their child is in theatre that parents, particularly of children with acquired deafness, relive their previous hospital experiences. Many parents still complain bitterly that they were not well informed about their children's illness, particularly in the case of meningitis, and many left the hospital with no knowledge or suspicion that their child's hearing was impaired in any way. Several parents recalled instances when they felt they knew their child could no longer hear before leaving the hospital, but their concerns were not believed by hospital staff. Many families waited months after their child's illness before the child's hearing was tested and even then they were reassured that the hearing loss might be temporary or only partial loss. One mother recalls being told she was 'neurotic' on many occasions because she would not accept the information that her child could hear. After two years of numerous appointments her son was declared profoundly deaf. Professionals have a duty to take note of information given by parents, and to listen to their concerns; they often know their children best.

Perhaps, surprisingly, many parents say very little about the actual time of operation except to make passing comment like James's mother:

> The operation itself is something you worry about from the beginning right up to the time they come out of theatre. Then suddenly it's gone and you get on with the job of helping them to get better, although they seem to do this remarkably quickly with very little help from mum and dad. Looking back I think that waiting for the results of the C.T. scans was just as traumatic as the operation. After all it might have been at this point when it was decided that it just was not possible to go ahead at all.

For Emily's father everything was running smoothly until Emily had her premedication just before her operation. In tears he told me:

> She just begged me to take her home with tears streaming down her face! Then she went to sleep! I was devastated and could quite easily have picked her up and taken her home. However, her mum was the sensible one, she just said 'Now we've come this far we're going through with it!' I just had to do as I was told.

Six months later Emily loves her 'behind-the-ear' speech processor. She says she can hear everything more clearly and her parents are confident about their decision.

Time spent in hospital for the surgery has decreased considerably over time. Ten years ago patients were hospitalized for 10 days; now many children are only in hospital for one or two days. This is often much better for the children and for the family as it means they are soon back at home, where children feel most comfortable and can relax and make a faster recovery. However, a few families have felt very nervous about taking a child home after a major operation, and have sometimes requested that they be allowed to stay for one further night, in order to feel better able to cope. Medical professionals need to take note that not all parents feel confident in managing postoperative care and are nervous about this aspect. A further consideration may be families' inability to keep the wound free from infection in their particular lifestyle.

Initial tuning sessions

Three to four weeks after the operation it is time for the family to return to the implant centre for the initial tuning of the device, described in Chapter 7. A visit is usually made to the family home between operation and initial tuning by the implant centre teacher of the deaf. This visit is most important for the child and family to see the equipment. The child tries on the dummy processor, reassuring parents that the magnet is working; this is often a source of great concern to parents.

This visit is a useful time to discuss how the child is going to wear the speech processor. Some families choose for the young child to wear a harness and some choose a bum bag. An older child might choose a belt clip. Some families choose to make their own pockets in vests or for teenage girls they might prefer a pocket attached to a bra. As the child is going to be wearing the speech processor all day and every day, how they wear it and what it looks like is of great importance, both to the child and to the parents, and it is helpful to deal with these practical issues before the initial tuning itself. With more and more 'behind-the-ear' processors being fitted, this issue is much less of a problem.

As with information about the operation, it is important to have an appropriate range of information for the child and the family about the initial tuning sessions (Figure 11.3).

On the first day of tuning everyone concerned is anxious, but perhaps the parents most of all. It is at this moment when many of them begin to question their decision to have an implant for their child and questions such as 'What if he doesn't like it? What if he won't wear it? What if it doesn't work?' fill their minds.

In Barbara's case there was no question about it; she definitely didn't like it and definitely was not going to wear it! Her mother wrote:

> On 24 September, with great anticipation, we went to the implant centre for Barbara to have her initial tuning. We had spent some time trying to tell Barbara what was going to happen and our excitement rubbed off on her. Dressed in her new outfit she had chosen specially for the occasion and full of smiles for everyone, she was 'switched on'. The first sensation of sound distressed Barbara and floods of tears were produced. I tried it on and daddy tried it on. The scientist tried it on and we all told her how great it was, but she refused to put it on. We came home feeling very flat and disappointed. The next day we tried again and she co-operated beautifully. She signed to me that she could hear a noise made by the man behind the window. We were all delighted.

Nine years later Barbara has just begun secondary school. She is a very efficient implant user, and a very keen horse rider who takes part in many local and national horse trials, with great independence.

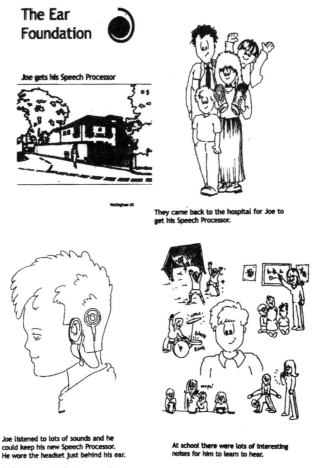

Figure 11.3. Joe gets his speech processor.

Not all initial tuning sessions are as fraught as the first one mentioned. Alice's parents were most concerned as their daughter had been deafened by meningitis nine years before her implant, and they wondered whether or not she would accept the new sensation of hearing. Alice's parents were both very nervous on the initial day of tuning. Alice too, was slightly nervous, but also very excited. Alice accepted the sounds from the computer quite happily and both parents were thrilled to realize that 16 electrodes had been tuned in a very short time. Over lunchtime she wore the speech processor happily and reacted to several loud environmental sounds and also to her father's voice, when he shouted as she stepped on his toe! In the afternoon session Alice responded to many different musical instruments, counting beats and copying rhythms, although she told us quite precisely what she could and couldn't hear. In the evening at the hotel where the family was staying, the hotelier played the electronic organ for Alice, at first beginning very quietly then increasing the sound until she could hear it. This completed a very happy and satisfying first day for all the family. Alice is now 17, attending her local college where she is studying to become a nursery nurse and she would like to work with young deaf children.

Christine's parents also found that they need not have worried quite as much as they did. Christine's father wrote:

> On the first day, she was quite happy to wear the processor until bath time at 7.30 p.m. She also said that her new 'hearing aid' was better than the old ones and wanted to wear it again after bath time, until bed time, which was another 30 minutes (something she had never done with her hearing aids!). On day two, after the tuning, she said the map was too loud at first, but then after 10 minutes of playing, everything was OK again. In the afternoon she had a listening session with the rehabilitation teacher of the deaf and responded to voice, drums and a variety of musical instruments, and was very happy with her speech processor. When we arrived home she played the piano, but complained that there was too much noise, took the coil off and went for a bath! (The TV had been switched on and with several people talking it may have all been too much.) After her bath Christine wanted to wear the processor again, she responded to voice from about 15 feet, heard the toilet flushing and was once again happy with the processor. On the third day of initial tuning Christine wore her processor all day until bath time, by which time we were all very tired!

Sadique was 16 when he made his decision to have a cochlear implant. He had normal hearing until he was seven years old, had a deteriorating loss between the ages of seven and 11, and struggled through secondary school with no useful hearing. Before his initial tuning he asked what the new hearing would sound like. We told him that adult implant users who had had normal hearing reported that hearing through an implant sounded a little bit like daleks (television robot-type characters) or Mickey Mouse (a cartoon character). Sadique said he could remember this type of 'talk'.

On the day of initial tuning Sadique's speech processor was tuned very quickly and he was pleased with the results. However, in the afternoon listening session he was keen to report that we were wrong! He said he could remember the daleks and his processor didn't sound anything like that. When listening to a tape of environmental sounds he took a long time to consider the first sound. The sound was played again; birds singing. He then commented: 'Oh I don't know whether they are sparrows or starlings. We don't get many different birds near my house!' he said. Having seven years of normal hearing had helped this young man to make extremely efficient use of his implant in a very short time.

Initial tuning sessions can be very stressful for implanted children and for their families. As many families have to travel some considerable distance to the implant centre it is extremely beneficial if the family can have somewhere to stay where they can feel relaxed, where the child has somewhere to play and where they are in the company of other families who have experienced the same circumstances. In Nottingham we are extremely fortunate to have such family accommodation and rooms designed specifically for listening activities, which can be made available to all our families (Figure 11.4).

The Centre is situated only a few minutes walk away from the hospital and was funded by our charity, The Ear Foundation. Children and their families are able to stay at the house whenever they have an appointment at the implant centre. The house is an invaluable asset to the programme as, working with many very young children, it is most important that the child arrives at the Centre refreshed after a good night's sleep, to enable him or her to co-operate well for the tuning and rehabilitation sessions. With long distances to travel, the Centre is an ideal place to stay.

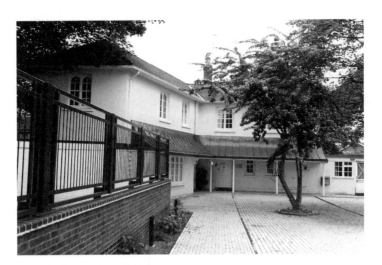

Figure 11.4. The Ear Foundation.

Before it was available, families had to stay in hotels or bed-and-breakfast facilities. As one family reports:

> Staying in a hotel room with a young deaf child was far from easy. There was nowhere for him to play and only the few small toys we brought from home for him to play with. When you are both anxious for everything to go well, being cooped up in one room does not help. Now when we stay at the implant centre house we look forward to our visits, as does our son. In the summer he can play with the toys in the garden and we can relax in the sunshine with him. In the winter the biggest problem is getting him out of the playroom to go to bed, whilst we can relax watching TV or talking with other parents. It has made stressful trips so much more relaxing and enjoyable.

Once families are home and able to return to their normal daily routine, their child having accepted the speech processor and wearing it set at the appropriate sensitivity setting, it then becomes a great temptation to 'test' their child's new sensation of hearing. This can be counterproductive.

Hayley's father had been so impressed with his young daughter's obvious pleasure at hearing a loud drum that he bought one on the way home from the initial tuning sessions. However, after several days of banging the drum each time his daughter wasn't watching him, she suddenly stopped responding! Panic stricken in case there was a problem with the speech processor he showed the drum to his daughter and asked, using sign language, if she could hear it? 'Yes' she signed 'noisy daddy, fed up, stop!'

Nigel's mother was well aware of the fact that she was continually asking her son if he had heard different sounds, even though she had been advised not to. One Sunday morning whilst they were in church a baby started crying loudly, out of Nigel's sight. As usual she asked him what he could hear. 'Nothing', he signed to her. She felt very disappointed and related the incident to her husband when they got home. Later that day Nigel signed to his father that he had heard a baby crying in church but he wouldn't tell mummy, because he was fed up with her always asking what he could hear.

Although the families are carefully counselled that they need to be very patient with their child, when they are first tuned some parents find it almost impossible to contain their curiosity to find out exactly what their child can hear, and they require continuing realistic support to enable them to encourage their child to listen and use the system in a sensitive way.

Learning to use the implant system

It is after the family has returned to their everyday routine that the work of supporting the child in using the system begins – by the child and families themselves, the local professionals and the implant team. All children progress at different rates and it is important to offer reassurance and to set sensible and achievable goals for everyone. Sometimes initial progress can seem very slow while the child begins to try to make sense of his new hearing, as Matthew's mother reports.

> At the time of writing, it is now over a year since Matthew had his operation and we could never have imagined the stress and worries of the past year. All of our problems have been made easier because we have had constant support and contact with a specialist team. We are lucky in that we are so near the doctors and scientists involved with Matthew, so any checks that Matthew has needed have not involved a plane flight. We know now that to have undertaken this abroad would have added more stress to our lives and especially to Matthew.
>
> The first six months after the operation for us were very difficult. Try as we could to keep our expectations realistic we were watching and wondering what he could hear, and looking for signs of him learning to talk again. It took Matthew three months before he could respond to his name, and his first attempt at 'mummy' came three months later. We have no regrets in making the decision to have a cochlear implant for Matthew at this crucial stage in his life. He is now saying two and three word phrases and understanding a lot of specific commands and questions. It is important to stress that it is not a magical cure for deafness. Matthew has come a long way during the past year, but he has a long way to go before he can understand general conversation.

Parents have also noticed that their children make good progress, then plateau for a while. Barbara's mother reports:

> We seem to have hit a quiet patch. Have tried for a few days to get Barbara interested in listening games, she made a half hearted attempt at them, but then suggested that we play something else that did not require her to listen. I have tried to think of new listening games, the only one she was enthusiastic about involved the doorbell (which has a very loud ring). I also think the past few days have seen less vocalizations.

Then only four days later: 'Barbara sang all morning non-stop. She handed me the newspaper and casually said "paper" (not a word we use a lot and not one I have tried to teach her).'

Keeping a good sense of humour is very important during the early days and Carol's father demonstrates this with the following comments:

Living where we do, beneath the flight path of Concorde, naturally we were excited when, whilst out walking, Carol looked up in response to the very loud noise made by an aeroplane and she signed aeroplane to us. The following week at around the same time we waited anxiously for a repeat performance as Concorde thundered over our heads, Nothing! No response! But then it was foggy!!

Many parents consider that their deaf children may be safer if they learn to use an implant. Angela's mother feels quite strongly that Angela's ability to hear saved her life.

The implant saved Angela's life today. We were crossing the road when a car came out of nowhere. I shouted at Angela to stop, as she was ahead of me. The car was travelling at about 80 or 90 mph. She stopped and was safe. She is taking a lot more care on the road now.

Six months later the same mother writes:

Angela phoned Jean (her taxi escort) to say that she was going to school tomorrow – she had been poorly since Tuesday. She dialled Jean's number and said, 'I'm going to school tomorrow Jean. What time will you pick me up?' Jean said, 'eight o'clock'. I asked Angela what time she said and Angela said 'eight o'clock'. Jean was thrilled, she said she understood every word that Angela had said, and went around telling everyone about it.

Learning how to use the telephone can take lots of patience and lots of practice, so we do encourage parents to allow their children to answer the telephone, when it rings, very soon after initial tuning. However, as Hayley's mum reports, this can sometimes create a few problems:

The telephone rang tonight. I told Hayley it was ringing and she ran to answer it. She 'talked' for three or four minutes non-stop and then replaced the receiver! Luckily it was a friend who telephoned straight back and was thrilled to hear Hayley trying to talk.

Advice from Barbara's mother is:

Make sure you inform all your family and friends that you are helping your child to learn to listen for the telephone ringing, because on several occasions when we have asked Barbara what she could hear, she has correctly said the telephone, but sometimes we have let it ring for so long, to see if she will tell us it is ringing, that people have rung off and we are still waiting for a call!

Learning how to use the telephone effectively can take a long time and requires lots of practice. David, one of our older children, did not enjoy telephone training, saying it was 'too difficult'. One morning he asked his mother if his friend could accompany him to a local football match. 'Yes, I suppose so,' she said, 'Why don't you ring and ask him?' Without thinking about it David picked up the telephone and rang his friend, whilst his mum waited anxiously in the kitchen. Five minutes later he appeared at the door saying, 'His mum says he can't come, because he's still in bed!' David had understood what had been said over the telephone, because the situation and the information were meaningful to him, quite different from a practice or test situation.

Parental questionnaires

Learning to listen and how to use the implant system effectively is something that goes on over a long period of time. In order to help us to ensure what parents expect from the implant system and to find out if their expectations have been realized, we used a series of pre-implant and post-implant parent questionnaires. A prospective longitudinal study was undertaken of the parents of a consecutive group of forty-three profoundly deaf children who all had cochlear implants (Nikolopoulos et al., 2001). The parents were asked to complete questionnaires before implantation and one, two and three years following implantation. The pre-implant questionnaire asked parents to answer questions about their expectations in three main areas:

- communication with others;
- listening to speech without lipreading;
- development of speech and language.

They were then asked the same questions at one, two and three years after implant. Parental expectations prior to implantation and the actual changes they perceived post-implant are demonstrated in Figures 11.5, 11.6 and 11.7.

Prior to implantation, parents were asked whether they expected the implant to give their child easier communication with others and 80% of parents said 'certainly yes', they expected the implant to give their child easier communication with others.

This figure was surpassed when parents were asked about what the implant had given their child at one year, two years and three years after implantation. Figure 11.5 shows that, three years after implantation, 98% of parents considered that the implant had given their child easier communication with others.

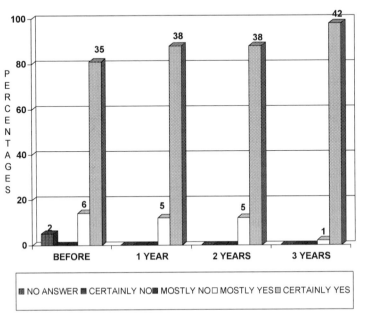

Figure 11.5. Parental questionnaire conducted pre-implant and annually post-implant: expectations – do you feel the operation will offer/has offered your child easier communication with others?

Prior to implantation parents were also asked whether they expected the implant would offer their child improvements in listening to speech without lipreading. These expectations were much more conservative, with only 35% of parents expecting a definite improvement. Figure 11.6 shows that, three years after implantation, 88% of parents considered that the implant had offered access to spoken language without lipreading, thus exceeding expectations.

Parents were also asked, prior to implantation, about whether they expected the implant to offer their child improved developments in their speech and language. Their expectations were high, with 86% of parents expecting that the implant would help with the child's development of speech and

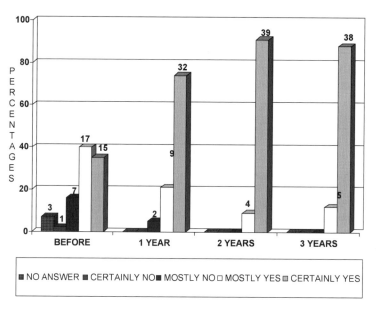

Figure 11.6. Parental questionnaire conducted pre-implant and annually post-implant: expectations – do you feel the operation will offer/has offered your child access to speech without lipreading?

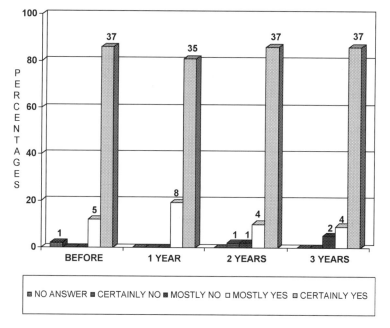

Figure 11.7. Parental questionnaire conducted pre-implant and annually post-implant: expectations – do you feel the operation will offer/has offered your child help to develop speech and language?

language. Post-implantation, parents felt their expectations were met, both at the two- and the three-year interval; however, speech development remained a major area of concern at all intervals.

These results suggest that outcomes of cochlear implantation largely satisfied parental expectations. Realistic expectations, fostered through the counselling and discussion in the early stages of a child being considered for implantation, are essential. For some children, for whom there may be other difficulties, we need to be cautious. Although the role of parents is so vital with regard to the implanted child, there is still little written from the parents' perspective to provide to other parents. It is recognized that repeated evaluation of patients' (or parental) views should become an integral part of routine healthcare (Richards, 1999), and thus provide this perspective.

Special moments

As any young child grows up there are many special moments that parents remember, and parents who have children with cochlear implants are no different.

Jamie's mother says: 'He is responding to many sounds, he turns to his name, he loves music, he's heard wind whistling in the trees, he's heard birds singing, he's constantly asking us what different sounds are, and his speech is improving all the time.'

David's mother reports: 'He can identify most household sounds, respond to his name immediately and can follow some conversation without lipreading. He is just learning to listen to music and his favourite is Tina Turner played at its loudest volume! He is part of a mainstream class and copes well with the demands of school.'

For Matthew's mother these words were very special: 'Last week as I was leaving Matthew's bedroom he said: "door, no leave it", which may not seem unusual, but they are words we thought we would never hear again, along with: "Night, night mummy, I love you".'

For Tania's parents it wasn't even a sentence:

The girls were washed and dressed this morning and had just cleaned their teeth. As always I said to Billie, 'open your mouth', (so I could inspect the teeth) 'and say aah'. On Tania's turn she obliged with the open mouth and out came a very high pitched 'aah' – we were overwhelmed. It was only a matter of months ago we took her to the doctors, he had asked her to say 'aah' and we had said to him, 'if only she could'!

Carol's mother witnessed an impromptu concert in her back garden one morning. When she asked her daughter what she was doing waving her arms around, she signed that she was listening to the birds singing and she was conducting their performance.

Barbara's mother writes: 'Tear jerker of the week coming up. Last week was my birthday and Barbara sang 'Happy Birthday' with no prompting. Although the words were not yet recognizable, the tune certainly was.'

For Emily's parents, although their 10-year-old daughter has only been implanted for three months, they say: 'The look on her face when she switches the processor on in the mornings is worth all the initial worries. She just loves it. She is also very proud of the fact that she can sing in time to her favourite pop songs, which she could only sign to, three months ago!'

For Neil's parents their special moment came five years after their son had been implanted:

> Neil made tremendous progress with his implant and local professionals felt he was ready to transfer from a primary school with a visit to our local primary school. At first he went a day a week for a term, to see if he liked it, then after the summer holidays he went full-time. We were both very nervous, but our special moment came at the end of his first full week when he came home with an invitation to his first party!

These parental memories are important, and may help others. In our yearly parental questionnaires we find it extremely useful to ask the parents of our implanted children to recall what they feel would be the most important considerations for other prospective parents of implanted children, before making the decision to go ahead with implantation for their child. Typical comments are:

- Obtain as much information, from as many different people, as possible.
- Have realistic expectations about the time it takes for progress to show.
- Make up your own mind in light of the information given.
- If there is anything of which you are unsure, ask.
- Try to satisfy every little doubt and worry; no question should be too trivial.

- Give the input following implantation and get information on how to do it.
- Try to attend an information day at the implant centre.

We also ask the same question of our older children. These are a few of their comments:

- Get it done, it helps a lot.
- The implant helps with talking and listening.
- It's best to get it done when you are little, then you don't worry about it.
- The operation goes quickly, then you have lots of fun.
- Don't waste any time; get the operation done and let the fun begin!

Families of children with cochlear implants come from great distances and meeting together with other families who have an implanted child is a great support for the children and the parents alike (Figure 11.8). Talking to parents who have shared a similar ex-perience can be extremely helpful; in the area of parental support, parents are the professionals. Support groups are required as numbers of implants grow, to enable parents to share mutual concerns and interests.

Teenage years bring forth many new issues related both to deafness and to cochlear implantation. A recently organized teenagers' day provided a group of young people with the

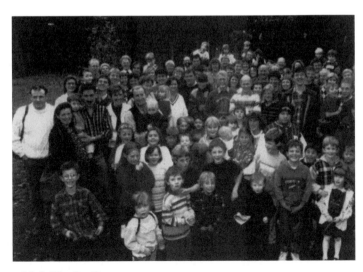

Figure 11.8. The families.

opportunity to come together to discuss many issues, both of a social and educational nature. Together they produced their first 'Teenz United' newsletter, which is now a regular feature and made plans for continuing 'get-together' days.

The child's family continues to provide the crucial link between the implanted child and all the professionals working with them. It is with great thanks to all our parents concerned that this chapter of the book has been possible.

References

Gregory S, Bishop J, Sheldon L (1995) Deaf Young People and their Families. Cambridge: Cambridge University Press.

Gregory S, Knight P (1998) Social development and family life. In S Gregory, P Knight, W McCracken, S Powers, L Watson (eds) Issues in Deaf Education. London: David Fulton Publishers.

Nikolopoulos TP, Lloyd H, Archbold S, O'Donoghue GM (2001) Pediatric cochlear implantation: the parents' perspective. Archives of Otolaryngology Head and Neck Surgery 127: 363–7.

Richards T (1999) Patients' priorities need to be assessed and taken into account. British Medical Journal 318: 277.

Tait M (1998) Cochlear Implants and Deaf Children: Implications for Education: Unit 3. Working with families. Distance Education: Hearing Impairment, School of Education, Birmingham University.

Index

SIR 362
video analysis 302
Pre-school Language Scale 346
pre-verbal skills 328, 339–40, 344
  FLLS 356
  PALS 347, 349–50
  TAPS 353
  video analysis 302–6, 313, 317–20,
    322, 323–5
primary auditory cortex 165, 183
Profile of Actual Linguistic Skills (PALS)
    345–50, 380
  Individual Profile 347–8
Profile of Actual Speech Skills (PASS)
    364–5, 368
programming 19, 34, 38, 198, 217–53,
    370
  EAT 366
  FLLS 357
  local support team 59, 64
  schedules 74
progressive (degenerative) hearing loss
    144, 341
  children under 5 years 99–100
  EAT 366
  family perspectives 397
  PALS 346
  rehabilitation 258, 268, 286
Prom-EABR waveform 193–6
promontory 140, 152
  electrophysiological measures 164,
    169, 171, 179, 184, 192–6
prosody 338
  PALS 348–9
  VSA 359–60, 368
pseudomonopolar stimulation mode 22,
    189–90, 237–9
psychology and psychologists 13, 56,
    108, 136, 148, 332
  assessment 76–8
  complex disabilities 143–4
  see also educational psychologists
psychophysical measurements 217,
    219, 231, 236, 240, 244–5
pulsatile waveforms 25–8
pure-tone audiometry 105, 111, 129–31

radiological assessment 56, 135–6,
    137–42
  children under 5 years 101
  complex disabilities 144
  counselling 147

monitoring by SLT 332–3
surgery 148, 157
receiver/stimulators 20, 22, 152, 155
  fitting and programming 219, 222,
    224, 236
receptive language 367, 371
  PALS 345, 348, 350, 380
  rehabilitation 274
  TROG 353–5
  video analysis 305
record keeping 330, 337
referrals 77, 97–9, 116–17
  schedule 74–5
rehabilitation 6, 17, 82–4, 257–301
  assessment 77–8, 261, 265, 283, 292
  children under 5 years 101, 114
  complex disabilities 83, 143, 266
  development of implants 49, 53
  electrophysiological measures 192
  etiology of deafness 145
  families 82–3, 266–7, 288, 289–90,
    292, 297, 388, 390, 397–8
  fitting and programming 249
  funding 85–6, 88
  hereditary deafness 146
  implant teams 57, 58–60, 62, 64, 70–2
  maintenance period 84
  monitoring by SLT 330, 335–7, 369,
    371, 374
  schedules 74–5
  surgery 82, 83
  video analysis 316
reimplantation 85, 122, 200, 244
repetitions 307, 312
reports by SLTs 331, 336–7
respiratory diseases 142
retrocochlear deafness 107, 168, 171,
    174–5
reverberation 250, 288, 305
reverse telemetry see back telemetry (BT)
Reynell Developmental Language Scales
    353, 367
  PALS 346
  TROG 354
research 323–4
  children under 5 years 116
  electrophysiological measures 204
  FLLS 357
  implant systems 14, 21, 28, 31, 32, 38
  monitoring by SLT 328, 335, 342–4,
    372–4
  PALS 349